Applied Ethics and Decision Making in Mental Health

To Alyson, Quentin, Delilah, and Emmeline—you are my inspiration.

—*Michael Moyer*

To Camille, my children Dáley and Charlie, my mother Susan, and other vibrant family—all of whom gave me more material from real life than could fit in a book.

—*Charles Crews*

SAGE was founded in 1965 by Sara Miller McCune to support the dissemination of usable knowledge by publishing innovative and high-quality research and teaching content. Today, we publish over 900 journals, including those of more than 400 learned societies, more than 800 new books per year, and a growing range of library products including archives, data, case studies, reports, and video. SAGE remains majority-owned by our founder, and after Sara's lifetime will become owned by a charitable trust that secures our continued independence.

Los Angeles | London | New Delhi | Singapore | Washington DC | Melbourne

Applied Ethics and Decision Making in Mental Health

Michael Moyer
University of Texas, San Antonio

Charles Crews
Texas Tech University

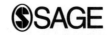

Los Angeles | London | New Delhi
Singapore | Washington DC | Melbourne

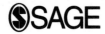

FOR INFORMATION:

SAGE Publications, Inc.
2455 Teller Road
Thousand Oaks, California 91320
E-mail: order@sagepub.com

SAGE Publications Ltd.
1 Oliver's Yard
55 City Road
London, EC1Y 1SP
United Kingdom

SAGE Publications India Pvt. Ltd.
B 1/I 1 Mohan Cooperative Industrial Area
Mathura Road, New Delhi 110 044
India

SAGE Publications Asia-Pacific Pte. Ltd.
3 Church Street
#10-04 Samsung Hub
Singapore 049483

Development Editor: Abbie Rickard
Editorial Assistant: Carrie Montoya
Production Editor: Bennie Clark Allen
Copy Editor: Pam Schroeder
Typesetter: C&M Digitals (P) Ltd.
Proofreader: Sue Schon
Indexer: Sylvia Coates
Cover Designer: Anupama Krishnan
Marketing Manager: Shari Countryman

Printed in the United States of America

Library of Congress Cataloging-in-Publication Data

Names: Moyer, Michael, author. | Crews, Charles, author.

Title: Applied ethics and decision making in mental health / Michael Moyer, Charles Crews.

Description: Los Angeles : SAGE, [2017] | Includes bibliographical references and index.

Identifiers: LCCN 2016000039 |
ISBN 978-1-4833-4975-6 (paperback : alk. paper)

Subjects: | MESH: Counseling—ethics | Mental Health—ethics | Professional-Patient Relations—ethics | Clinical Decision-Making—ethics | Confidentiality—ethics

Classification: LCC RC455.2.E8 | NLM WM 21 | DDC 174.2/9689—dc23 LC record available at http://lccn.loc.gov/2016000039

This book is printed on acid-free paper.

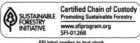

16 17 18 19 20 10 9 8 7 6 5 4 3 2 1

Brief Contents

Detailed Contents

Editors' Preface: Introduction to the Series

Counseling and Professional Identity in the 21st Century

Applied Ethics and Decision Making in Mental Health by Dr. Michael Moyer and Dr. Charles Crews is a textbook that targets ethics courses in graduate programs in mental health counseling. The text distinguishes itself from all other books on professional ethics in that it addresses not only ethical and legal issues but also professional issues and ethical decision making related to the profession's code of ethics. There are a number of distinctions between this text and many others on ethical and legal issues in counseling.

The first distinction is that *Applied Ethics and Decision Making in Mental Health* has integrated into the text the newest code of ethics of the American Counseling Association (ACA, 2014). Since the ACA Code of Ethics significantly impacts the counseling profession and all counseling professionals, this timely integration of the most recent version will assist both graduate students in counseling and counseling professionals to abide by the ACA Code of Ethics and practice using professional standards.

The second distinction is that this text has a unique dimension of internal focus on readers. Dr. Moyer and Dr. Crews challenge the readers to understand their own morals, values, and beliefs and how those beliefs interact with their interpretation of the ACA Code of Ethics. As a result, the book will help readers develop self-awareness and promote their critical thinking.

The third distinction is that unlike many other books on ethical and legal issues in counseling, which mainly focus on the readers' understanding of the code of ethics, *Applied Ethics and Decision Making in Mental Health* not only emphasizes the dimensions of the readers' understanding the code of ethics but also promotes an understanding of their personal ethics in the process of ethical decision making through numerous case illustrations and ethical dilemmas along with guided discussion questions.

The final distinction is that this book also includes a dimension on the development of counseling professional identity. It is more than a text that provides knowledge and skills; it will inform readers about the most recent ethics codes, research, theory, and practice and facilitate readers in developing their professional identity.

While we are proud of the content and topics covered within this text, we are more than aware that one text, one learning experience, will not be sufficient for the development of a counselor's professional competency. The formation of both your professional identity and practice will be a lifelong process. It is a process that we hope to facilitate through the presentation of this text and the creation of our series: *Counseling and Professional Identity in the 21st Century.*

Counseling and Professional Identity in the 21st Century is a new, fresh, pedagogically sound series of texts targeting counselors in training. This series is *not* simply a compilation of isolated books matching those already in the market. Rather each book, with its targeted knowledge and skills, is presented as but a part of a larger whole. The focus and content of each text serves as a single lens through which a counselor can view his/her clients, engage in his/her practice, and articulate his/her own professional identity.

Counseling and Professional Identity in the 21st Century is unique not just in the fact that it packages a series of traditional texts but that it provides an *integrated* curriculum targeting the formation of the readers' professional identity and efficient, ethical practice. Each book within the series is structured to facilitate the ongoing professional formation of the reader. The materials found within each text are organized to move the reader to higher levels of cognitive, affective, and psychomotor functioning, resulting in his/her assimilation of the materials presented into both his/her professional identity and approach to professional practice. While each text targets a specific set of core competencies (cognates and skills), competencies identified by the professional organizations and accreditation bodies, each book in the series emphasizes each of the following:

1. The assimilation of concepts and constructs provided across the text found within the series, thus fostering the reader's ongoing development as a competent professional

2. The blending of contemporary theory with current research and empirical support

3. A focus on the development of procedural knowledge with each text employing case illustrations and guided practice exercises to facilitate the reader's ability to translate the theory and research discussed into professional decision making and application

4. The emphasis on the need for and means of demonstrating accountability

5. The fostering of the reader's professional identity and with it the assimilation of the ethics and standards of practice guiding the counseling profession

We are proud to have served as coeditors of this series feeling sure that all of the texts included, just like *Applied Ethics and Decision Making in Mental Health,* will serve as a significant resource to you and your development as a professional counselor.

Richard Parsons, PhD
Naijian Zhang, PhD

Authors' Preface

This book is targeted as the primary textbook for ethics or ethics-related courses in mental health and counseling programs. The content covers professional issues in mental health fields and ethical decision making related to the ACA Code of Ethics. As one of many textbooks focused on ethical concerns in this field, we hope to set this one apart by focusing primarily on the practical application of codes of ethics and ethical decision-making processes. It is our belief that there is more to being an ethical mental health professional than simply memorizing codes of ethics. Ethical guidelines change, and most ethical codes are vague and offer broad guidelines to assist professionals in determining how to best act in specific situations. We believe it is imperative that professional counselors and other mental health professionals know how to critically examine ethical guidelines and interpret standards in ways that best provide for the client. Therefore, readers will see numerous case illustrations throughout every chapter to allow them to apply these codes and ethical decision-making skills in realistic situations. Our goal is to challenge readers to understand their own morals, values, and beliefs and how those beliefs interact with their interpretation of ethical codes. This book emphasizes the development of self-awareness and the promotion of student critical thinking.

While this text is primarily written from a professional counseling point of view, other ethic guidelines (American Psychological Association [APA] and American Association for Marriage and Family Therapists [AAMFT]) have been infused into the text to broaden the scope of the materials. Incorporating multiple perspectives allows the reader to appreciate the similarities and differences of various mental health professions. Ultimately, understanding the subtleties of each profession will aid the reader in strengthening his/her own professional identity.

Our goal in writing this text is to provide real-world ethical situations for students and faculty to discuss. Ideally, faculty will use the ethical dilemmas to enhance small- and large-group discussions within their classrooms. Our hope is that students will respond to the dilemmas as they would if they were facing the dilemma as a practicing professional, and not as a student sitting in a classroom, to best prepare them for the ethical challenges they are likely to face in the field.

Acknowledgments

T his book would not have been possible without the support and encouragement of many who have been with us throughout this journey. First, we would like to thank our friends and family who have stood by us. You have acted as reviewers, editors, and sounding boards throughout the process and provided encouragement all along the way. There is no way to express our full appreciation for all that you have done to support our efforts. We would like to thank Drs. Naijian Zhang and Richard Parsons, who provided us the opportunity to author this book. To Dr. Jerry Juhnke and Dr. Jeremy Sullivan, your friendship and mentorship continues to be a blessing. Thank you for all your feedback and suggestions. Thank you to our graduate students over the years who have helped us organize our thoughts and shape the way this book is presented. Finally, we want to especially thank Abbie Rickard and Kassie Graves at SAGE Publications for their patience and guidance through the process.

SAGE gratefully acknowledges the following reviewers for their kind assistance:

Barbara G. Leavy, *Rutgers, The State University of New Jersey*

Djuradj Stakic, *Pennsylvania State University, Brandywine Campus*

Elizabeth O' Brien, *University of Tennessee at Chattanooga*

Jo Ann Jankoski, *Pennsylvania State University, The Eberly Campus*

Julie M. Koch, *Oklahoma State University*

Kristi Gibbs, *University of Tennessee at Chattanooga*

Mona Robinson, *Ohio University*

Susan A. Adams, *Texas Woman's University*

Eugenie Joan Looby, *Mississippi State University*

Rochelle Caroon-Santiago, *University of the Incarnate Word*

Susan L. Williams, *National University*

About the Authors

Michael Moyer, PhD, LPC-S, is an associate professor in the Department of Counseling at the University of Texas at San Antonio (UTSA). He received his master's in counseling and doctorate in counselor education and supervision from Texas A&M University–Corpus Christi. While at UTSA, Dr. Moyer has taught various courses, however, most often enjoys teaching courses in ethics, practicum, and development of counseling skills. Some of Dr. Moyer's primary research interests include ethical decision making, non-suicidal self-injury, and school counselor education. In addition to his teaching and research at UTSA, Dr. Moyer maintains a small private practice in San Antonio and specializes in working with individuals who self-injure. Outside of work, Dr. Moyer enjoys exercising, being outside, and spending time with his wife, Alyson, and three children, Quentin, Delilah, and Emmeline.

Charles Rutledge Crews, PhD, LPC-S, is an associate professor in the graduate educational psychology and leadership department for the counseling program at Texas Tech University, where he has served as the coordinator of the school counseling program since 2007. Dr. Crews is a licensed professional counselor and a board-approved supervisor. He is also a certified school counselor in New Mexico. He works with schools, districts, and universities in designing interventions to best meet the needs of students. Dr. Crews also maintains a private practice treating children and adolescents using creative interventions. He currently provides clients with interventions pertaining to compulsive technology use, school achievement, intensive outpatient programs, veterans issues, school planning, prison rehab, hospital rehab, and church spiritual discernment and through the court system.

Dr. Crews keeps busy authoring numerous journal articles on technology-related issues and opportunities in counseling. He is frequently invited to present on a wide range of topics for local, state, regional, national, and international associations and organizations. He has been interviewed by national associations on topics related to technology overuse and suicide prevention, intervention, and postvention.

Born in El Paso, Texas, Charles graduated from El Paso High School, one of the oldest high schools in the region. He ventured from the comfort of home to travel south, arriving in Seguin, Texas, where he earned a BA degree in psychology and theology from Texas Lutheran University. After graduation, he went back home to El Paso and completed his master's of education at UT–El Paso in guidance and counseling. He didn't stop there; he left home once again to attend Texas A&M University–Commerce, where his lifelong dream to complete his PhD in counselor education and supervision came true.

Charles worked as a school counselor in Burnet, Texas, before completing his dissertation and earning a tenure-track position at Texas Tech University. At Texas Tech he was awarded the President's Excellence in Teaching Award, was inducted into the Texas Tech Teaching Academy, and was named one of the top five professors at Texas Tech by the student body. He was also awarded the Dean's Excellence in Teaching award.

Dr. Crews is married to Camille Frost; they have one little girl and a little boy on the way. Charles loves outdoor activities and blends them into his counseling work as much as possible. Camping, hiking, cooking, and fishing make for the perfect workday away from academia.

1

Introduction to Ethics

In order to properly understand the big picture, everyone should fear becoming mentally clouded and obsessed with one small section of truth.

—Xunzi

Chapter 1 introduces ethics and the various codes of ethics pertinent to professional counselors. The authors will discuss the reasons and need for ethical codes and how they impact both practitioners and the general public. The authors will also discuss ethics as philosophy, in addition the concepts of relativism and absolutism, and introduce methods of knowing along with how individuals are motivated to act. The main purpose of this chapter is to introduce ethics and get students to begin reflecting on and evaluating the ways in which they make decisions in their lives. Specifically, after reading Chapter 1, students will be able to do the following:

1. Define what it means to be an ethical professional counselor.

2. Explain the purpose of professional organizations' codes of ethics.

3. Discuss the principles on which the ACA Code of Ethics is based.

4. Explain the difference between relativism and absolutism.

5. Describe how counselors' motivations may affect their interpretation of ethical standards.

6. Explain the Socratic method and ways to apply it when facing ethical dilemmas.

Codes of ethics are living, changing documents and continue to change over time. Thus, it is more important to understand how to interpret a code of ethics and make

▶ 1

ethical decisions than it is to memorize specific ethical standards. Throughout this text you will find many case illustrations and ethical dilemmas along with guided discussion questions to help you identify your own values and personal ethics. The combination of providing (1) an in-depth review of ethical codes, (2) ethical dilemmas, and (3) review questions geared toward challenging students to understand how morals, values, and beliefs affect one's interpretation of codes of ethics will engender vibrant discussions throughout any ethics course. Although you are most likely reading this text as a part of your graduate course and not actually faced with the dilemmas presented, the authors encourage you to think about them and respond to the dilemmas as if you were in a real-life scenario. In responding, think about how you might act, what you might say, and the impact your words or actions might have on your client and others.

Defining Ethics

Before delving into ethical codes, the authors believe it to be important to first understand what we are talking about when we use the term "ethics." Merriam-Webster's (2013) online dictionary defines ethics as "the principles of conduct governing an individual or a group." Others (Cottone & Tarvydas, 2007; Ford, 2006; Remley & Herlihy, 2014) describe ethics as a practice that protects clients, practitioners, and the general public; guidelines for acceptable behavior within a profession; and a field of study seeking to understand right and wrong. Ethics, in general, refers to the study of acceptable behaviors and standards governing the conduct of those within a profession. For our profession, ethics encompasses everything you do as a professional counselor. When you begin your training, ethics is included in your education and the acquisition of your licensure. As a practicing counselor, ethics is involved in everything from the way you conduct your practice and interact with clients and other professionals to the way you keep records and bill for services. Ethics encompasses every action and interaction.

Codes of Ethics

Codes of ethics are the building blocks for professional organizations, their morals, their values, and what they find to be important. In our own personal ethics, it is our own morals, values, and what we find to be important in interacting with others. Personal ethics include what we find to be important in ourselves and how we put value to those we interact with and the actions we take. When we talk about professional ethics, we're talking about the values and the important aspects of a profession—in this case counseling and counselor education. One of the most difficult aspects of being a professional counselor is keeping personal ethics separate from professional ethics. It is critical for professional counselors to understand their own personal ethics and avoid imposing personal values onto the values of the profession. Consider Case Illustration 1-1 as Becky struggles with keeping her personal ethics separate from professional ethics.

CASE ILLUSTRATION 1-1

Becky is a clinical mental health counseling student currently enrolled in her program's practicum class. As part of the class, she spends three days a week at her university's free counseling clinic. The clinic offers free counseling services to the surrounding community and is primarily comprised of practicum students. One of Becky's first clients is a 35-year-old female experiencing symptoms related to anxiety. The client is recently divorced and has sole custody of her two children (ages 10 and 14).

During the first few sessions Becky's client reports confusion related to her current relationships. Becky's client claims that she entered into a relationship with a new partner shortly after her divorce was finalized. However, the client reports having intimate encounters with both her new partner and her ex-husband, and she describes feeling invigorated by being able to string along both people.

In hearing her client describe her new relationships, Becky feels the urge to talk to her client about how moving back and forth between two relationships may be negatively impacting her children. Becky knows the client's children stay with aunts, uncles, and cousins while their mom goes out to party with her husband and partner and are never exposed to their mother's escapades. Still, Becky believes her client has a duty to be at home with her children and raise them properly rather than pawn them off on family members.

What can you surmise about Becky's values from this case illustration?

How should Becky handle her strong feelings about her client's parenting choices?

Case Illustration 1-1 is an example of how a counselor's values can get in the way of his/her work with clients. Becky has strong beliefs about her client's behaviors and how her client raises her children. In response to the first question posed in Case Illustration 1-1, the reader is able to determine that Becky has strong beliefs in favor of parents staying at home with their children rather than sending them to other family members' houses. One might also deduct from the illustration that Becky believes in monogamous relationships and may not approve of her client's lifestyle.

In response to the second question, there are many ways Becky might respond. Whichever she chooses it is critical that she separates her own values from the values of the counseling profession. There are no ethical standards guiding counselors to instruct parents on assumed proper parenting styles.

Various professional organizations, licensure boards, and agencies have developed codes of ethics to help guide their members' decisions. For example, the ACA developed the ACA Code of Ethics (2014), the American Psychological Association (APA) developed ethical principles of psychologists (2010), and the AAMFT developed the AAMFT Code of Ethics (2015). Each of the previously mentioned associations developed ethical standards to act as a guide of best practices for their respective professions. In the preamble, the ACA identifies five main purposes of the code of ethics: (1) to clarify the nature of the ethical responsibilities held by the members of the organization; (2) to help support the mission of the organization; (3) to establish principles, best practices, and ethical behaviors for members; (4) to serve as an ethical guide to members in making decisions about practice; and (5) to serve as a basis for processing ethical complaints (ACA, 2014). Even with these five main purposes, the ACA and other codes of ethics do not provide a cure-all or dictate specific guidelines for practice. Ethical standards cannot be applied in a prescription-type manner (Freeman, 2000). Rather, codes of ethics provide a broad, general guide to what is generally considered "best practice." See Case Illustration 1-2 as an example of how the ACA Code of Ethics guides a counselor without providing strict, prescription-type instruction.

CASE ILLUSTRATION 1-2

Faisal is a newly licensed professional counselor who works at a community mental health clinic. He has been meeting with Mr. and Mrs. Vasquez for almost two months due to some minor marital conflict. In the past few sessions, the Vasquezes have made tremendous progress and are considering terminating the counseling relationship because they have accomplished the goals set at the onset of services. At one of their last counseling sessions, Mr. and Mrs. Vasquez express their extreme gratitude to Faisal for his help in strengthening the couple's relationship. Mrs. Vasquez invites Faisal to a dinner at the couple's house. Mr. and Mrs. Vasquez both describe the dinner as a "celebration of their rejuvenated love for each other." There will be many friends and family members attending, and they would be honored to have Faisal attend as he played such a large role in their marital success.

How should Faisal respond to the couple's request?

How does the ACA Code of Ethics direct Faisal's response?

As stated previously, codes of ethics do not offer prescription-type guidelines; therefore, in Case Illustration 1-2 Faisal has many options. The only action he "should" take is to engage in an ethical decision-making model. In response to the second question in Case Illustration 1-2, the ACA Code of Ethics offers Faisal guidance in ethical Standard A.6.b. (Extending Counseling Boundaries). Standard A.6.b. requires Faisal to consider risks and benefits of extending boundaries with the Vasquez family and directs Faisal to discuss possible concerns with his clients. Ethical Standard A.6.b. does not direct Faisal to either attend or not attend the dinner. Rather, it guides him on "best practices" for making a thoughtful choice of how to respond to the Vasquez's invitation.

Professional ethical codes provide assistance and protection to both practitioners and the general public. For practitioners, codes of ethics provide some backing and support if your actions are ever called into question. When responding to an ethics complaint, counselors must show they acted in an ethical or "appropriate" manner. This means they acted in a way others with similar training would act if they were put in a similar situation. The code of ethics also provides some assistance in guiding one's decisions related to his/her counseling practice (Freeman, 2000; Meara, Schmidt, & Day, 1996).

Using the example provided in Case Illustration 1-2, the ACA Code of Ethics could provide support to Faisal if anyone were to make a complaint about his decision, for example, if Faisal attended the dinner, and someone at the dinner did not agree with his attendance and decided to make a complaint to Faisal's state licensure board. The ACA Code of Ethics could offer support to Faisal if he acted according to the ACA Code of Ethics Standard I.1.b. (Ethical Decision Making), Standard A.6.b. (Extending Counseling Boundaries), and A.6.c. (Documenting Boundary Extensions). By following the ACA Code of Ethics, Faisal would be able to show he acted as other counselors would act if placed in a similar situation.

For the general public and clients, the codes of ethics provide assurance than services will adhere to certain standards. Clients who visit a professional counselor can expect their counselors to have a certain level of training and act or behave in a professional manner.

Principle Ethics

Professional counseling codes of ethics are strongly based on the moral principles of autonomy, beneficence, non-maleficence, justice, fidelity, and veracity. The principles of autonomy, non-maleficence, beneficence, and justice were first discussed by Beauchamp and Childress (1979). Kitchener, in Urofsky, Engles, and Engebretson (2008), expanded on the original four, adding fidelity, and Meara et al. (1996) again expanded the principles by adding veracity. For information on the APA's and AAMFT's principles of ethics, see Text Box 1-1.

Autonomy

Autonomy is the right to self-determination. As a professional counselor, it is important for students and clinicians to remember that clients have the right to choose their own path and make their own decisions. This means they have the freedom to choose what they wish to talk and not talk about. They also have the choice to pursue or discontinue counseling services. Oftentimes respecting a client's autonomy is straightforward and relatively easy to observe. Consider Case Illustration 1-3 as an example of when counselors might find it easy to respect a client's autonomy.

CASE ILLUSTRATION 1-3

A counselor is meeting with her client Cheryl. Cheryl first initiated counseling due to her discontent with her current working conditions. Cheryl reports to her counselor that she is unhappy with her current work hours and the wages she is paid. Cheryl and her counselor decide to set "finding a new job" as the primary goal for counseling.

In Case Illustration 1-3, Cheryl sought out counseling to help her find a new job. The authors believe it is likely Cheryl's counselor will have little trouble respecting Cheryl's decision to work on finding a new job. Cheryl's counselor will not likely challenge her to stay in the same job or avoid changing jobs. In other situations respecting a client's autonomy may be more difficult for counselors. Consider Case Illustration 1-4 as an example of when it may be more difficult for some counselors to respect a client's autonomy.

CASE ILLUSTRATION 1-4

Conner is a 35-year-old married male and the father of two young boys. Conner reports that both he and his wife work, and their family lives quite comfortably. Conner meets with his counselor and tells her he is not happy with the way his life has turned out. Conner further reports that he never wanted to have children and wants to run away from his family and go to live in a cabin in the middle of the mountains by himself.

In a situation such as the one presented in Case Illustration 1-4, it may be more difficult for counselors to respect the client's autonomy. Counselors may not tell Conner he shouldn't leave his family or move to a secluded cabin, but the questions counselors may ask might hinder his autonomy. For example, counselors might be more inclined to ask "Why do you want to do that and how will your choice affect your family?" more in Case Illustration 1-4 than in Case Illustration 1-3. Case Illustration 1-4 may also bring about more negative remarks from the counselor than Case Illustration 1-3 (e.g., "You moving away and just disappearing are going to seriously affect your kids.").

In some of these cases, counselors may be ethically or legally required to notify a third party (e.g., child abuse, elder abuse, or clear and foreseeable harm); still, clients have a right to make their own choices free from judgment from their counselors. Clients are able to choose their own path and are responsible for their own behaviors.

Non-Maleficence

Sperry (2007) described non-maleficence as the "most fundamental ethical value across all helping professions" (p. 26). It means, as counselors, we do not harm our clients. Counselors may not always aid in improving clients' situations, some may stay the same. However, clients should not be worse off or harmed by their interactions with or the services provided by professional counselors. Doing no harm involves actions that are both intentional and unintentional. While very few counselors may intentionally harm their clients, many may unintentionally cause harm. Incompetence in working with a particular client or population may be a form of causing harm to clients (Meara et al., 1996). Review case illustration 1-5 and the examples of how counselors may unintentionally cause harm to clients.

CASE ILLUSTRATION 1-5

Example 1

A counselor typically goes out with friends on Wednesday nights and stays out late. As a result the counselor finds himself yawning and feeling tired during his Thursday morning sessions; oftentimes fighting the urge to fall asleep during session.

Example 2

A new professional working in an agency setting is trying to build her caseload and notoriety with referral sources. As a result, she takes on many referrals of clients with a broad range of concerns; some that may be outside of her competence area.

In example one of case illustration 1-5 the counselor certainly is not acting maliciously toward his clients. However, in going out late and failing to recognize how the lack of sleep or late night activities may affect the next mornings' sessions this counselor is possibly unintentionally harming his clients. Counselors never know how clients may interpret yawning or lack of attention during session. Some may understand and others may take it as a sign that their issues are unimportant or boring.

Example two in case illustration 1-5 describes a new counselor trying to build her caseload. Many professional counselors begin their careers in agency settings and it is common to want to take on as many clients as possible to gain notoriety and maximize financial gain. However, while doing so, counselors must also always monitor their own effectiveness and take care to not expand the boundaries of competence too quickly. Doing so may lead to symptoms of burnout and unintentional harm to clients.

Beneficence

Beneficence is doing good or active kindness toward others. Beneficence involves counselors helping their clients and members of society who could benefit from their expertise (Houser & Thoma, 2013). This also means counselors sometimes act in a way to prevent harm from coming to their clients. In some situations counselors have the duty to intervene in order to try and prevent that harm from occurring. Examine case illustration 1-6 as an example of how a counselor might practice beneficence.

CASE ILLUSTRATION 1-6

Amy is a professional school counselor working at a large urban high school. One of her students approaches her at the end of the school day appearing to be very distraught. The student describes her plans to go home and seriously injure herself because of a recent breakup with a longtime friend. The student shares a "good-bye" letter she wrote during the school day and describes her plans to hurt herself in great detail.

Hearing her student's concerns and understanding the imminent harm, Amy talks with her student and finds a safe place for her student to wait while her parents come to pick her up. Upon hearing of their daughter's plans, the parents make arrangements for her to be assessed by a psychiatrist and physician.

Case illustration 1-6 describes Amy's actions to protect her student in a time of distress. By talking with her student, contacting the student's parents, and facilitating a referral to the psychiatrist/physician, Amy was acting with beneficence in mind.

Justice

Justice is being fair and consistent with services. For counselors, this can involve many things. If counselors are going to offer *pro bono* or reduced rate services, they make the criteria to receive such services consistent among all clients. Additionally, counselors work to make sure the offices and institutions they work within do not discriminate against others. Review case illustration 1-7, which exemplifies a counselor's struggles with Justice.

CASE ILLUSTRATION 1-7

Alyson has been working in private practice for over 10 years. Over the ten years, she has worked with many clients for various lengths of time. Jennifer, one of her weekly clients, called and left a message earlier today saying she would not be able to make her appointment due to being sick with the flu. Since Alyson has developed a close working relationship with Jennifer and they have a very strong rapport, Alyson writes a short get well note and drops it in the mail to Jennifer. It simply says "I hope you are feeling better soon and I look forward to scheduling our next visit." In addition to the card, Alyson also sends a small Edible Arrangements bouquet to Jennifer.

If Alyson does not write and mail a get well card to all of her clients and send a fruit bouquet, could it be seen as unethical? Is she acting with justice in mind?

Similar to some of the previous examples, Alyson may not be acting maliciously toward her clients; regardless, she may be guilty of ignoring the principle of justice. If Alyson does not write a get well card and send a fruit arrangement to all of her clients when she knows they are sick, she may be sending the wrong message to Jennifer (i.e., that her relationship with Jennifer is more important or different than the relationship she has with other clients).

Fidelity

Fidelity is faithfulness, being honest, loyal, and keeping the commitments you make to others (Sperry, 2007). Welfel (2010) indicates that a key to fidelity is counselors putting the best interests of their clients in front of their own even in situations when it puts the counselor in an uncomfortable situation. In short, counselors are honest and truthful in their interactions with others. Trust is of immense importance in the counseling relationship. Without trust, very few clients would be willing to enter into a counseling relationship and share their concerns with a stranger. See Case Illustration 1-8 and the two examples of counselors' fidelity to their clients.

CASE ILLUSTRATION 1-8

Example 1

Paul is a licensed professional counselor and is currently working with Kevin. At the end of this week's session, Paul indicates he will bring an article to the next session that he thinks may be helpful to Kevin. During the week, things get busy, and Paul forgets to print and bring the article. When Kevin asks about the article at their next session, Paul says he forgot and will try to remember for next week.

Example 2

Steven is a counselor working in private practice. He sees clients back-to-back throughout the day and typically writes his case notes in the short time he has between clients. Even though his clients are scheduled on the hour (e.g., 2 p.m., 3 p.m., etc.), he typically keeps his clients waiting 10 to 15 minutes past the start of the hour, while he finishes his notes from the previous session.

In Example 1 of Case Illustration 1-8, Paul is not acting with fidelity in mind. When counselors tell clients they will provide information, it is critical that they follow through on those commitments. As previously stated, counselors must put the best interests of the client ahead of their own. In Example 1 Paul is still obligated to bring articles for his client, even though it may cause him to work overtime through a busy week.

In Example 2 of Case Illustration 1-8, Steven must also follow through with his commitments to clients. If Steven schedules an appointment for 2 p.m., he should be ready to begin the session at 2 p.m. unless there is an unforeseen event preventing him from starting on time (e.g., extreme traffic conditions, illness, family emergency, or crisis with a previous client).

Veracity

Discussed in depth by Meara et al. (1996), the authors have argued for elevating veracity to an ethical principle rather than simply a rule. Veracity means to be truthful and honest in working with clients and other professionals (Remley & Herlihy, 2014). For counselors, this means being truthful about our qualifications and credentials. Examine Case Illustration 1-9 as an example of how the principle of veracity might affect counselors.

CASE ILLUSTRATION 1-9

Betty is a licensed professional counselor who has been invited to a middle school in her town to talk about non-suicidal self-injury. Betty has been asked to speak to parents and teachers about how to recognize signs of distress in students due to her reputation around town and knowledge of the topic. As the principal introduces her as the speaker, Betty hears that she is being introduced as "a psychologist who is an expert in self-injury."

What should Betty do in this situation?

In Case Illustration 1-9, Betty is put into what could be an awkward situation. It is Betty's responsibility to make sure she clearly identifies her credentials and educational background according to the principle of veracity and according the ACA Code of Ethics Standards C.4.a. and C.4.b. (ACA, 2014).

TEXT BOX 1-1

American Psychological Association

The APA's Ethical Principles of Psychologists and Code of Conduct (2010) uses similar language to the ACA when describing the principles on which their ethical codes are based. The APA's general principles include the following:

Principle A: Beneficence and Non-Maleficence

Similar to the ACA's principles of beneficence and non-maleficence, psychologists work to do no harm to those with whom they work. Additionally, APA includes specific wording urging psychologists to "guard against personal, financial, social, organizational, or political factors that might lead to misuse of their influence" (APA, 2010, p. 3). Simply stated, to understand the power that goes along with the title of "psychologist" means being conscientious and thoughtful about your relationships and business practices to avoid the abuse of your power.

Principle B: Fidelity and Responsibility

Again, similar to the ACA Code of Ethics, fidelity means being faithful and trustworthy. Psychologists are encouraged to be honest and build trusting relationships with those with whom they work. Principle B also includes the notion of responsibility. Psychologists are responsible for clarifying their roles, cooperating with others, and gatekeeping for the profession. Finally, Principle B includes the obligation for psychologists to dedicate a portion of their time to providing pro-bono services. The ACA Code of Ethics obliges professional counselors to do the same in Standard C.6.e. (Contributing to the Public Good; ACA, 2014).

Principle C: Integrity

Integrity equates to being honest and truthful and is similar to the ACA principle of veracity. Psychologists are honest in their reporting and do not "steal, cheat, or engage in fraud, subterfuge, or intentional misrepresentation of fact" (APA, 2010, p. 3).

Principle D: Justice

The principle of justice is one that is included in both the ACA and APA Codes of Ethics. Justice is being fair and consistent in services provided to consumers. Professional counselors and psychologists are cautious to make sure personal biases do not interfere with their ability to provide quality services.

Principle E: Respect for People's Rights and Dignity

The principle of respect for people's rights and dignity is in line with ACA's principle of autonomy. Psychologists respect their clients' right to privacy, confidentiality, and self-determination. Similarly, psychologists respect cultural diversity and avoid imposing their own values and biases onto clients.

American Association of Marriage and Family Therapy

AAMFT does not include general principles such as the ACA or APA. Instead they include "core values." The AAMFT core values are as follows:

(Continued)

(Continued)

1. Acceptance, appreciation, and inclusion of a diverse membership

2. Distinctiveness and excellence in training of marriage and family therapists and those desiring to advance their skills, knowledge, and expertise in systemic and relational therapies

3. Responsiveness and excellence in service to members

4. Diversity, equity, and excellence in clinical practice, research education, and administration

5. Integrity evidenced by a high threshold of ethical and honest behavior within association governance and by members

6. Innovation and the advancement of knowledge of systemic and relational therapies

Ethics as Philosophy

Self-awareness and understanding why we do the things we do are critical competencies for counselors. Therefore incorporating some philosophical constructs of decision making seems appropriate in understanding our own decision making. The philosophy of ethics includes reasoning and using processes to determine which actions are most appropriate in given situations (Freeman, 2000). Beginning and seasoned counselors often strive to do what is "best" for clients or make the "right" decision when finding themselves in ethical dilemmas. However, before counselors are able to determine what is right and wrong, they must first understand how we, as individuals, understand right and wrong.

Relativism Versus Absolutism

Where do you stand firm, and where do you have room for flexibility? Do you believe there is always a right and wrong answer? Do you believe there are absolute rights and absolute wrongs? These are just a few questions that may be helpful in understanding where you stand on certain issues and begin to bring awareness to how you may interpret codes of ethics.

Cultural relativists believe there are rights and wrongs; however, what is right and wrong is determined by those in a particular culture. If it is right for the culture or society one lives in, then it is right (Freeman, 2000). For example, a community or culture that believes in sharing and ownership belongs to everyone. If everyone in the community has equal access to all assets and supplies within the community, then a cultural relativist may argue that it is right for someone in the community to take and use things they need or wish to take without asking the permission of others. However, if one lives in a community that does not believe in shared ownership and community supplies, then a cultural relativist would argue that it is not ethical to take and use materials without asking. On the contrary, someone who is an ethical absolutist would most likely argue the community you live in or the beliefs of those around you do not matter in determining the ethicality of your actions. An absolutist would argue that taking things without asking is unethical or wrong in all situations. Review Case Exercise 1-1 and reflect on how you feel about the topics presented.

CASE EXERCISE 1-1

Think about issues or areas in which your beliefs may be more relativistic or absolutist. When thinking about these areas, consider what you believe is "right" or "wrong" and not necessarily what you believe your obligations are as a professional counselor. Consider your feelings related to the following:

Education and the importance of school

Multiple relationships

Premarital or extramarital sexual relationships

Gang activity

Suicide

Alcohol or drug usage

How might your own personal beliefs about these areas influence your reading and understanding of ethical codes?

Motivation

Freeman (2000) asks, "What motivates individuals to act or choose one action over another?" and "Do we always act for the sake of our own self-interest or do we sometimes act for the sake of others?" (p. 34). Counselors are encouraged to always look out for their clients and act in a way promoting the best interests of clients. The ACA Code of Ethics (2014) Section A.1.a specifically points out that the top priority and responsibility for counselors is the welfare of their clients. However, in everyday life and especially as counselors, there is a continuous balancing act between our altruistic and egotistic selves—altruistic meaning the part of us motivated to do things purely for the benefit of others and egotistic meaning the things we do for our own self-interests. Consider Case Illustration 1-10 as an example of the pull between altruism and egoism.

CASE ILLUSTRATION 1-10

Look at the decisions and actions you make on a daily basis and even as a counselor in training. Are your motivations altruistic or egotistic?

When driving your car, do you follow the speed limit (assuming that you do) because you are looking out for others on the road and want to drive safely or because you want to avoid getting a speeding ticket and having to pay a fine?

When making your choice to pursue a counseling degree, was it so that you could be trained to help and use your learned skills to improve the lives of others or because you wanted a better job, to make more income, or simply the status of having an advanced degree?

When working with a client who indicates she has had recent thoughts about harming herself, do you break confidentiality and notify the proper authority because you want to keep your client safe or because you don't want to possibly be held accountable?

As a school counselor, you are meeting with a student who indicates he is sexually active with other students at the school, and you know your student is under the legal age of consent. Do you break confidentiality and notify others? If so, what is your motivation? Is it the student's safety and well-being or your own concern that you may be held accountable if it is found out that you knew about these behaviors and did not report them?

In all of the situations presented in Case Illustration 1-10 and possibly many others, your motivations are most likely a mix of altruism and egoism. For example, in the first scenario presented in Case Illustration 1-10, readers are asked to reflect on their reasons for driving the speed limit. Most would probably agree that they drive the speed limit as a way to avoid being stopped by the police and looking out for the safety of others on the road. Therefore individuals follow the speed limit for both altruistic and egotistic reasons. Similarly, the third scenario in Case Illustration 1-10 asks about breaking confidentiality when a client reports wanting to hurt herself. Counselors might choose reporting as a way to avoid any legal repercussions (i.e., counselor could be held liable if the client does hurt herself) and because the counselor genuinely does not want any harm to come to the client—again a mix of altruistic and egotistic motivations.

In the upcoming chapters the authors will discuss ethical decision making and how individuals interpret ethical codes. For right now we stress understanding and being aware of your motivations. The authors believe it is not unethical or wrong to have egotistic or altruistic motivations; however, it is critical counselors understand the motivation behind their actions.

Socratic Method

The Socratic method is a way of seeking knowledge. It seeks to determine what is opinion and what it truth through the use of questions and answers. Socrates argued that knowing the truth or right, no one would ever choose the wrong. He believed that when people make an incorrect choice or act in a hurtful way, they do so believing it will have some benefit (Freeman, 2000).

For counselors and counselors in training, the Socratic method is helpful in making decisions based on fact and reason rather than on assumption. Counselors may be tempted to fall into the trap of making quick decisions based on what they believe to be true or what they have heard from others to be true rather than seeking the truth themselves. The Socratic method may also be helpful for counselors when looking to clarify their own personal values as opposed to a value of the counseling profession. Examine Case Illustration 1-11 and how Sarah and her clinical supervisor work through an ethical dilemma.

CASE ILLUSTRATION 1-11

Sarah has recently graduated with her master's degree in counseling and started working toward completing the supervised experience hours needed to become a licensed professional counselor. In her most recent supervision session, she shared information about a new client she is seeing, Mark. She described Mark as a 19-year-old male who lives at home with his parents. He does not have a job and does not go to school anymore. Sarah is concerned about Mark because during their last session, he described an incident in which he needed some money for gas, and his parents would not lend him any. As a result, he went to a local convenience store and robbed the store (threatening the clerk with a fake gun he had). During session, Mark joked about how easy it was and said he would maybe do it again sometime if he needed the money. He also seemed to show little remorse for his actions.

In her conversations with her supervisor, Sarah mentions that she feels like she needs to do something; she should call the police to report the behavior. She describes feeling as though stealing is wrong, and Mark must be held accountable for his actions. Sarah knows she is not ethically able to report past criminal behavior but still feels like it needs to be reported. After some thinking and looking over the code of ethics, Sarah mentions that she feels like Mark may be a danger to himself because he might get hurt if one of his future robberies does not go well. She also states that he might be dangerous to others if he does another robbery because he showed little remorse for the first one. She asks, "Who is to say he won't do more or actually hurt someone the next time he robs a store for money?" Sarah rationalizes her decision to break confidentiality and report Mark's behavior based on the ACA Code of Ethics Section B.2.a. (Serious and Foreseeable Harm and Legal Requirements).

If Sarah chooses to report her client's behavior to the police, would her actions be considered ethical?

What should Sarah do in this situation and why?

How might Sarah's supervisor use the Socratic Method in this situation to help her clarify her decision?

The first question associated with this case illustration asks about the ethicality of Sarah's actions if she were to report Mark's past criminal history to the police. In response, it is difficult to say for sure whether reporting Mark's robbery would be considered ethical. However, Sarah was correct in stating there is no part of the ACA Code of Ethics requiring her to report clients' past criminal behavior. Hence, it would most likely be seen as unethical and an inappropriate breach of confidentiality if she were to call the police unless Mark specifically indicated he was going to commit another crime.

The second question in Case Illustration 1-11 inquires as to what Sarah should do given the situation. Simply stated, Sarah would want to engage in an ethical decision-making process (e.g., identify the problem; identify relevant ethical codes and legal statutes; consult with others; consider her own morals, values, and beliefs; identify possible courses of action; consider the consequences of all possible courses of action; and finally make a decision on how best to move forward). The ACA Code of Ethics Standard I.1.b. (Ethical Decision Making) directs counselors to engage in an ethical decision making process when faced with an ethical dilemma.

Question 3 associated with Case Illustration 1-11 asks how Sarah's supervisor might use the Socratic method to help Sarah clarify her decision. Her supervisor might ask her questions to challenge her own thought processes. Review the dialogue between Sarah and her supervisor in Case Illustration 1-12 as one example of how Sarah's supervisor might use Socratic questioning to help her identify a best course of action.

CASE ILLUSTRATION 1-12

Supervisor: Sarah, I understand you are having trouble deciding on whether or not you should report your client's behavior to the police based on the ethical standard related to Serious and Foreseeable Harm. Please help me understand how you interpret that standard.

Sarah: My understanding is I have to report behaviors if I think someone is going to hurt someone else or be seriously harmed themselves. I feel like it's possible Mark could hurt someone if he ever gets desperate for money again. Things might not go the way he planned, and he might get hurt, or he might do something drastic and hurt someone else.

Supervisor: I understand your worry, and if you did call the police, I'm wondering what you might tell them? For example, would you be calling the police to report a past crime, or would you be calling to tell them about a "foreseeable crime," with foreseeable meaning likely, predictable, or probable?

Sarah: I would probably be reporting his past crimes because I don't know when, how, or even if the future crime may occur.

Supervisor: Therefore you would be reporting a serious past crime instead of a serious and foreseeable crime? Do you see any standards in the ACA Code of Ethics or any legal requirements obligating you to report serious past crimes?

Sarah:	No, I guess not.
Supervisor:	Sarah, I can see you are struggling with this issue because you have very strong values about theft, robbery, and taking things that don't belong to you. Still, it seems like those are your values and not necessarily the values of the counseling profession or the values of your client.
Sarah:	I see what you mean, but it's still very difficult for me to separate the two. I don't know if I will be able to sleep knowing I'm staying quiet and letting my client get away with his crime.
Supervisor:	I understand, and I think we might want to explore your values and ways in which you might be more easily able to separate your own personal values from the values of the counseling profession.

Conclusion

Chapter 1 introduces readers to the ACA Code of Ethics and its six principles: autonomy, beneficence, non-maleficence, veracity, justice, and fidelity). It acts as a basis for the remaining 13 chapters and encourages counselors to question their own decision making. We believe self-reflection and self-evaluation are critical components of developing into a counselor and address issues related to motivation and relativism. The authors describe Socratic questioning in hopes that counselors will begin to challenge their own beliefs and natural tendencies to choose one action over another. Johann Wolfgang von Goethe said there is nothing more frightful than ignorance in action. Related to counseling, there is nothing more dangerous than a counselor who acts without knowing the basis for his or her actions. Chapter 1 and the remainder of this text are geared toward counselors not only understanding the ACA Code of Ethics but also how they monitor their own ethical interpretations. Use the information you have learned in this chapter to address the ethical dilemma presented in Case Exercise 1-2 and the corresponding discussion questions.

CASE EXERCISE 1-2

You are a counselor who recently began working with Kevin, a 33-year-old male who is married and a father of two young children. He was referred to you by a social worker at the hospital where he was recently diagnosed with a serious but treatable form of lung cancer. During your most recent session with Kevin, he shared with you his struggles with depression since losing his job over a year ago. As the months went by and he was unable to find a new job, he began to lose hope and now feels as though he is "a failure and unable to support his wife and kids like any good man should." He feels as though this new diagnosis is just another way he is letting

(Continued)

(Continued)

his family down and causing more problems than doing good. He mentions that against his doctor's recommendations, he believes he will not seek treatment for his cancer or fight it in any way. In addition, he says he has decided to keep his diagnosis a secret from his wife, kids, and family. He doesn't want to cause them any additional stress. Kevin says that after he dies, his wife won't be held down anymore, and she can find a "real man" to support her and his kids. At the end of your session, Kevin states that he likes talking with you and would like to keep meeting with you until his medical condition deteriorates to the point he is physically no longer able to. He says talking with you helps as he doesn't want to share his diagnosis with anyone else.

As the counselor working with Kevin, are there any ethical dilemmas that you may need to address?

Explore your own personal values. How might your own values affect the way that you work with Kevin?

How might your personal values affect the types of questions you ask or other interactions you have with Kevin?

How do the principles of autonomy, justice, fidelity, non-maleficence, beneficence, and veracity relate to Kevin's case?

How might you proceed in working with Kevin? What is your motivation for the actions you choose?

Discussion Questions

How do you understand what is right and what is wrong? What do you use as your guide? Laws? Ethical codes? Other guides?

Do you believe it is possible to separate our own personal ethics from our professional ethics?

Do you consider yourself to have more absolutist or relativist views?

Keystones

- Ethical codes are living, changing documents, therefore understanding how to interpret ethical codes is more critical than memorizing them.
- Ethics is the study of acceptable behaviors governing the conduct of those in a particular profession.
- It is critical for counselors to separate personal ethics from professional ethics.
- Codes of ethics do not provide prescriptive cures for all ethical dilemmas. Instead they provide general guidelines for all practice.
- Principles on which the ACA Code of Ethics are built include autonomy, non-maleficence, beneficence, fidelity, veracity, and justice.

- Counselors should always be aware of their motivations and understand the influence of egoism versus altruism.
- Socratic questioning helps counselors make decisions based on fact rather than opinion.

Additional Resources

Amada, G. (2010). Mandatory counseling: Clinical beneficence or malevolence? *Journal of College Student Psychotherapy, 24*(4), 284–294. doi:http://dx.doi.org/10.1080/87568225.2010.509225

Elliott, G. R. (2011). When values and ethics conflict: The counselor's role and responsibility. *Alabama Counseling Association Journal, 37*, 39–45.

Fialkov, E. D., Jackson, M. A., & Rabinowitz, M. (2014). Effects of experience and surface-level distraction on ability to perceive ethical issues. *Training and Education in Professional Psychology, 8*(4), 277–284. doi:http://dx.doi.org/10.1037/tep0000067

Lambie, G., Ieva, K., & Ohrt, J. (2012). Impact of a counseling ethics course on graduate students' learning and development. *International Journal for the Scholarship of Teaching and Learning, 6*, 1–15.

Wolf, A. W. (2009). Comment: Can clinical judgment hold its own against scientific knowledge? Comment on Zeldow. *Psychotherapy: Theory, Research, Practice, Training, 46*(1), 11–14. doi:http://dx.doi.org/10.1037/a0015133

References

American Association for Marriage and Family Therapy. (2015). *Code of ethics*. Retrieved from https://www.aamft.org/iMIS15/AAMFT/Content/legal_ethics/code_of_ethics.aspx

American Counseling Association. (2014). *Code of ethics*. Alexandria, VA: Author.

American Psychological Association. (2010). *American Psychological Association ethical principles of psychologists and code of conduct*. Retrieved from http://www.apa.org/ethics/code/principles.pdf

Beauchamp, T. L., & Childress, J. F. (1979). *Principles of biomedical ethics*. New York: Oxford University Press.

Cottone, R. R., & Tarvydas, V. M. (2007). *Counseling ethics and decision making* (3rd ed.). Upper Saddle River, NJ: Pearson Merrill Prentice-Hall.

Ethics. (n.d.). In *Merriam-Webster online* (n.d.). Retrieved from http://www.merriam-webster.com/dictionary/ethics

Ford, G. G. (2006). *Ethical reasoning for mental health professionals*. Thousand Oaks, CA: Sage.

Freeman, S. J. (2000). *Ethics: An introduction to philosophy & practice*. Belmont, CA: Wadsworth.

Housa, R. A., & Thoma, S. (2013). *Ethics in counseling & therapy*. Thousand Oaks, CA: Sage.

Meara, N. M., Schmidt, L. D., & Day, J. D. (1996). Principles and virtues: A foundation for ethical decisions, policies, and character. *Counseling Psychologist, 24*, 4–77.

Remley, T. P., & Herlihy, B. (2014). *Ethical, legal, and professional issues in counseling* (4th ed.). Upper Saddle River, NJ: Pearson.

Sperry, L. (2007). *The ethical and professional practice of counseling and psychotherapy*. New York: Pearson.

Urofsky, R. I., Engles, D. W., & Engebretson, K. (2008). Kitchener's principle ethics: Implications for counseling practice and research. *Counseling and Values, 53*, 67–78.

Welfel, E. R. (2010). *Ethics in counseling & psychotherapy: Standards, research, and emerging issues*. Belmont, CA: Brooks/Cole.

2

The Counselor as a Person and Professional Identity

Price is what you pay. Value is what you get.

—Warren Buffett

Chapter 2 will build on the self-awareness introduced in the first chapter. Readers will examine their motivations in entering the counseling profession, how they handle stress, and their own values. The chapter will then examine the counseling profession and values within it. The authors will differentiate counseling from other mental health professions. The latter half of the chapter will discuss the process of becoming a professional counselor. Students will be introduced to the various degrees and credentialing standards along with professional organizations. Ethical dilemmas in this chapter will encourage students to reflect on themselves as professionals and their identity as professional counselors.

In your training to become a professional counselor, you have no doubt learned or will learn many different theories and techniques to aid you in your practice. However, the primary tool that you will use in working with others is yourself. Therefore, understanding yourself or becoming clear about self-awareness is critical in developing yourself as a competent and ethical counselor. Similar to gaining a full understanding of a chosen theory before using it in practice (i.e., the background, history, basic concepts, techniques, view of the counseling relationship, etc.), it is best to have a full understanding of yourself before working with others. In this chapter the authors address issues related to self-awareness in addition to professional identity. After reading this chapter the reader will be able to accomplish the following:

1. Explain the differences in various mental health professions including the difference between wellness and medical models.

2. Describe the educational requirements and overall process in becoming a professional school or clinical mental health counselor.

3. Define the purpose of professional counseling associations.

4. Discuss the effect personal values have on interactions with clients.

5. Explain the relationship between counselor values and being an ethical counselor.

Counselor Self-Awareness

What brings you to this profession? How did you decide to enter a counseling program? In Chapter 1, we discussed what motivates individuals to choose one action over another. With that in mind, was your decision to seek out a counseling degree more egocentric or altruistic? Whatever the reason, it is important to be aware of your motivations and understand how they may affect your ability to work with certain clients. Counseling is a profession involving intimate relationships between counselors and the clients they serve. As you begin working with clients, you will often gain a very detailed understanding of clients' behaviors and the way they view life. Some clients may have beliefs very similar to your own, and some may have beliefs that are polar opposites. Certainly all clients will have some effect on you as a counselor. Knowing yourself, your values, how you handle stress, and your own unresolved issues is critical to your development as an ethical counselor.

In Chapter 1 the authors discussed values of the counseling profession. Later, in Chapter 5, they will discuss the ethical responsibility counselors have to avoid imposing values onto clients. Before counselors are able to avoid imposing values onto clients, they must first be self-aware and fully understand their own morals, values, and beliefs. Take a look at the counselor in case Illustration 2-1 to see how motivation and values affect Neelam and the way in which she works with her client Fred.

CASE ILLUSTRATION 2-1

Neelam, a graduate student in a clinical mental health program, is near the end of her course work and this semester is completing her practicum. As a part of the class, she meets with clients at her university's counseling clinic and receives supervision from both a site supervisor and the faculty teaching the class. Prior to starting her graduate studies, Neelam struggled

(Continued)

(Continued)

with addictions, and she is still very active in her Alcoholics Anonymous (AA) group. Neelam spent many years trying to get sober, and the only thing she feels helped her maintain her sobriety was her dedication to AA and following the 12-step program. Since getting sober, Neelam has also helped many others in her AA group maintain sobriety. Her career goal after graduation is to primarily work with adults who are struggling with addictions. Neelam feels as though she has a special connection with those individuals and can help them by sharing some of her own successes. As a result of her interest in working with addictions and her confidence in working with that population, Neelam specifically requests to work with anyone coming into the clinic who is dealing with addictions.

Recently, Neelam started working with Fred, a 56-year-old male, who claims to be struggling with relationships. He also admits to having a minor drinking problem that he believes may contribute to his anger outbursts. At the end of the first session, during the session summary and closure, Neelam suggests that Fred find an AA group to attend and ultimately seek out a sponsor. Neelam also provides Fred with some AA-related pamphlets and says she looks forward to seeing him again next week.

The following week Fred does not show up for his appointment, and he calls in later to say that he is no longer interested in counseling at this time. During her supervision session, Neelam explains Fred's discontinuation of services as his not wanting sobriety bad enough yet. When asked more about it, Neelam explains in her experience, alcoholics have to hit rock bottom before they can get better. Fred simply has not hit rock bottom yet, and he won't be able to get sober until he does.

What is Neelam's motivation in becoming a professional counselor?

What are Neelam's values related to sobriety and how individuals gain and maintain sobriety?

How might Neelam's references to AA have affected Fred's decision to seek out counseling?

In Case Illustration 2-1, Neelam is a counseling student who has fairly strong beliefs about AA and its importance in gaining sobriety. In response to the first two questions in Case Illustration 2-1, it seems clear Neelam was drawn to the counseling profession to help others who are struggling with addiction. Neelam struggled with addictions herself and wants to share her story with others as a way to help them "get sober." Additionally, Neelam feels as though the most effective way to maintain sobriety is to closely follow the 12-step program. Neelam knows the 12-step program was and is the only thing that has helped her gain and maintain sobriety.

Neelam's motivations and values are not necessarily a concern in this scenario. There are many people who likely join the counseling profession for similar reasons. Concern arises only when Neelam's own personal beliefs and values become an imposition on her clients. The third question related to Case Illustration 2-1 is likely the most important one (i.e., How did her actions affect her client?). Neelam has very strong beliefs about the

12-step program, but what does her client think about it? Neelam may have viewed her suggestions and informational pamphlets as an honest effort to provide her client with "helpful" information. However, what if Fred does not believe in the 12-step program or AA? What Neelam saw as a genuine way of providing the best help may have come across to Fred as her being pushy and wanting to force her agenda onto him.

With that said, it is not unethical or inappropriate to share possibly helpful information with clients. The unethical or inappropriateness is not in the information shared but rather how the information is shared. Review the following interactions and two different ways of sharing information.

#1 Neelam:		We are getting close to the end of our session today, and I know you talked some today about your struggles with alcohol. I highly recommend you seek out an AA group and start attending. The groups are wonderful, and even though they may seem a bit uncomfortable at first, I think you will really benefit from attending. I also have some general information about 12-step programs in these pamphlets (hands materials to Fred). Would you like to reschedule for the same time next week?
Fred:		Sure that's fine.
#2 Neelam:		We are getting close to the end of our session today, and I know you talked some today about your struggles with alcohol. I'm wondering if you have any experience with any programs or if you would be interested in learning more about programs that may be helpful to you?
Fred:		I appreciate you asking, and yes, I would be interested, but I don't particularly agree with the teachings of AA. It hasn't been very successful for some of my other family members, and I don't have much faith in it. If you have any other ideas, I would love to have any handouts or information you have.
Neelam:		I will be happy to look up information for you, and I will bring whatever I'm able to find to our next session if that will be alright with you. Would you like to meet again next week at the same time?
Fred:		Sure, that will be great.

In Interaction 1, Neelam shares information about AA and 12-step programs without checking with Fred. Neelam leads the conversation and uses words and phrases such as "highly recommend" and "groups are wonderful" without first knowing Fred's feelings about the subject. As a result, Fred lost his connection with Neelam and felt as though she was pushing her agenda on him. In the second interaction, Neelam let Fred lead. She let him tell her what would be helpful and not helpful.

In terms of knowing one's own values and motivations, Neelam must understand her values related to AA. Most important, Neelam must understand her values and beliefs about AA are not everyone's beliefs. For Neelam, self-awareness includes understanding the significance of 12-step programs in her own life and realizing those are her personal experiences. Self-awareness means Neelam is careful not to let her beliefs about 12-step programs become an imposition on her clients. She must let her client lead and understand her clients' beliefs and values instead of pushing her own. Review the following case illustration as another example of how self-awareness is a key ethical issue for professional counselors.

CASE ILLUSTRATION 2-2

Wes is a 36-year-old male and decided to pursue a degree in counseling after spending the past 10 years as the director of an outdoor adventure camp. Wes has always enjoyed working with people, and now as his kids (two sons age 11 and 14) are getting older, he would like to get a job with more conventional hours. He wants to spend more time with his kids and family. He recently completed his graduate program and is currently working as a counseling intern and accruing his licensure hours at a fairly small community agency. Because he is unable to bill insurance, Wes typically works with individuals who lack insurance or the financial means to pay for services.

One of Wes's current clients is a 19-year-old female, Robin. Robin has been living with a friend for the past six months and trying to "make it" as an adult. Her parents and family still live in the same city, but Robin works hard to prove she can be independent. She has her own job making just above minimum wage and has been able to fully support herself.

Robin self-referred to counseling due to a recent fight with her friend. The official fight happened at Robin's work, while she was on the clock, and subsequently Robin was fired. Robin is not sure what to do or where to stay now that her friend has kicked her out of the apartment. She feels downtrodden by the recent turn of events. Consider the following interaction between Wes and Robin as they discuss her housing situation.

Wes: So I know you were living on your own, and now you find yourself without a place to live due to this fight. What do you think you might do?

Robin: I'm not sure. I'm thinking about maybe just living in my car for a while or even moving to a different city.

Wes: Yes, those are definite options. Also, I know your parents still live here. What about staying some with them until you get yourself another job?

Robin: I'm not sure. I don't want to go crawling back. I mean I don't even really want to tell them about the whole thing. It will just show them how I failed.

Wes: I know you feel like you would be crawling back, but I'm pretty sure your parents would love to have you at home. Parents are just like that. They want to take care of their kids. It will also probably be good for you to be around people who care about you.

Robin: I don't know; maybe you're right.

> Wes: I think that would be good, and then they can also help you look for another job. Do you think you might want to work in the same business or move on to something else? Also, there is the possibility of going back to school to get your degree. The more education you have, the better the job you can get.
>
> *Knowing the small amount of background information provided and after reading the interaction between Wes and Robin, what are you able to conclude about Wes's values?*
>
> *Why is it important for Wes to understand his own morals, values, and beliefs?*

After reading the interaction in Case Illustration 2-2, the entirety of Wes's values and beliefs may not be clear, but some information is available. First, one of the reasons Wes gave for pursuing a counseling degree was so he could have a career that allowed him to spend more time with family. Therefore, it might be safe to assume Wes values family and spending time with them. Second, Wes made the choice to go back to school and further his education. One might also conclude Wes values education and believes education is important.

The second question related to Case Illustration 2-2 asks why it is important for Wes to understand his own morals, values, and beliefs. According to ACA (2014) Standard A.4.b. counselors "are aware of" values (p. 5). Even though the primary focus of Standard A.4.b. is on avoiding imposing values on clients, the standard still includes awareness as a prerequisite for avoiding imposing one's values (i.e., a counselor must first be self-aware to avoid imposing his/her values onto clients).

The importance of a counselor knowing his/her own morals and values is rooted in Standard A.1.a., which speaks to counselors promoting the welfare of clients. Standard A.1.a. requires professional counselors to promote the client's welfare based on the thoughts, views, and ideas of the client as opposed to what the counselor feels is best. A counselor without self-awareness may lack the ability to separate his/her own values and beliefs from what is "best" for the client. In Case Illustration 2-2, Wes genuinely believes it is in Robin's best interest to stay with her parents, while she figures out her next move in life. Wes believes this in part because he believes in family unity. He believes families protect and encourage their members. Wes also believes pursuing an education is in Robin's "best interest." He believes it based on his own beliefs and values about education. This is not to say education and family unity are immoral and to be avoided. The vast majority of clients may agree with those values. Still, the vast majority is not everyone, and if a counselor is to avoid harming clients, he/she must avoid using value-based statements as universal truths. If Wes was more self-aware, he might use his words more strategically, avoiding questions, statements, and comments encouraging Robin to act in one way or another. Instead he would use his words and nonverbal actions in a way to encourage Robin to realize her own course of action based on what she believes is in her best interest. Review the following interaction between Wes and Robin in which Wes shows self-awareness and avoids imposing his own values or beliefs onto Robin.

Wes: I know you were living on your own, and now you find yourself without a place to live due to this fight. What do you think you might do?

Robin: I'm not sure. I'm thinking about maybe just living in my car for a while or even moving to a different city.

Wes: It seems like you're at a loss right now and not sure what to do. Based on how you said that, it sounds like the only options you can think of are sleeping in your car or moving to another city and starting over there.

Robin: Yeah, there is just too much on my mind right now, and I haven't been able to think straight—so many things just going on in my head.

Wes: What do you think may be helpful to you today during our session? You've talked some about your fight with your roommate, losing your job, possibly moving to a new city, and the overall chaos it has caused in your life. Is there one area that sticks out above the others where you think, if we addressed it, it may have a positive impact on other areas?

Robin: I think that if I had a place to stay, that would probably make things easier. My car is nice and all, but I would like to have other options.

Wes: So you have your car right now as an absolute last resort, but you would like to have some other options, possibly more comfortable options. As you're talking I notice you looking up, almost as if you are thinking about it right now and trying to figure things out. I'm wondering if you might share what you're thinking.

Robin: Nothing really, I keep thinking about my parents. They live pretty close, and I guess moving back home is an option, but I want to try and do this on my own. I don't want them to think I'm a failure.

Wes: Your parents live here, and that is an option, but not one at the top of your list right now. You would like to exhaust all other possibilities first.

Robin: Yeah, I just wouldn't know how to talk to them or what to say without feeling like a failure. I guess I would really like to go back home, but I wouldn't know how to even call or talk to them.

Wes: Going back home is what you would like to do, at least for a little while, but the main thing standing in your way is how to approach your parents and talk to them about what happened. Is that something you might want to talk more about and see if we can maybe figure out some possibilities for you to try?

In this interaction, Wes keeps his values and beliefs to himself and does not suggest Robin act in one way or the other. Wes uses his counseling skills to promote Robin figuring out her own course of action rather than simply following Wes's suggestions and ideas about what he thinks is best. In keeping his values out of the interaction, Wes is promoting the welfare of his client.

Self-awareness involves small nuances in the interactions between counselors and clients. By asking a question a certain way, encouraging a client to act one way or another, or simply putting value to a statement that previously had none, counselors reveal their personal values. Without self-awareness, counselors may easily fall into imposing their own values and beliefs onto clients without realization. See Text Box 2-1 for the APA's and AAMFT's perspectives on self-awareness.

TEXT BOX 2-1

While the ACA Code of Ethics emphasizes the importance of counselor self-awareness and avoiding imposing values onto their clients, the APA and AAMFT do not place an emphasis on values in their ethical codes. The APA (2010) encourages psychologists to be aware of and respect cultural diversity and avoid letting differences (e.g., gender identity, race, age, religion, national origin, etc.) bias their work. However, this topic is only covered under the "General Principles" section in which it is made clear "general principles, in contrast to ethical standards, do not represent obligations and should not form the basis for imposing sanctions" (p. 3). Therefore, avoiding bias may be seen as an aspiration rather than an obligation. Similarly, the AAMFT Code of Ethics (2015) does not address the imposition of values either. In summary, while the actions of Wes and Neelam in Case Illustration 2-1 and 2-2 may be an ethical concern for professional counselors, their actions would likely not be a concern if they were psychologists or marriage and family therapists.

Stress in Counseling

The ACA Code of Ethics instructs counselors to be aware of and "monitor themselves for signs of impairment from their own physical, mental, or emotional problems and refrain from offering or providing professional services when impaired" (2014, p. 9). Text Box 2-1 describes how the APA and AAMFT deal with counselors' personal problems. What follows are a few questions that may be helpful to your understanding of yourself and becoming aware of potential issues that may cause impairment if not addressed. These questions are important not only as you begin your counseling career but also throughout your career as a professional counselor. Continued reflection will aid in preventing any future impairment. In Case Illustration 2-3, you are asked to consider the case of Buddy and how he handles stress associated with his new job as a professional counselor.

CASE ILLUSTRATION 2-3

Buddy is a new licensed professional counselor and works as a contract counselor at a local agency. Because he is the newest counselor at the agency and a newly licensed counselor, the agency office staff members give him many cases with a variety of different concerns. Wanting

(Continued)

(Continued)

to fit in and show that he is capable of handling the work demands, Buddy gladly accepts all the cases he is offered. His caseload consists of clients with issues related to an assortment of concerns, including addictions, domestic violence, self-injury, general anxiety, and depression.

As the weeks go on, some of Buddy's clients begin to show minor improvements; however, many either show no improvement or discontinue services after a short time. Buddy begins to have some self-doubt and questions his ability to help his clients. He starts to take his work home with him and thinks about his clients over the weekends. Buddy has also noticed that he has trouble sleeping at night; he worries about the well-being of his clients, his own competency, and capabilities as a counselor.

Do you see any ethical concerns that may need to be addressed in this dilemma?

How might issues such as the inability to help clients, self-doubt, and seeing too many clients affect a counselor's overall stress level and competency?

How would you know if you were overly stressed or burned out?

In answering the first question in Case Illustration 2-3, you may have several concerns that need to be addressed. However, one of the main concerns is Buddy losing sleep over his clients, thinking about his clients over the weekends, and possibly even showing some countertransference toward his clients. Understanding only the information given, you may believe Buddy is showing signs of impairment and may need to narrow his scope of practice or take some time for wellness activities. If Buddy continues on his current course, he will be likely to do more harm than good to his clients.

Issues such as those listed will no doubt add extra stress to an already stressful occupation. Counselors must limit their scope of practice and implement wellness activities to avoid impairment and eventual burnout.

Answering Question 3 requires counselors to practice self-awareness. Consider ways that you may be able to monitor yourself in accordance to Standard C.2.g., "Counselors monitor themselves for signs of impairment" (ACA, 2014, p. 9).

Stress in counseling is inevitable. The nature of the job requires counselors to listen and be empathic to others' concerns and worries on a day-to-day basis. Similarly, counselors may often feel a sense of responsibility for their clients' personal well-being (similar to Buddy in the case illustration). While small amounts of stress may not negatively affect a counselor's ability to work with clients, stress that is built up over time and not addressed may be an ethical concern. Take a few moments to address the following questions to see how you might prevent stress from negatively impacting your ability to provide adequate services.

How do you determine if you are a competent counselor?

Do you depend on your clients' success or feedback, or is there another way that you evaluate your effectiveness?

To what degree do you see yourself as responsible for your clients' behaviors and actions or their success or lack thereof in counseling?

How do you handle stress?

TEXT BOX 2-2

American Psychological Association

APA Ethical Standard 2.06 (Personal Problems and Conflicts) requires psychologists to refrain from entering into a professional relationship when there is a "substantial likelihood that their personal problems will prevent them from performing" (APA, 2010, p. 5). Part two of Standard 2.06 requires psychologists to "take appropriate measures" to address their personal concerns before continuing their practice.

In summary, psychologists must monitor themselves for signs of stress, burnout, or other conditions that may interfere with their ability to perform work-related duties. If there is impairment, psychologists must address those issues prior to continuing work-related activities.

American Association for Marriage and Family Therapists

The AAMFT Code of Ethics addresses impairment in Standard 3.3. Similar to the expectations set forth by ACA and APA, marriage and family therapists must seek assistance when faced with issues (e.g., stress or burnout) having the potential to impair their performance. AAMFT Standard 3.3 implies that marriage and family therapists should monitor themselves for signs of impairment. If they determine there is impairment, then they must seek assistance.

Wellness Model

One of the things differentiating professional counselors from other mental health providers is the model that counselors follow when working with clients. Professional counselors follow a "wellness model," which is different from psychologists and psychiatrists, who follow a "medical model" or "illness model." According to Remley and Herlihy (2014), counselors follow four basic beliefs:

1. The best perspective for assisting individuals in resolving their emotional and personal issues and problems is the wellness model of mental health.

2. Most of the issues and problems that individuals face in life are developmental in nature.

3. Prevention and early intervention are far superior to remediation in dealing with personal and emotional problems.

4. The goal of counseling is to empower individual clients and client systems to resolve their own problems independently of mental health professionals and to teach them to identify and resolve problems autonomously in the future. (pp. 26–27)

The authors add the idea that the wellness model follows the belief that clients and students have the ability to make changes they see as appropriate or beneficial to bettering their life circumstances within themselves. It is the counselors' role to work with clients and students to help them better understand themselves and how to go about making those identified changes.

On the contrary, the goal of the medical or illness model is to identify the illness or problem that is causing discomfort, diagnose the problem, and then fix the problem. In the medical model, the mental health professional is responsible for "fixing" the problem or curing the person. If another problem arises, the client is dependent again on having the professional "fix" the problem. Using the wellness model, clients are able to work with professionals to identify and make changes to address ailments. If other ailments arise, clients have the skills learned previously to work toward making needed changes to address the new ailment. Take a look at Case Illustration 2-4 exemplifying the differences in how a clinician practicing from a medical model may conceptualize a case as opposed to that of a clinician practicing from a wellness model.

CASE ILLUSTRATION 2-4

An adult client visits a counseling office for the first time. During the course of the intake and over the first several sessions, the client discusses some anxiety issues and wanting to find better ways to handle anxiety. The client says currently the only thing that helps with the anxiety is making several cuts on his/her upper arm, but that is not something he/she wants to continue doing.

A clinician practicing from a medical or illness model may suggest or give professional advice to the client about how he/she may better handle anxiety. If the clinician has prescription privileges, he/she may prescribe some medication to aid in lessoning the anxiety. The clinician's actions would most likely follow the idea that the client has a concern, and it is the clinician's role and responsibility to tell the client how to get better.

A clinician practicing from a wellness model would most likely work in tandem with the client to determine (depending on the clinician's theoretical model) ideas for change and what type of change the client would like to see. The clinician may work with the client to identify activities that have been more or less helpful, triggers to the anxiety, and possible strategies for change. The clinician's actions would most likely follow the idea that the client has a concern, and it is the clinician's role and responsibility to work with the client and through many interactions help the client to identify strategies for change.

The ACA Code of Ethics reiterates the wellness model in the introduction of Section A, The Counseling Relationship. "Counselors facilitate client growth and development in ways that foster the interest and welfare of clients and promote formation of healthy relationships" (ACA, 2014, p. 4). Further, in the same introductory paragraph, professional counselors are instructed to "actively attempt to understand the diverse cultural backgrounds of the clients they serve" and "explore their own cultural identities and how these affect their values and beliefs about the counseling process" (p. 4). Through this paragraph it is clear that counseling is about understanding clients and helping them determine how to make changes the client feels are necessary. Counselors are directed to be self-aware and keep their own motives and initiatives out of the counseling process. Simply stated, counseling is not about the counselor; it is about the client or student. As was discussed in Chapter 1, for counselors to keep from imposing on his/her clients, he/she must first have a thorough understanding of him/herself.

Counselor Credentialing

In Chapter 1, the authors discussed the foundation on which codes of ethics are often built and, specifically, the foundation for the ACA Code of Ethics. Throughout this chapter, the authors discuss the process of transitioning into the counseling profession and the right to call oneself a "professional counselor." There are many people who may call themselves "counselors" (e.g., camp counselors, spiritual counselors, legal counselors, etc.). However, the term "professional counselor" is a protected term, meaning that to identify yourself as a professional counselor, you must possess certain licensure or certification. Those who represent or advertise themselves as professional counselors who do not possess the necessary qualifications are subject to ethical and legal ramifications (specific penalties will vary based on state law). Consider the case of Roman and his issues concerning practicing without a license.

CASE ILLUSTRATION 2-5

Roman recently graduated with his master's degree in clinical mental health counseling and has made several attempts to pass his state's licensure exam but has failed on three separate occasions. As a result, he is required by his state board of licensure for professional counselors to enroll in an additional nine hours of graduate work prior to taking the exam again. Feeling frustrated with the licensure process and knowing that he already has a job waiting for him at his church's counseling center, Roman decides to postpone the licensure process and start working as a counselor and case manager.

Several months into his new job, Roman has built up a good reputation within the center and his clients often recommend him to others outside the congregation. Due to his success, Roman decides to open up a small private practice in addition to his work at the church counseling center. He knows he is not able to bill insurance due to lacking the required licensure, so he accepts only clients who are able to pay cash. As his private practice begins to grow,

(Continued)

(Continued)

Roman has business cards made and even develops a webpage, all of which identify him as a professional counselor.

Is Roman acting unethically in opening a private practice and advertising as a professional counselor?

Would it be considered more appropriate if Roman were to use the term "counselor" rather than "professional counselor" in his advertisements?

What might be the legal and/or ethical ramifications for Roman?

In regard to the first question of Case Illustration 2-5, the answer is yes; Roman is acting unethically in identifying himself as a professional counselor when he does not hold the proper licensure. As mentioned earlier, "professional counselor" is a protected term, and only those possessing the necessary education and licensure are able to identify and advertise themselves as professional counselors.

Question 2 related in this case may be a bit trickier as Roman would no longer be using a protected term if he were to adjust his advertising to use the term "counselor" rather than "professional counselor." However, he would still most likely be seen as acting in an unethical and illegal manner. Standard C.3.a. (Accurate Advertising) of the ACA Code of Ethics (2014) requires counselors to advertise "in an accurate manner that is not false, misleading, deceptive, or fraudulent" (p. 9). By practicing counseling and opening up a business that offers counseling-type services, Roman would most likely be seen as misleading or being deceptive to his clients and the general public. By continuing to operate his practice in the current manner, Roman would be opening himself up to legal and ethical ramifications. Ethically, Roman's ability to become fully licensed in the future may be in jeopardy if his state's licensure board were to determine his actions egregious enough to ban him from licensure. Depending on state laws, Roman may legally be subject to fines and other penalties.

Because you will need to acquire necessary credentialing (i.e., licensure and/or certification) prior to practicing or identifying as a professional counselor, it is critical to discuss the credentialing process. In Chapter 12 the authors will discuss ethics related to counselor education programs and specific standards addressing actions and behaviors of counselor educators along with requirements of counselor education programs. However, counselor education is only one component or "piece of the puzzle" in becoming licensed as a professional counselor. The following paragraphs examine the full licensure and certification process.

In most states, becoming a licensed professional counselor requires a master's degree in counseling or a related field (a related field is often determined by specific state licensure boards). Degree requirements and course offerings vary from state to state; however, the majority of graduate programs in counseling require students to acquire either 48 or

60 hours, the trend being that most counseling programs will require students to acquire 60 hours to be eligible for licensure. In addition to a graduate degree, you will most likely be required to pass a state licensing exam. Finally, every state requires the completion of a set number of supervised experience hours prior to receiving full licensure status. Please see the specific licensure requirements of each state at http://www.counseling.org/ knowledge-center/licensure-requirements/state-professional-counselor-licensure-boards.

Similar to state standards for acquiring licensure as a professional counselor, each state has its own standards for becoming certified as a professional school counselor. To view school counselor certification requirements for each state, please visit the following site: http://schoolcounselor.org/school-counselors-members/careers-roles/state-certification-requirements.

Professional Associations

Professional associations serve as places where individuals within a profession are able to share common attitudes and beliefs about the profession and address concerns of the profession as a group. Professional associations also provide leadership to those within the profession (Meany-Walen et al., 2013). The ACA provides leadership to all professional counselors by developing and distributing a code of ethics for professional practice, but the ACA is not the only entity providing ethical guidance to counselors. Many divisions of the ACA (e.g., Association for Specialists in Group Work, American School Counseling Association [ASCA], International Association of Marriage and Family Counselors [IAMFC], etc.) also provide their own ethical codes. These other ethical codes provide more specific guidance to counselors working with distinct populations. For example, the ASCA Code of Ethics guides school counselors' behaviors and addresses issues that may pertain only to school counselors. Regional and state counseling associations often have their own codes of ethics tailored to state and regional expectations.

Because there are many codes of ethics for professional counselors, with each sharing commonalities as well as distinctions, there is opportunity for confusion when discrepancies arise between these codes and legal requirements. Consider Case Illustration 2-6 below and how Rhonda may handle her ethical dilemma.

CASE ILLUSTRATION 2-6

Rhonda is a counselor with almost 10 years of experience in working with couples and families. She is a member of several counseling associations, including the ACA, and her state counseling association. However, she has been most active and identifies most closely with the IAMFC, which is a division of the ACA.

Rhonda is single and enjoys playing sports and going dancing with friends in her spare time. Recently, Rhonda has recognized a man on her co-ed soccer team, Jeremy, as one of her

(Continued)

(Continued)

past clients from about three years ago. After some reflection and using an ethical decision-making model, Rhonda determines that because Jeremy is a past client, there is no reason for concern that he is on her team. The two continue to talk and become closer friends over the course of the season, and Rhonda really enjoys Jeremy's company. As the weeks go by, the two become closer, and Rhonda worries that she may be acting unethically if she were to pursue a romantic relationship with Jeremy. In going through another ethical decision-making process, Rhonda determines there are some discrepancies in the codes of ethics for each of her professional associations. The ACA Code of Ethics (2014) requires that Rhonda wait a minimum of five years prior to pursuing a relationship with a past client, whereas the IAMFC Code of Ethics does not include anything related to the number of years a clinician must wait. Instead, the IAMFC Code states, "Couple and family counselors are responsible for demonstrating there is no harm from any relationship with a client or family member. The key element in this ethical principle is the avoidance of exploitation of vulnerable clients" (Hendricks, Bradley, Southern, Oliver, & Birdsall, 2011). To complicate the situation more, the laws in Rhonda's state do not address relationships with past clients at all.

Which code of ethics should Rhonda abide by?

If Rhonda were to disregard the code of ethics, what might be the penalty, and how might it affect her licensure?

The general consensus related to Question 1 for Case Illustration 2-6 is that Rhonda should follow the most stringent requirements. Therefore, Rhonda would want to abide by the ACA Code of Ethics and wait a minimum of five years prior to pursuing a relationship with her past client.

Question 2 asks about possible repercussions or penalties Rhonda might face if she were to disregard ethical guidelines. For any repercussions to take place, a complaint must first be made. In this example, a complaint might be made by Jeremy if he feels as though he has been wronged or taken advantage of. A complaint may also be made by another professional counselor if Rhonda were to share her exploits with a friend or colleague. If the complaint is made to the counseling licensure board in the state where Rhonda lives, the licensure board would likely conduct an investigation and enforce penalties (see your state licensure board for specific processes). If the complaint is made to a professional association (e.g., ACA, IAMFC, state counseling association, etc.), a different process would likely take place as professional associations do not have the power to directly suspend, revoke, or otherwise affect a clinician's licensure status.

According to the *ACA Policy and Procedural Manual* (2013), all ethical complaints are handled by the ACA ethics committee. The committee is charged with investigating the complaint, voting on whether or not the complaint is valid, and finally determining an appropriate penalty (if necessary). At the conclusion of the process, the ethics committee is charged with notifying all involved parties of the outcome. Additionally, the committee forwards copies of the complaint, process, and outcome to all counseling associations and licensure boards the clinician is associated with.

Related to Case Illustration 2-6, if a complaint was made to the ACA about Rhonda's suspect behaviors, the ACA ethics committee would investigate the claim and determine whether further action was needed. If the ethics committee determined Rhonda was indeed acting in an unethical manner, they would then determine an appropriate punishment (e.g., reprimand, suspension of membership to the association, or lifetime ban from the association). In addition to notifying Rhonda of her punishment, the ethics committee would also send letters to Rhonda's state licensure board and the IAMFC, notifying both entities of the complaint against Rhonda and the ACA ethics committee's resolution.

Not all professional counselors or counselors in training belong to professional organizations. Therefore, the question remains: Does a professional counselor have to follow the ACA Code of Ethics or any code of ethics if he/she is not a member of a professional organization? Consider Case Illustration 2-7 related to professional ethics for Melanie, who is a professional counselor but does not see the importance of joining professional organizations.

CASE ILLUSTRATION 2-7

Melanie is a licensed professional counselor with two years of experience being fully licensed. She works in private practice in a relatively large city and is an active participant in a "consultation group" that she and several other counselors started. The group serves as a way for private practitioners to stay connected with other professionals and is a place where each can consult on cases and share referral sources. Today Melanie talks about her frustration with all the paperwork she is required to do by insurance companies. Melanie shares her concern that the paperwork takes away from her productivity. Melanie further states that she is planning on removing herself from insurance panels and will only take private-pay clients. That way, she doesn't have to play by their rules and "can be a counselor instead of a secretary." Melanie explains that she plans to continue keeping small notes to help her remember clients but will no longer be completing treatment plans or intake packets or worrying about how long to keep files after she stops seeing clients. Upon hearing this, another member of the group expresses concern that Melanie may be acting in an unethical manner according to the ACA Code of Ethics (2014). Melanie responds by saying that she isn't a member of ACA anymore and plans to drop her state counseling association membership as well. Melanie rationalizes that if she isn't a member of any professional counseling associations, she doesn't have to follow any of their codes of ethics.

Is Melanie correct in her belief that because she is not a member of a professional organization, she does not have to abide by the association's code of ethics?

The simple answer to the question in Case Illustration 2-7 is no. Even if counselors are not members of specific organizations, they must follow a code of ethics. Earlier, the authors discussed the term "professional counselor" and how it is a protected term that only individuals possessing certain licensures and certifications may use. Melanie may no longer be an active member of the ACA or other associations, but she is still a professional

Table 2-1 Divisions of the American Counseling Association

Association for Adult Development and Aging (AADA)	Chartered in 1986, AADA serves as a focal point for information sharing, professional development, and advocacy related to adult development and aging issues and addresses counseling concerns across the lifespan.
Association for Assessment and Research in Counseling (AARC)	Originally the Association for Measurement and Evaluation in Guidance, AARC was chartered in 1965. Its purpose is to promote the effective use of assessment in the counseling profession.
Association for Child and Adolescent Counseling (ACAC)	Association for Child and Adolescent Counseling aims to focus on the training needs of counselors who work with children and adolescents, while also providing professional support to those counselors, whether they are school counselors, play therapists, or counselor educators.
Association for Creativity in Counseling (ACC)	The ACC is a forum for counselors, counselor educators, creative arts therapists, and counselors in training to explore unique and diverse approaches to counseling. ACC's goal is to promote greater awareness, advocacy, and understanding of diverse and creative approaches to counseling.
American College Counseling Association (ACCA)	ACCA is one of the newest divisions of the ACA. Chartered in 1991, the focus of ACCA is to foster student development in colleges, universities, and community colleges.
Association for Counselors and Educators in Government (ACEG)	Originally the Military Educators and Counselors Association, ACEG was chartered in 1984. It is dedicated to counseling clients and their families in local, state, and federal government or in military-related agencies.
Association for Counselor Education and Supervision (ACES)	Originally the National Association of Guidance and Counselor Trainers, ACES was a founding association of ACA in 1952. ACES emphasizes the need for quality education and supervision of counselors in all work settings.
The Association for Humanistic Counseling (AHC)	AHC, formerly C-AHEAD, a founding association of ACA in 1952, provides a forum for the exchange of information about humanistically oriented counseling practices and promotes changes that reflect the growing body of knowledge about humanistic principles applied to human development and potential.
Association for Lesbian, Gay, Bisexual and Transgender Issues in Counseling (ALGBTIC)	ALGBTIC educates counselors about the unique needs of client identity development and a nonthreatening counseling environment by aiding in the reduction of stereotypical thinking and homoprejudice.
Association for Multicultural Counseling and Development (AMCD)	Originally the Association of Non-White Concerns in Personnel and Guidance, AMCD was chartered in 1972. It strives to improve cultural, ethnic, and racial empathy and understanding by developing programs to advance and sustain personal growth.
American Mental Health Counselors Association (AMHCA)	Chartered in 1978, AMHCA represents mental health counselors, advocating for client access to quality services within the health-care industry.

American Rehabilitation Counseling Association (ARCA)	ARCA is an organization of rehabilitation counseling practitioners, educators, and students who are concerned with enhancing the development of people with disabilities throughout their life span and in promoting excellence in the rehabilitation counseling profession's practice, research, consultation, and professional development.
American School Counselor Association (ASCA)	Chartered in 1953, ASCA promotes school counseling professionals and interest in activities that affect the personal, educational, and career development of students. ASCA members also work with parents, educators, and community members to provide a positive learning environment.
Association for Spiritual, Ethical, and Religious Values in Counseling (ASERVIC)	Originally the National Catholic Guidance Conference, ASERVIC was chartered in 1974. It is devoted to professionals who believe that spiritual, ethical, religious, and other human values are essential to the full development of the person and to the discipline of counseling.
Association for Specialists in Group Work (ASGW)	Chartered in 1973, ASGW provides professional leadership in the field of group work, establishes standards for professional training, and supports research and the dissemination of knowledge.
Counselors for Social Justice (CSJ)	CSJ is a community of counselors, counselor educators, graduate students, and school and community leaders who seek equity and an end to oppression and injustice affecting clients, students, counselors, families, communities, schools, workplaces, governments, and other social and institutional systems.
International Association of Addictions and Offender Counselors (IAAOC)	Originally the Public Offender Counselor Association, IAAOC was chartered in 1972. Members of IAAOC advocate the development of effective counseling and rehabilitation programs for people with substance abuse problems, other addictions, and adult and/or juvenile public offenders.
International Association of Marriage and Family Counselors (IAMFC)	Chartered in 1989, IAMFC members help develop healthy family systems through prevention, education, and therapy.
National Career Development Association (NCDA)	Originally the National Vocational Guidance Association, NCDA was one of the founding associations of ACA in 1952. NCDA inspires and empowers the achievement of career and life goals by providing professional development, resources, standards, scientific research, and advocacy.
National Employment Counseling Association (NECA)	NECA was originally the National Employment Counselors Association, chartered in 1966. The commitment of NECA is to offer professional leadership to people who counsel in employment and/or career development settings. See more at http://www.counseling.org/about-us/divisions-regions-and-branches/divisions#sthash.WIIAftXH.dpuf.

counselor and therefore must abide by the laws in her state that govern professional counselors. Concomitantly, all states have ethics as a part of the rules and regulations governing licensees. For example, some states (e.g., Texas, North Carolina, Illinois, etc.) have their own codes of ethics written into state law. Other states (e.g., Arkansas) simply refer to the ACA Code of Ethics rather than developing their own.

Ward v. Wilbanks (2011) offered additional guidance related to students' ethical requirements and whether or not students must abide by professional codes of ethics. Students are not yet licensed and many may not be members of any professional counseling associations (especially those in the earliest stages of their graduate program). *Ward v. Wilbanks* (2011) found that students who are enrolled in graduate programs that abide by professional codes of ethics must abide by those same ethical codes even if they are not members of the association.

Even though the ACA is the most commonly referenced professional association in this and many other texts and journal publications, there are numerous local, state, and national professional counseling associations. Each professional counseling association provides key resources for the counselors it serves. The ACA alone has 20 different divisions, each catering to counselors in various work settings and specific populations. For example, the Association for Child and Adolescent Counseling (ACAC) is the newest division of the ACA. ACAC caters to professional counselors internationally who have an interest in working with children and/or adolescent populations. Similar to other divisions of ACA, the ACAC provides discussion forums, continuing education opportunities, and an opportunity for those who serve or have an interest in serving child and adolescent populations to collaborate and share concerns and successes.

In addition to the 20 divisions of ACA, many states and regions have their own professional counseling associations that act as subsidiaries of the ACA; within state organizations there are divisions and chapters dedicated to more local interests and concerns.

Table 2.1 shows the ACA's 20 divisions. In addition to the information listed in the table, the authors suggest that you review your own state and local professional associations in determining which may be appropriate for you.

Conclusion

This chapter discusses the transition into professional counseling. At the onset, readers are asked to consider their motivations in wanting to be a professional counselor. The authors also examine stress related to counseling and differentiate counseling from other mental health professions. Further, they explore professional identity, professional associations, and both legal and ethical aspects of calling oneself a professional counselor. Finally, the authors provide licensing and credentialing requirements for all 50 states and list the 20 divisions of the ACA. The chapter was placed early in the book because it covers professional identity and the role professional associations and licensure boards play in governing the behaviors of anyone practicing as a professional counselor.

Counselors have little choice pertaining to the licensure board with which they associate (e.g., counselors in Texas must follow the rules set forth by the licensure board for Texas professional counselors). Once licensed, counselors have more options when considering which professional associations to join but nevertheless are ethically obligated to join and actively participate. The introductory paragraph to Section C of the ACA Code of Ethics (2014) requires counselors to "actively participate in local, state, and national associations that foster the development and improvement of counseling" (p. 8). Therefore, we ask you to answer the questions in Exercise 2-1 with the information you have learned in this chapter to help you begin to think about how you might be able to start getting involved in professional counseling organizations.

EXERCISE 2-1

At the beginning of this chapter, the authors discussed values and self-awareness. Take a few minutes to reflect on your own values and beliefs. How do you think your values may affect your choice of words and/or phrases when interacting with clients?

In this chapter the authors listed the 20 divisions of the ACA; however, there are many other state and regional professional organizations. Discuss with your classmates and colleagues all of the other professional organizations in your area.

Considering the many diverse local, state, and national professional organizations, which one(s) seem most appropriate for you?

Now that you have determined which professional organization(s) may be most appropriate for you and your interests, discuss with your classmates and colleagues ways in which you may be able to become an active member in your identified professional organizations.

Keystones

- Stress in counseling is inevitable. As such, professional counselors must learn self-awareness and monitor their own wellness.
- Counselors work from a wellness model as opposed to a medical or illness model, focusing on the strengths of each client.
- "Professional counselor" is a protected term, and only those possessing appropriate licensure or certification may advertise as professional counselors.
- Requirements for becoming a professional counselor are determined by state licensure boards and typically consist of a 48- or 60-hour graduate program, successfully passing a state licensure exam, and supervised experience hours.
- Professional counseling associations serve as a hub for professional counselors and offer a place where professional counselors are able to discuss concerns of the profession.
- Many professional counseling associations develop and maintain professional codes of ethics to govern the behaviors of professional counselors.
- Professional associations impose sanctions on membership to the associations (e.g., suspension of membership); licensure boards impose sanctions related to licensure to practice counseling (e.g., suspension of license, reprimand, etc.).

- When discrepancies exist in professional codes of ethics, professional counselors should follow the most stringent guidelines.
- The ACA Code of Ethics (2014) requires professional counselors to join and be active participants in professional counseling associations.

Additional Resources

Brennan, C., Eulberg, J. E., & Britton, P. J. (2011). Improving awareness of vulnerabilities to ethical challenges: A family systems approach. *Journal of Systemic Therapies, 30*(3), 73–85. doi:http://dx.doi.org/10.1521/jsyt.2011.30.3.7

Croft, M. A. (2015). *Mandated reporting: The effects of self-care and professional help seeking behavior on mental health care providers' levels of distress.* (Order No. 3619520, The Chicago School of Professional Psychology). *ProQuest Dissertations and Theses*, 158. Retrieved from http://search.proquest.com/docview/1532773582?accountid=7122

Gibson, D. M., Dollarhide, C. T., & Moss, J. M. (2010). Professional identity development: A grounded theory of transformational tasks of new counselors. *Counselor Education and Supervision, 50*(1), 21–38.

Jennings, L., Sovereign, A., Bottorff, N., Mussell, M. P., & Vye, C. (2005). Nine ethical values of master therapists. *Journal of Mental Health Counseling, 27*(1), 32–47. Retrieved from http://search.proquest.com/docview/620641735?accountid=7122

McLaughlin, J. E., & Boettcher, K. (2009). Counselor identity: Conformity or distinction? *Journal of Humanistic Counseling, Education and Development, 48*(2), 132–143.

Pompeo, A. M., & Levitt, D. H. (2014). A path of counselor self-awareness. *Counseling and Values, 59*(1), 80–94. doi:http://dx.doi.org/10.1002/j.2161-007X.2014.00043.x

Shapiro, S. L., Jazaieri, H., & Goldin, P. R. (2012). Mindfulness-based stress reduction effects on moral reasoning and decision making. *The Journal of Positive Psychology, 7*(6), 504–515. doi:http://dx.doi.org/10.1080/17439760.2012.723732

References

American Association for Marriage and Family Therapy. (2015). *Code of ethics*. Retrieved from https://www.aamft.org/iMIS15/AAMFT/Content/legal_ethics/code_of_ethics.aspx

American Counseling Association. (2013). *ACA policy and procedural manual*. Retrieved from http://www.counseling.org/docs/leadership-resources/policies-and-procedures-manual—march-2013.pdf?sfvrsn=2

American Counseling Association. (2014). *Code of ethics*. Alexandria, VA: Author.

American Psychological Association. (2010). American Psychological Association ethical principles of psychologists and code of conduct. Retrieved from http://www.apa.org/ethics/code/principles.pdf

Hendricks, B. E., Bradley, L. J., Southern, S., Oliver, M., & Birdsall, B. (2011). Ethical code for the International Association of Marriage and Family Counselors. *The Family Journal, 19*, 217–224.

Meany-Walen, K. K., Carnes-Holt, K., Barrio Minton, C. A., Purswell, K., & Pronchenko-Jain, Y. (2013). An exploration of counselors' professional leadership development. *Journal of Counseling & Development, 91*, 206–215. doi:10.1002/j.1556-6676.2013.00087.x

Remley, T. P., & Herlihy, B. (2014). *Ethical, legal, and professional issues in counseling* (4th ed.). Upper Saddle River, NJ: Pearson.

Ward v. Wilbanks, No. 10-2100, Doc. 006110869854 (6th Cir. Court of Appeals, Feb. 11, 2011). Retrieved from http://www.counseling.org/resources/pdfs/EMUamicusbrief.pdf

3

Ethical Decision Making

Not everything that can be counted counts and not everything that counts can be counted.

—Albert Einstein

Chapter 3 introduces ethical decision-making models and the importance of having a process in making ethical decisions. Readers will be introduced to the importance of using a process when making ethical decisions and encouraged to examine various decision-making strategies while comparing and contrasting each model. The authors will discuss differences in ethical and legal decision making and describe ways in which counselors can best avoid ethical and legal troubles. At the conclusion, readers will be encouraged to choose an ethical decision-making model and practice moving through each of the steps while responding to an ethical dilemma. After reading this chapter the reader will be able to do the following:

1. Discuss the importance of using an ethical decision-making model when working through an ethical dilemma.

2. Name ways in which he/she is best able to protect him/herself from ethical complaints.

3. Explain best practice strategies for making legal decisions.

4. Describe several decision-making models.

5. Define the steps of his/her own preferred ethical decision-making model.

Overview of Ethical Decision Making

Making an ethical decision requires counselors to take into consideration numerous bits of information and come to some conclusion as to how to move forward. Depending on the surrounding circumstances and the severity of the dilemma, counselors' decisions may result in a myriad of outcomes. Each outcome may be similar or quite different from the others with the "ethicality" of the decision based more on the process with which the counselor used to determine the outcome than the actual outcome itself. Thus, the decision-making process is more of an art than a science.

Dilemmas often arise when there is "a problem for which no course of action seems satisfactory. The dilemma exists because there are good, but contradictory ethical reasons to take conflicting and incompatible courses of action" (Kitchner, 1984, p. 43). As such, there will always be situations in which counselors are forced to choose one action over another, and regardless of how one sets up his/her practice and clientele, there will always be ethical dilemmas. When dilemmas arise, it is the counselors' responsibility to go through an ethical decision-making process to choose the "best" course of action. It is the authors' belief that in making ethical decisions, there may be many appropriate and, likewise, inappropriate courses of action. For example, there are numerous standards in the ACA, ASCA, and other codes of ethics that indicate counselors "may" act in one way or another.

"Counselors may barter only if the relationship is not exploitive or harmful and does not place the counselor in an unfair advantage, if the client requests it, and if such arrangements are an accepted practice among professionals in the community" (ACA, 2014, A.10.e.).

If all conditions are met (i.e., if not an exploitive or harmful relationship, if the client requests, and if such practices are acceptable in the community), then counselors are able to choose whether they wish to barter with a client. In this case, it would be considered ethical to barter or not barter. It is not the end decision that matters most; instead, it is the process in making the decision.

"When clients disclose that they have a disease commonly known to be both communicable and life threatening, counselors may be justified in disclosing information to identifiable third parties, if they are and known to be at demonstrable and high risk of contracting the disease" (ACA, 2014, B.2.c.).

Similar to this example, this standard does not direct counselors to act or not. It gives counselors the option to act if certain conditions are met. Again, it is the author's belief that the decision-making process is more important in determining the ethicality of the response than the actual response.

"Recognize the complicated nature of confidentiality in schools and consider each case in context. Keep information confidential unless legal requirements demand that confidential information be revealed or a breach is required to prevent serious and foreseeable harm to the student" (ASCA, 2010, A.2.c.).

This standard in the ASCA Code of Ethics (2010) is a bit different from the other examples. Rather than giving the option to act or not, it requires counselors to interpret the meaning of "serious and foreseeable harm" and judge a client's or student's behavior as serious enough to break confidentiality. In some situations (e.g., a second grader reports using drugs or alcohol on a daily or weekly basis), the decision may be easier, and in others (e.g., a 17-year-old student who reports smoking marijuana), it may be more difficult. For the latter example, arguments could be made to back up either decision (i.e., to maintain or break confidentiality). Therefore it is the process the counselor uses to make the decision that is oftentimes more important that the actual, final decision.

Most, if not all, ethical decision-making models require counselors to navigate through steps (e.g., identify the problem, review applicable ethical codes, review applicable laws, consulting with others, tune into your own feelings, etc.) prior to making their decision. Throughout your training and career, you will find yourself in situations where you must go through a decision-making process almost instantaneously (e.g., choosing whether to accept a gift from a client when he/she presents it to you at the end of a session) and other times when you have more time to think about your decision (e.g., if you receive an invitation in the mail to attend a client's birthday party). Because of this, it is the authors' belief that counselors should have a preferred decision-making model, be mindful of the steps, and be able to go through them almost automatically when called upon by the situation. The ACA Code of Ethics specifically addresses the need for a process in making ethical decisions in two areas. First, in the opening pages when discussing the purpose of the code of ethics, it states:

> When counselors are faced with ethical dilemmas that are difficult to resolve, they are expected to engage in a carefully considered ethical decision-making process. Reasonable differences of opinion can and do exist among counselors with respect to the ways in which values, ethical principles, and ethical standards would be applied when they conflict. While there is no specific ethical decision-making model that is most effective, counselors are expected to be familiar with a credible model of decision-making that can bear public scrutiny and its application. (ACA, 2014, p. 3)

And toward the latter part of the document, when discussing ways in which counselors should act when resolving ethical issues, it states:

> Standard I.1.b.—Ethical Decision Making—When counselors are faced with an ethical dilemma, they use and document, as appropriate, an ethical decision-making model that may include, but is not limited to, consultation; consideration of relevant ethical standards, principles, and laws; generation of potential courses of action; deliberation of risks and benefits; and selection of an objective decision based on the circumstances and welfare of all involved. (ACA, 2014, p. 19)

See Text Box 3-1 for the role of ethical decision-making models in APA and AAMFT.

TEXT BOX 3-1

American Psychological Association

The APA Code of Ethics (2010) does not include standards requiring psychologists to engage in ethical decision-making models when faced with ethical dilemmas. However, it does encourage psychologists to seek consultation concerning ethical problems.

American Association for Marriage and Family Therapists

The AAMFT Code of Ethics, like the APA Code of Ethics, does not address ethical decision making within specific standards. Instead, marriage and family therapists are directed to "take reasonable steps to resolve conflicts in a way that allows the fullest adherence to the Code of Ethics" and "encouraged to seek counsel from consultants, attorneys, supervisors, colleagues, or others" when unsure about the ethics of a particular situation" (AAMFT, 2015).

Throughout this chapter the authors will discuss various ethical decision-making models and how they might be used to address different ethical dilemmas. Consider Case Illustration 3-1 and how Charles might respond when he is caught off guard by one of his coworkers.

CASE ILLUSTRATION 3-1

Charles is a certified school counselor and a licensed professional counselor. He is a high school counselor and also has a small private practice where he meets with clients primarily on weekends. Charles has had his private practice for several years and works mainly with adults who have been involved with domestic violence. Over the years he has worked with many adults and families with varying degrees of success. At the beginning of this school year, Charles was recruited to move to a newly built school and be the head counselor. Although he enjoyed his old school, Charles is excited to move to a new building and have the opportunity to build the counseling program there.

As part of settling into his new position and meeting all of his new colleagues, Charles schedules times to introduce himself and meet all of the teachers. At the beginning of his meeting with Sandra, one of the science teachers, Charles is caught off guard when she gives him a big hug and says how glad she is to finally be able to meet him. Sandra describes herself as the sister of one of Charles's past clients from his private practice. She talks in-depth about all of the hardships that her sister went through and tells Charles what a great help he was to her. Sandra goes on to say that her sister is doing well now thanks to his help. Sandra hands Charles a small envelope and says that her sister asked her to give it to him. It is just a small thank-you note from his client and a few pictures that the children illustrated to show how appreciative they are of his help.

In Case Illustration 3-1, Charles finds himself in what could potentially be an awkward situation. One of his new colleagues (Sandra) is the sister of one of his past clients. At their first meeting, Sandra openly discusses the progress that her sister has made and how Charles played a large role in her success. Charles has a number of ways he can respond; however, he is in a situation in which he must respond immediately and does not have the luxury of taking time to go through a long decision-making process. He must think on his feet and be genuine in his response to Sandra. He does not have the option of saying, "Hold on, I need to go and consult with my supervisor or colleagues on how best to respond." He must take into consideration several areas of the code of ethics, weigh the potential positive and negative outcomes of each, and respond to Sandra before it becomes an awkward situation.

Charles may accept the thank-you note and begin talking to Sandra about her sister, engaging her in conversation about his past client.

Even though it is clear Charles's past client has shared her experiences with her sister and is comfortable with her sister knowing about her experiences in counseling, it is her right to disclose information and not Charles's right to disclose for her. If Charles chooses to acknowledge he knows Sandra's sister or discuss his past client with his new colleague, he is clearly breaking the counselor/client confidentiality he had with his previous client.

Charles may say, "I'm sorry, but I'm not able to either confirm or deny that I know your sister or that she has been my client in the past."

If Charles chooses to respond in this manner, he may be acting in a way he sees as ethical and avoiding breaking the confidentiality or privacy he had with his previous client. However, in the situation presented, it is clear that Sandra knows Charles had a counseling relationship with her sister. She is not asking if he knows her sister or curious as to whether he is the same counselor her sister met with. Sandra is clear and knows Charles has helped her sister and has been "looking forward to meeting him." In choosing to "neither confirm nor deny" he had a relationship, Charles may be hurting his relationship with Sandra as a coworker. Although Sandra may understand or know the ethical justification for Charles's response, she may still view him as lacking genuineness, and this ultimately may make for an awkward relationship between the two.

How Would You Respond If You Were in Charles's Situation?

In many situations counselors may know what they want to say or how they would like the client or other person to which they are talking to hear them. However, it is the authors' belief that one of the more difficult aspects of learning to be a professional counselor is getting words to come out of your mouth and be heard in the way they are intended. Readers are encouraged to practice with a friend, classmate, or colleague on how you might respond to this situation.

Ethical Decision-Making Models

In the previous paragraphs, the authors discussed the importance of having an ethical decision-making model, and there are multiple ethical decision-making models from which to choose. However, there is not one model that is considered the best or most appropriate for working through ethical dilemmas. The following is a review of some ethical decision-making models that are most commonly used by professional counselors and how those models may look when applied to specific situations. Some of the models presented have similar if not identical steps within the entire process. In your own practice, you may choose to use one of the models described in the pages that follow, combine several models together to form a unique decision-making process, or look to a different model. However you choose, it is critical to have a decision-making process to aid you in making difficult decisions. In Case Illustration 3-2, the authors share an example of how an ethical decision-making process may look when applied to a real situation.

CASE ILLUSTRATION 3-2

Brooke is a professional school counselor in a middle-class high school and has been working with Sofia, a 17-year-old female student, for both academic and personal reasons. Sofia's parents recently divorced, and she is not coping well as shown by her drop in grades and change in social behaviors. Sofia was referred by one of her teachers, and because Brooke's school policy dictates that she contact parents prior to initiating long-term individual meetings with students, Brooke has spoken to and received consent from Sofia's mother. During Brooke's meeting with Sofia's mother, it was fairly clear that both parents are supportive of Sofia and want the best for her. However, they are minimally interested in Sofia's interactions with the counselor and don't see a huge benefit to counseling.

As Brooke begins to meet with Sofia, she is able to build rapport and trust quickly. Sofia discusses her recent change in peer groups and that she has started hanging out with an older crowd (18- and 19-year-olds), including some recent dropouts. During one session Sofia tells Brooke that she is sexually active with her new boyfriend, who is 19. She says they don't use any type of protection because they feel it is unnatural. Sofia acknowledges Brooke's concerns about her safety but does not seem to be the least bit concerned for herself. Later in the session Sofia discusses her desire to become pregnant and have a baby. She sees this as a way to get away from all the things that are going on with her parents and move on with her life. Sofia further describes that her boyfriend does not know of her desire to get pregnant and that she is not going to tell him until she is sure she is. Sofia mentions that she doesn't consider her relationship with her boyfriend as a long-term thing; she just knows his family has money, and he will be able to financially support both her and the baby. As the session comes to a close, Sofia thanks Brooke for letting her talk so much about all the stuff that is going on in her life and keeping things between the two of them. Sofia says she could never tell her parents these things as they would just not understand.

See how Case Illustration 3-2 may be addressed using the Corey, Corey, and Callanan (2011) ethical decision-making model.

1. *Identify the problem.*

   a. The potential problem or dilemma in this situation is that the school counselor (Brooke) is now aware of a 17-year-old (minor) student who is sexually active with an adult (19-year-old) partner. Additionally, the student has indicated her goal in the relationship is to become pregnant without her partner's knowledge.

2. *Identify potential issues involved.*

   a. There are several *potential* concerns in this situation. We emphasize the potential nature of these concerns because depending on Brooke's morals, values, beliefs, and the way she interprets the code of ethics, some of these may be more concerning than others. However, when making a thoughtful ethical decision, it is important to look into all potential issues involved.

      i. Brooke is aware her client (Sofia) is 17 and is sexually active with a 19-year-old partner. Depending on where she lives and age of consent laws in her state, this may or may not be a potential concern.

      ii. Brooke is aware her 17-year-old client (Sofia) is sexually active and is trying to get pregnant. This may be a situation in which Brooke feels ethically obligated to notify Sofia's parents or maybe even a school official (depending on school policy).

      iii. Brooke's client (Sofia) has indicated that she has plans to become pregnant without her partner's knowledge and is potentially using him due to his family's financial status. Brooke may feel an obligation to notify Sofia's partner.

3. *Review relevant ethical guidelines.*

   a. In reviewing the ethical guidelines, Brooke should first determine which ethical guidelines to review. Because she is a school counselor, she will need to look at the ASCA and ACA Codes of Ethics. If there is any discrepancy in the codes, the common belief is that Brooke should follow the more stringent of the two guidelines.

      i. Relevant ethical guidelines from the ASCA Code of Ethics (2010) for this scenario may include the following:

         1. ASCA Standard A.1.a.: Professional school counselors have a primary obligation to the students, who are to be treated with dignity and respect as unique individuals.

         2. ASCA Standard A.2.c.: Professional school counselors recognize the complicated nature of confidentiality in schools and consider each case in context. Keep information confidential unless legal requirements demand that confidential information be revealed or a breach is required to prevent serious and foreseeable harm to the student.

         3. ASCA Standard A.2.d.: Professional school counselors recognize their primary obligation for confidentiality is to the students but balance that obligation with an understanding of parents' or guardians' legal and inherent

rights to be the guiding voice in their children's lives, especially in value-laden issues. Understand the need to balance students' ethical rights to make choices, their capacity to give consent or assent, and parental or familial legal rights and responsibilities to protect these students and make ethical decisions on their behalf.

4. ASCA Standard A.2.e.: Professional school counselors promote the autonomy and independence of students to the extent possible and use the most appropriate and least intrusive method of breach.

5. ASCA Standard B.2.d.: Professional school counselors provide parents and guardians with accurate, comprehensive, and relevant information in an objective and caring manner, as is appropriate and consistent with ethical responsibilities to the student.

6. ASCA Standard D.1.b.: Professional school counselors inform appropriate officials, in accordance with school policy, of conditions that may be potentially disruptive or damaging to the school's mission, personnel, and property while honoring the confidentiality between the student and the school counselor.

ii. Relevant ethical guidelines from the ACA Code of Ethics (2014) for this scenario may include the following:

1. ACA Standard B.2.a. Serious and Foreseeable Harm and Legal Requirements: The general requirement that counselors keep information confidential does not apply when disclosure is required to protect clients or identified others from serious and foreseeable harm or when legal requirements demand that confidential information must be revealed.

2. ACA Standard B.5.b. Responsibility to Parents and Legal Guardians: Counselors inform parents and legal guardians about the role of counselors and the confidential nature of the counseling relationship, consistent with current legal and custodial arrangements. Counselors are sensitive to the cultural diversity of families and respect the inherent rights and responsibilities of parents and guardians regarding the welfare of their children or charges according to law.

3. ACA Standard B.1.c. Respect for Confidentiality: Counselors protect the confidential information of prospective and current clients. Clients disclose information only with appropriate consent or with sound legal or ethical justification.

4. *Know applicable laws and regulations.*

a. In this situation Brooke will need to know her school policies that may be relevant.

b. Additionally, Brooke will need to know state and federal laws that may be relevant to this situation. While it would be helpful for Brooke to be familiar with some laws related to counseling, she is not expected to be an expert in all legal matters. Brooke is a professional counselor and is expected to be an expert in counseling; attorneys are experts in legal matters. Therefore it might be helpful for Brooke to contact an attorney if she suspects there may be some state or federal laws that might influence her actions.

5. *Obtain consultation.*

   a. If Brooke's decision is ever challenged and she must defend her decision, she will need to demonstrate that other counselors with similar training would make a similar decision if put in a similar situation. Therefore, Brooke should consult with colleagues, supervisors, and other professionals. Consulting with others will help her determine if her intended actions are in line with how others in her profession may act if put in the same situation.

6. *Consider possible and probable courses of action.*

   a. Brooke could decide to keep all of Sofia's information confidential.

   b. Brooke could decide to inform Sofia's parents about her behaviors.

   c. Brooke could decide to inform Sofia's partner about her intentions to get pregnant.

7. *Enumerate consequences of various decisions.*

   a. Brooke could keep information confidential.

      i. There is the possibility Sofia does not get pregnant.

      ii. There is the possibility that Sofia does get pregnant and her parents and partner are very upset with her and Brooke.

      iii. There is the possibility that Sofia does get pregnant and her parents and partner are not upset about her decision or Brooke's in keeping information confidential.

   b. Brooke could inform Sofia's parents about her behaviors.

      i. If Sofia's parents are notified, they may be supportive of Sofia, and everything may work out wonderfully.

      ii. If Sofia's parents are informed, they may get very upset and take out their anger on Sofia and/or the boy with whom Sofia is in a relationship.

   c. Brooke could decide to inform Sofia's partner about her behaviors.

      i. If Brooke notifies Sofia's partner, everything might work out well, and the two may mutually agree to continue the relationship or split apart.

      ii. If Brooke notifies Sofia's partner, he may get very upset and take out his anger on Sofia.

8. *Decide on the best course of action.*

   a. At the conclusion of the decision-making process, Brooke must ultimately make a decision about her course of action. Based on the information listed, which course of action do you believe would be best for Brooke?

This dilemma was processed using one of many ethical decision-making models. What follows are two other commonly used models.

Welfel's Model (2010)

Develop ethical sensitivity.

Clarify facts, stakeholders, and the sociocultural context of the case.

Define the central issues and the available options.

Refer to relevant laws and regulations.

Search out ethics scholarship.

Apply ethical principles to the situation.

Consult with a supervisor and colleagues.

Deliberate and decide.

Inform a supervisor and take action.

Reflect on the experience.

Cottone and Tarvydas Integrative Model (2007)

Stage I: Interpreting the Situation Through Awareness and Fact Finding

Component 1: Enhance sensitivity and awareness.

Component 2: Determine the major stakeholders.

Component 3: Engage in the fact-finding process.

Stage II: Formulating an Ethical Decision

Component 1: Review the problem or dilemma.

Component 2: Review applicable ethical codes, laws, ethical principles, and institutional policies and procedures.

Component 3: Generate courses of action.

Component 4: Consider potential positive and negative consequences.

Component 5: Consult with supervisors and peers.

Component 6: Select a course of action.

Stage III: Selecting an Action

Component 1: Engage in reflective recognition and analysis of competing, nonmoral values, personal blind spots, or prejudices.

Component 2: Consider contextual influences on values selection at all levels.

Component 3: Select a course of action.

Stage IV: Planning and Executing a Course of Action

Component 1: Figure out a sequence of actions.

Component 2: Anticipate and work out barriers to effective execution.

Component 3: Carry out a course of action.

Summary of Decision-Making Models

Each model presented and many models available in the literature (Forester-Miller & Davis, 1995; Hill, Glaser, & Harden, 1995; Keith-Spiegel & Koocher, 1985; Rest, 1984; Stadler, 1986; Steinman, Richardson, & McEnroe, 1998) have common steps but also include their own uniqueness. As previously mentioned, the specific model used is of minimal importance. Instead, emphasis should be put on going through the steps in a meaningful way. The authors offer the following process and steps to aid readers in the decision-making process.

Identify the Problem

What is the dilemma? What makes you think something needs to be done? In this first step, the focus is on understanding the concern, gathering information, and understanding the stakeholders involved. Some dilemmas may be more straightforward or simplistic, and others may be quite complex. Gaining a full understanding of the issues and entities involved is inherent.

Review Relevant Ethical Codes and Laws

Go to the code of ethics (ACA, ASCA, ASGW, IAMFC, state ethical codes, etc.) or multiple codes of ethics (depending on your area of practice) to determine which standards may be helpful or offer some guidance. The ACA, ASCA, and other professional counseling codes of ethics provide standards. They are the basis for how professional counselors must act. As previously mentioned, there are some situations (i.e., a client presents you with a gift at the end of a session) in which you might be unable to physically look at the code of ethics; in those times having a general understanding of ethical codes will be imperative. In other times, when you have the ability, the authors encourage you to review the actual codes of ethics rather than depend on previous knowledge or understanding of their wording. Ethical codes change from time to time, and thus standards and guidance may change to influence your decisions in one way or another. See Case Illustration 3-3 for examples of how small changes to codes of ethics may affect interpretations.

CASE ILLUSTRATION 3-3

ASCA Standard A.2.b. (2004): Keeps information confidential unless disclosure is required to prevent clear and imminent danger to the student or others or when legal requirements demand that confidential information be revealed. Counselors will consult with appropriate professionals when in doubt as to the validity of an exception.

ASCA Standard A.2.c. (2010): Recognize the complicated nature of confidentiality in schools and consider each case in context. Keep information confidential unless legal requirements demand that confidential information be revealed or a breach is required to prevent serious and foreseeable harm to the student. Serious and foreseeable harm is different for each minor in schools and is defined by students; developmental and chronological age, the setting, parental rights and the nature of the harm. School counselors consult with appropriate professionals when in doubt as to the validity of an exception.

ACA Standard B.2.b. (2005): Contagious, Life-Threatening Diseases: When clients disclose that they have a disease commonly known to be both communicable and life threatening, counselors may be justified in disclosing information to identifiable third parties, if they are known to be at demonstrable and high risk of contracting the disease. Prior to making a disclosure, counselors confirm that there is such a diagnosis and assess the intent of clients to inform the third parties about their disease or to engage in any behaviors that may be harmful to an identifiable third party.

ACA Standard B.2.c. (2014): Contagious, Life-Threatening Diseases: When clients disclose that they have a disease commonly known to be both communicable and life threatening, counselors may be justified in disclosing information to identifiable third parties, if the parties are known to be at serious and foreseeable risk of contracting the disease. Prior to making a disclosure, counselors assess the intent of clients to inform the third parties about their disease or to engage in any behaviors that may be harmful to an identifiable third party. Counselors adhere to relevant state laws concerning disclosure about disease status.

In Case Illustration 3-3, you can see how small changes might influence your interpretation. In the first example, the ASCA standard related to clear and foreseeable harm was slightly changed. The 2004 version was less precise and allowed for greater discrepancies in interpretation. The 2010 version still allows room for interpretation; however, additional guidelines were added. The second example involves the ACA Code of Ethics and the standard related to contagious and life-threatening diseases. The 2014 standard lacks the statement "counselors confirm there is such a diagnosis," therefore eliminating one of the counselor's responsibilities when determining whether to break confidentiality.

Similar to ethical codes, it is recommended that counselors have some general knowledge of state and federal laws that relate to your job as a counselor. Instead of burdening yourself with trying to be an expert in two different fields (counseling and law), the authors encourage professional counselors to focus efforts on counseling and depend on legal experts for assistance in legal matters. The ACA, many ACA divisions, and some state counseling associations offer free legal care with paid membership. Counselors should use those services as aids in making ethical and legal decisions.

Understand Your Own Morals, Values, and Beliefs and How They Might Influence Your Interpretation of the Code of Ethics and Laws

Socrates said, "The unexamined life is not worth living." Concomitantly, Goethe added, "There is nothing more frightful than ignorance in practice." The authors encourage counselors to understand their own morals, values, and beliefs and take ownership of them. It is the authors' belief that all people (those in the counseling profession or any other) have beliefs and values that are held onto tightly and shape individual personalities. Those beliefs are not to be judged as good or bad but are our own individual beliefs and not necessarily the values or beliefs of the counseling profession. Professional counselors are encouraged to challenge tendencies in ethical decision making to determine if individual values are influencing one's decisions and, if so, in which ways.

Identify Possible Courses of Action

What are your options, and what can you do? A critical component of this step is to look at many courses of action, even those that may not be a top choice. In most situations counselors will have multiple options as to which course of action to choose (e.g., in cases of breaching confidentiality, counselors have the option to keep information confidential or share information with another party).

Identify Benefits and Consequences of Possible Courses of Action

What might happen if you choose one course of action over another? As counselors, we want to have a full understanding of the impact of our decisions and make fully informed decisions. By looking at the potential benefits and consequences of actions, counselors are better able to weigh all options and identify significant drawbacks or benefits that may influence a counselor to choose one action over another.

Consult With Others

Ethical dilemmas are, at their foundation, dilemmas. This means there may be multiple ways to act, with each action having its own potential negative and positive consequences. If a counselor's decisions are ever called into question, he/she will need to demonstrate that someone with similar training, put in a similar situation, would act in a similar way. Consulting with others will help counselors determine if in fact the intended actions are in line with how other counselors might act if put in a similar situation.

Decide on a Course of Action and Implement

Finally, professional counselors must take action, and in some cases a lack of action will be the course of action. Taking all of these steps in mind, counselors must ultimately choose a course of action and implement his/her decision.

Legal Decision Making

Ethical and legal decision making are often lumped together as similar processes. However, there are distinct differences in the two. Ethical decision making involves following the guidelines set forth by a specific profession or organization. For professional counselors, that typically means following the code of ethics of the ACA, ASCA, and/or other state or regional counseling codes of ethics. Failing to follow such ethical guidelines may result in having to pay fines, suspension of one's license, or even having one's license revoked. Conversely, legal decision making involves following the guidelines set out by the local, state, and/or federal government. Failing to follow legal guidelines may result in having to pay fines or jail time.

Similar to ethical codes, state and federal laws are updated and change over time. While it is recommended that professional counselors be familiar with general laws as they relate to the counseling profession, counselors are not expected to be experts in legal matters. When counselors are faced with making decisions that may have legal ramifications, the authors recommend acquiring legal representation or speaking with an attorney (the ACA, ASCA, and some state counseling associations offer free legal care to all paid members).

CASE ILLUSTRATION 3-4

Chelsey is a counselor who has her own private practice and has been practicing on her own for almost 15 years. Because Chelsey has a relatively small practice, she does not have the resources available to hire any administrative help. She relies on a voice-mail system at her office to catch any calls she misses while in session. One day during her lunch break, Chelsey checks her messages and is surprised to hear that she has received a call from an attorney who claims to be representing Greg, a past client. The attorney states that she is representing Greg in a custody hearing, and Greg recommended that she contact Chelsey. The attorney mentions she would like to talk to Chelsey about her sessions with Greg and get a copy of all of her case notes and treatment plans. The attorney ends the message by leaving her phone number and asking Chelsey to return her call.

What are the possible pros and cons if Chelsey decides to return her call (or not return her call)?

If Chelsey decides that she does not want to get involved in the mentioned custody battle, does she have to talk to the attorney?

What if Chelsey doesn't have a signed release of information form from Greg? Does she need one before returning the attorney's call?

How would you proceed if you were in Chelsey's situation?

In this situation, Chelsey has several different options. Ultimately she will need to decide what to share with the attorney, if she decides to share any of her notes at all. However, first she must decide whether she will return the call. The ACA Code of Ethics (2014) offers some guidance to help Chelsey in determining what and how much to share with the attorney (i.e., Standard B.2.e. [Minimal Disclosure], B.2.d. [Court-Ordered Disclosure], and B.1.c. [Respect for Confidentiality]) but is limited in its assistance on what to do about returning the call. In this situation it might be helpful for Chelsey to contact an attorney herself to find out about the legal repercussions of her actions.

In response to the first question after the dilemma, there is no doubt of many possible pros and cons to both returning the attorney's call and choosing not to. Possible advantages to returning the call are that Chelsey would be able to find out more information about the attorney's inquiry. Chelsey may also avoid any possible legal trouble that may arise if she chooses to ignore the attorney's request for an extended time. Possible drawbacks to returning the call or positives of not returning the call include avoiding a complaint from her client that she inappropriately breached confidentiality without having the proper consent.

In response to the second question, it is unlikely that Chelsey "has to" talk to the attorney as there are very few absolutes. However, it is likely that Chelsey will need to talk to the attorney at some time if the call was valid and Greg did request that his attorney contact her. It is not an option for Chelsey to claim privilege on behalf of her client. If Chelsey intends to avoid legal repercussions, she will most likely need to talk to the attorney.

Related to Question 3 and according to the ACA Code of Ethics (2014) Standards B.2.c. (Court-Ordered Disclosure) and B.2.d. (Minimal Disclosure), Chelsey should work to obtain a signed written release of information from Greg prior to returning the attorney's phone call. Chelsey would also want to discuss with Greg the types of information he would like Chelsey to reveal to the attorney.

Avoiding Ethical Problems

Still the question remains: How can counselors avoid ethical dilemmas, and are counselors able to avoid dilemmas altogether? While there is no way to completely avoid all ethical problems, there are some things professional counselors can do to reduce their risk. The authors offer the following suggestions for ways to avoid ethical problems.

Restrict Your Area of Practice

Limit the clients with whom you work and the concerns with which you work to your areas of competence. This seems like a fairly simple concept and one that might be fairly easily followed; however, counselors of all experience levels can easily find themselves in situations where they are overwhelmed with caseloads and/or practicing outside of their competence area. The authors recommend that counselors be cognizant of their time and balance their professional and personal life. Counselor self-care and wellness are critical parts of being an effective practitioner. Similarly, counselors must know when to refer clients to others. Recognizing one's own limitations and referring when a client is outside of one's competency may sometimes be difficult but, again, critical in being an effective and ethical professional counselor.

Maintain Professional Boundaries

Maintaining appropriate boundaries with clients may be one of the more difficult or easier things to uphold, depending on the client. Counselors will most likely have some clients with whom they get along better and find more likable. With these clients, professional boundaries may become more blurred at times. Likewise, counselors will possibly have some clients with whom they have very little in common and may find less amiable. In these cases boundaries may be more easily held firm. In either case, when counselors enter into a counseling relationship with another person, they enter into a professional relationship. As a professional counselor, you are *not* your client's friend, client's family member, parent, guardian, sibling, romantic partner, buddy, and so on. Rather, you are your client's professional counselor and, as such, must maintain a professional relationship with them.

Consult With Others

When a counselor finds him/herself in a difficult situation, he/she must consult with other professional counselors. Consultation is a listed step in almost every ethical decision-making model and is useful in determining how one's decision making compares to others in the profession.

Connect With Other Professional Counselors

Connecting with other professional counselors means joining a professional association or associations, attending conferences and professional development workshops, and staying abreast of new trends in the profession. Connecting with others also means that counselors move outside of their own comfort zones to understand the counseling profession as a whole. Maintaining an ethical practice means continually growing in one's own skills and sharing one's knowledge with other professionals.

Strive for Self-Awareness

Strive to understand yourself and why you make the decisions you make. The authors recognize complete self-awareness may be difficult to achieve; however, we view it similar to that of aspirational ethics and always hoping to achieve the highest standards. Continually looking inward at one's own morals, values, motivations, and beliefs may prevent complacency and stagnation as a professional. Doing so may also reduce the chance of counselors imposing their own morals and values on clients, as stated in Standard A.4.b. (ACA, 2014).

Be Transparent With Clients

Continuously involve clients in the entire counseling process (e.g., record keeping, diagnosis, treatment planning, referrals, and consultation). Having open communication with clients throughout the counseling relationship may help counselors avoid some potential ethical dilemmas. Open communication will make the counseling process a joint effort rather than counselors acting on their own.

Conclusion

Ethical decision making is the foundation for any ethics class. It is not enough for counselors to simply memorize specific codes of ethics or be able to talk about the "right" way to handle ethical dilemmas. Professional counselors must be able to apply knowledge to real-life situations. Chapter 3 introduces ethical decision-making models and highlights the importance of using a model when resolving ethical dilemmas. Throughout the chapter, the authors described various ethical decision-making models, provided examples, and described how they might be applied to specific situations. As stated previously, the specific model is not important; instead the depth of the process a counselor uses when working through the steps is most important. Use the information you have used in this chapter to work through Exercise 3-1. Please choose an ethical decision-making model that you find to be helpful, and use it to determine how you might respond to the corresponding questions.

EXERCISE 3-1

You are a professional counselor working at a local agency. Overall, you see a wide range of clients for various reasons; however, most of your current clients are referred from the Department of Child and Family Services and have been court ordered to see you due to allegations of abuse or neglect.

(Continued)

(Continued)

You have been seeing Mr. Shefland for about four weeks due to allegations of family violence and drug use. During sessions, Mr. Shefland has let you know that he has been court ordered to have no contact with his wife or two children (ages 10 and 14) unless it is a supervised visit authorized by the state. Mr. Shefland also has let you know that he has been sober from drugs and alcohol for about three months and is doing everything required of him from the state so that he and his wife can move back in together and carry on with their lives without the intrusion of the state. Overall, Mr. Shefland has presented as a fairly straightforward person. He has been very open and honest during his sessions and is generally very likable.

However, just yesterday you and your family were out at a local city park for a weekend barbecue with friends. During the course of the afternoon, many other groups were also at the park. One group at the picnic area next to yours was excessively loud to the point that some individuals in your own group began to take notice and make comments. As you turned to look, you noticed that one particular person seemed familiar. After taking a closer look, you noticed it was Mr. Shefland with what looked to be his wife and kids. For the remainder of the afternoon, you wondered how you should handle what you saw. Not only do you know that Mr. Shefland has broken his court order in being with his wife and children, but you now know that he has not been honest with you about his drinking habits.

How would you handle this at your next meeting with Mr. Shefland?

What might you take into consideration as you make your decision?

How might your own morals, values, and beliefs influence your decision to act in one way or another?

Keystones

- Understanding and using an ethical decision-making model when resolving ethical issues is a requirement for professional counselors.
- The process used when making an ethical decision is often more important than the actual outcome of the decision.
- There are many subtleties in the wording of ethical codes, and wording often changes over time. Therefore it is critical to review codes of ethics for oneself and not rely on a previous understanding or others' interpretations.
- When faced with a legal decision, professional counselors should seek out and consult with an attorney or other legal expert.
- Ways to best insulate yourself from ethical problems include: restricting your area of practice, maintaining professional boundaries, ongoing consultation, connecting with other professionals, being transparent with clients, and striving for self-awareness.

Additional Resources

Ametrano, I. M. (2014). Teaching ethical decision making: Helping students reconcile personal and professional values. *Journal of Counseling & Development, 92*(2), 154–161. doi:10.1002/j.1556-6676.2014.00143.x

Cottone, R. R., & Claus, R. E. (2000). Ethical decision-making models: A review of the literature. *Journal of Counseling & Development, 78,* 275–283.

Garcia, J. G., Cartwright, B., Winston, S. M., & Borzuchowska, B. (2003). A transcultural integrative model for ethical decision making in counseling. *Journal of Counseling and Development, 81*(3), 268–277.

Lambie, G. W., Hagedorn, W. B., & Ieva, K. P. (2010). Social-cognitive development, ethical and legal knowledge, and ethical decision making of counselor education students. *Counselor Education and Supervision, 49*(4), 228–246. doi:http://dx.doi.org/10.1002/j.1556-6978.2010.tb00100.x

Oddli, H. W., & Halvorsen, M. S. (2014). Experienced psychotherapists' reports of their assessments, predictions, and decision making in the early phase of psychotherapy. *Psychotherapy, 51*(2), 295–307. doi:http://dx.doi.org/10.1037/a0029843

Zhong, C. (2011). The ethical dangers of deliberative decision making. *Administrative Science Quarterly, 56*(1), 1–25. doi:http://dx.doi.org/10.2189/asqu.2011.56.1.001

References

American Association for Marriage and Family Therapy. (2015). *Code of ethics.* Retrieved from https://www.aamft.org/iMIS15/AAMFT/Content/legal_ethics/code_of_ethics.aspx

American Counseling Association. (2005). *Code of ethics.* Alexandria, VA: Author.

American Counseling Association. (2014). *Code of ethics.* Alexandria, VA: Author.

American Psychological Association. (2010). *American Psychological Association ethical principles of psychologists and code of conduct.* Retrieved from http://www.apa.org/ethics/code/principles.pdf

American School Counselor Association. (2004). *Ethical standards for school counselors.* Alexandria, VA: Author.

American School Counselor Association. (2010). *Ethical standards for school counselors.* Alexandria, VA: Author.

Corey, G., Corey, M. S., & Callanan, P. (2011). *Issues and ethics in the helping professions* (8th ed.). Belmont, CA: Brooks/Cole, Cengage Learning.

Cottone, R. R., & Tarvydas, V. M. (2007). *Counseling ethics and decision making* (3rd ed.). Columbus, OH: Pearson.

Forester-Miller, H., & Davis, T. E. (1995). *A practitioner's guide to ethical decision making.* Alexandria, VA: American Counseling Association.

Hill, M., Glaser, K., & Harden, J. (1995). A feminist model for ethical decision making. In E. J. Rave & C. C. Larsen (Eds.). *Ethical decision making in therapy: Feminist perspectives* (pp. 18–37). New York: Guilford.

Keith-Spiegel, P., & Koocher, G. P. (1985). *Ethics in psychology: Professional standards and cases.* New York: Random House.

Kitchner, K. S. (1984). Intuition, critical evaluation and ethical principles: The foundation for ethical decisions in counseling psychology. *Counseling Psychologist, 12,* 43–55.

Rest, J. R. (1984). Research on moral development: Implications for training counseling psychologists. *Counseling Psychologist, 12*, 19–29.

Stadler, H. A. (1986). Making hard choices: Clarifying controversial ethical issues. *Counseling and Human Development, 19*, 1–10.

Steinman, S. O., Richardson, N. F., & McEnroe, T. (1998). *The ethical decision-making manual for helping professionals*. Pacific Grove, CA: Brooks/Cole.

Welfel, E. R. (2010). *Ethics in counseling & psychotherapy: Standards, research, and emerging issues*. Belmont, CA: Brooks/Cole.

4

Ethics and Diversity

We become what we think about.

—Earl Nightingale

Chapter 4 explores the ethics of diversity and how diversity and multicultural competence affect counselors' interactions with their clients. The various facets of diversity and understanding the differences are a continual concern facing all counselors in all settings (Shallcross, 2013). As such, multiculturalism and diversity are infused throughout the 2014 ACA Code of Ethics as a notice to the counseling field of the importance of counselor competency. Throughout the chapter, the authors will highlight and discuss the areas of multiculturalism and diversity from the ACA Code of Ethics. At the conclusion of Chapter 4, readers will be encouraged to examine their own diversity, such as cultural bias, in addition to understanding how their own morals, values, and beliefs affect the ways in which they work with these diverse populations. After reading this chapter, the reader will be able to do the following:

1. Discuss the importance of understanding diversity and how multicultural competency correlates with being an ethical counselor.

2. Describe areas of the ACA Code of Ethics in which diversity is specifically addressed.

3. Explain the importance of considering culture when determining the appropriateness of accepting gifts.

4. Describe culturally appropriate ways for making referrals.

5. Name multicultural considerations for counselors when maintaining websites.

6. Define multicultural issues when choosing and administering assessments.

7. List their own potential biases and areas for continued self-awareness.

8. State the importance of cultural sensitivity when providing diagnoses.

9. Explain diversity issues in counselor education and supervision.

Multicultural Competence and Understanding Diversity

In Stephen Covey's (1989) book *The 7 Habits of Highly Effective People*, habit number five is to seek first to understand and then to be understood. Although important for all individuals regardless of age or chosen profession, this habit is particularly critical for counselors. Starting with the preamble and continuing throughout the document, diversity and the importance of understanding cultural differences are stressed in the ACA Code of Ethics. The preamble states, "Counseling is a professional relationship that empowers diverse individuals, families, and groups to accomplish mental health, wellness, education, and career goals" (ACA, 2014, p. 3), and further, "honoring diversity and embracing a multicultural approach and support of the worth, dignity, potential, and uniqueness of people within their social and cultural contexts" (p. 3) is listed as one of five core values of the counseling profession. On subsequent pages, the introduction of Section A, The Counseling Relationship, sets the tone for how counselors are expected to behave in relationships with clients.

The ACA multicultural competencies were first explored by Sue, Arredondo, and McDavis (1992) by calling for the profession to take action. Next, multicultural competencies were written for the ACA by Arredondo et al. (1996). These competencies have made their way into every facet of professional counseling from accreditation standards to the rubrics used to assess program proposals for professional counseling conferences. A lack of knowledge about these multicultural competencies not only creates a less effective counseling experience for the clients counselors serve, but this deficiency in counselors is unethical.

In the opening section of the ACA Code of Ethics, professional counselors receive direct guidance connected to diversity and multicultural competence: "Counselors actively attempt to understand the diverse cultural backgrounds of the clients they serve" (ACA, 2014, p. 4). Consider Case Illustration 4-1 related to understanding a client's cultural background and how understanding this background may affect counseling treatment.

CASE ILLUSTRATION 4-1

Brenda, a Native American, is a 12-year-old female who is referred to your counseling center because she has anxiety issues. The first time you meet, you ask her about her family. She states that her family is too involved in her life, and she just wants to be left alone. You build rapport over time, and she reveals that she pulls out her hair when she is nervous, and her family is starting to notice. She says she is now even more concerned that her family will find out that she picks her hair out because she is starting to create bald spots underneath her long, jet-black hair. To meet the treatment plan developed with her, you call her mother and ask her (mom) to bring the rest of the family to the next session. When the next session arrives, you hear a knock on your office door; it is the office administrative assistant and billing coordinator. She has a blank stare and states, "Come here now. We have a problem." The direct tone in her voice prompts you to drop what you are doing and quickly go to the waiting room. There is standing room only. You see Brenda wearing a white hat and sitting between two women. You recognize one of the women as her mother, and you assume the lady on the other side is her grandmother.

Why is the waiting room full?

How might you proceed in working with this client?

In response to the first question, the waiting room is full possibly due to Brenda's cultural background. Brenda belongs to a Native American (Indigenous Peoples) tribe. The whole family unit, which includes siblings, aunts, uncles, cousins, and even in-laws in some cases, typically deals with problems all together as a cohesive unit. In this case, Brenda is so important to the tribe that when Brenda's mother asked the family to come to the counseling session, they all participated as a natural practice in their culture. Possibly a definition of family may have helped the counselor here.

In regard to the second question associated with Case Illustration 4-1, there are likely many ways to proceed with this client. The diversity issue here is awareness of the family beliefs and customs. Sometimes referred to as "family of origin," asking questions about clients' family relationships is vital to a better understanding of the unique diversity this client experiences inside and outside of her home. Although there is no specific prescription as to how to move forward with this particular client, it would be important for the counselor to seek to understand and follow the guidance of the client rather than trying to fit the client into the counselor's general treatment strategy. One technique would be to use clarifying statements to address the cultural background of the client and check for understanding.

As mentioned before, the client in Case Illustration 4-1 belongs to a Native American tribe and being a part of this tribe is a part of her culture. With the diffusion of genetics in the Native American populations, one cannot tell the cultural background of a person based on appearance alone. The question about culture must be addressed in every counseling relationship. It is the author's belief that all too often when discussions take place about culture, the central focus of understanding culture or being "multiculturally competent" is focused on race, religion, sexual orientation, language, socioeconomic status, and so on. However, culture involves so much more than race, religion, language, sexual orientation, and economic status. Culture is every part of every individual. It includes a rich chronicle of a person's life from city of birth to which schools the client attended to even how the client views the world. As you continue to read, take time to consider the finer intricacies of culture and diversity.

Diversity Considerations
in the Counseling Relationship

ACA Standard A.2.c. (2014) Development and Cultural Sensitivity: Counselors communicate information in ways that are both developmentally and culturally appropriate . . . counselors consider cultural implications of informed consent procedures and where possible, counselors adjust their practices accordingly.

The authors believe "developing cultural sensitivity" is a critical and essential component of Standard A.2.c. Developing sensitivity includes understanding differences in people and clients and the counselor making needed adjustments rather than expecting the client to make adjustments. Cultural sensitivity may be garnered from participating in culturally diverse events. Examples of culturally diverse events may include Dia de Los Muertos, Juneteenth, Lunar New Year, Thanksgiving, Boxing Day, and a Native American Death Ceremony among other celebrated cultural events. This list is by no means exclusive or comprehensive. The challenge to the ethical counselor is to get outside of his/her own culture and view the world from the lives of other culturally diverse people.

Examine Case Illustration 4-2, and determine whether you believe Trevor's actions are ethical.

CASE ILLUSTRATION 4-2

Trevor, a licensed professional counselor, primarily works with adolescents and young adults in his small private practice. Today Trevor has a new client, Raul, who is a 16-year-old student enrolled in the 10th grade. During the intake session Trevor realizes that Raul and his mother have recently moved to the United States from Mexico. Although Raul speaks fluent English and Spanish, his mother is monolingual and speaks only Spanish. Because Trevor does not speak Spanish, he asks Raul if he will translate the consent form and describe it to his mother in Spanish.

Would Trevor's behaviors be considered communicating in developmentally and culturally appropriate ways?

Trevor's behaviors in Case Illustration 4-2 would most likely be considered inappropriate according to Standard A.2.c. Instead of asking Raul to translate, Trevor would want to "develop cultural sensitivity" and be sure to have all of his consent forms and other vital documents in both the English and Spanish languages. Developing such sensitivity indicates Trevor more fully understands his diverse community and knows there may exist a possibility his clients from diverse cultures would reach out to him for counseling services. Being a culturally sensitive professional counselor, Trevor would want to set up his counseling practice, and all associated forms, to accommodate the needs of all potential clients. An examination of the various languages spoken in his geographic location may help him decide the languages to use for his counseling forms and marketing. In addition to translating his printed forms, Trevor might also consider locating and contracting with a Spanish language interpreter. Trevor would also want to be sure to develop a comprehensive list of referral sources, being cognizant to include counselors who are English/Spanish bilingual. Understanding language differences increases the success of counseling for the client, thus producing a more culturally sensitive approach to counseling.

ACA Standard A.4.b. (2014) Personal Values: Counselors respect the diversity of clients, trainees, and research participants and seek training in areas in which they are at risk of imposing their values onto clients.

Professional counselors are to respect diversity and seek further training in the areas they may feel are most needed in their own professional development. Professional development may consist of workshops, conference programs, online trainings, courses at institutions of higher education, and for some, reading books. The most important characteristic of professional development is to understand a person is never done developing and must actively seek out more knowledge over his or her lifetime. Many of the state licensure or certification boards require annual continuing education as a part of renewal processes. According to Standard A.4.b., counselors should seek out training in understanding diverse populations. Also, the latter part of this standard encourages counselors to seek out training when they are "at risk" of imposing their personal values on the client. To avoid this risk, counselors must first be self-aware and acknowledge feelings and values present in themselves. In Chapter 2 the authors emphasized the importance of self-awareness and understanding values. It is the author's opinion that all counselors have values, which are neither good nor bad. Values become disruptive (and unethical) when counselors let their own personal values become an imposition on their clients. In meeting with clients, the counselor's values do not matter and should not interfere with the client's growth. The ethical counselor, to increase the empathic experience of both the counselor and the client, must remove values from the counseling formula.

Correspondingly, the authors have yet to meet a professional counselor who openly admits or acknowledges he/she consciously or purposely imposes personal values on clients. A counselor who considers him/herself to be a person to change all of his/her client's worldviews would not have a client's best interests in mind. Instead, this counselor is putting his/her own best interests first. This would obviously be a counselor who lacks self-awareness and does not fully understand and acknowledge that imposing his/her own values on the client may indirectly cause harm. Consider Case Illustration 4-3 related to counselors understanding their own values.

CASE ILLUSTRATION 4-3

Dennis is a school counselor working at a high school located in a middle/upper-middle-class neighborhood. He has been there for almost five years and feels a special connection to the school and neighborhood because he lives in the area and graduated from the same high school.

(Continued)

(Continued)

Earlier this week, Dennis talked to Charlie, a new student, about his goals for after high school. Charlie is a junior this year, and Dennis typically makes a point to meet with all juniors to discuss college applications and career goals. During the meeting, Charlie seems disinterested in going to college and says he would rather work in construction than go to college. Charlie continues his explanation by stating that college is something other people do, but he would like to start making money right away rather than spend it on college. In response, Dennis says, "You have great test scores and really high grades. I'm sure we could get you a scholarship to any college or university. You don't really want to do construction. It may sound fun now, but eventually you are going to want a real job, and the only way to do that is to go to college." Charlie reluctantly agrees and says he will think about it and come back the following week.

Then, Dennis receives a call from Charlie's mother asking about his conversation with Charlie earlier in the week. Charlie's mom expresses her concern because Charlie came home from school and talked about his father not having a real job. Somehow, she says, Charlie was given the idea that construction was not a "real job." Charlie's mom went on say that for the past four generations, Charlie's relatives have worked in construction and have enjoyed their work. At the conclusion of the call, Dennis apologizes for his choice of words and tries to explain that he did not mean anything negative. He stresses that he always encourages all students to go to college because he wants them to be successful in life rather than to have to work minimum-wage or low-paying jobs all their lives.

How did Dennis's values affect his choice of words in this situation?

What might Dennis have done differently if he were more self-aware?

It is impossible to determine Dennis's complete list of values from the brief scenario provided, but there is enough to gain some insight as to Dennis's beliefs. Dennis seems to value education; specifically he seems to believe a college education is vital to becoming "successful" in life. It may also be fair to say Dennis values "white-collar" over "blue-collar" jobs. There is an inherent bias present in how Dennis is interacting with Charlie, although Dennis may not purposely be out to hurt the client. The biased comments made by this counselor are called micro-aggressions and should be explored.

Dennis certainly did not mean to offend his student or Charlie's parents. In addition, he did not intend to imply that the student's father was not successful. Most likely, Dennis was acting and speaking in a way he thought would be most helpful to his student. Nevertheless, through his choice of words, Dennis's values were very clear to his student and were also very offensive. Being offended causes a client to typically shut down emotionally, or resort to aggression, or terminate counseling. Dennis would be well served by examining his implicit bias.

Question 2 asks what Dennis might have done differently given the same circumstances. Dennis may have chosen his words more conscientiously. Rather than trying to force Charlie into his idea of "success," Dennis might have listened and *respected the diversity* of his student. He could have encouraged Charlie to explore his own values and ideas of success. See the following dialogue as one possible example.

Dennis: Hi, Charlie, I'm talking to all juniors this month about college applications and everyone's ideas about what to do after high school. I noticed you have really high test scores, which will certainly be helpful to you in whatever you choose. Have you thought about what you might like to major in and which college you plan to attend?

Charlie: I really don't have any interest in going to college. I would rather start making money right away and go into the construction business.

Dennis: You have very little interest in going to college and don't really see it as a viable option for you? You would rather go into construction and start making money right away? How did you decide on construction?

Charlie: My dad does construction, and my grandfather did the same thing. I guess it's something I grew up with, and it seems really interesting and fun to me. I know the work is hard labor, but I get to work outside all the time, and the money can be pretty good.

Dennis: It sounds like something you know quite a bit about, and it runs in your family. I'm wondering if there is a certain type of construction you would want to do. How do you plan on getting a construction job doing what you want?

ACA Standard A.10.f. (2014) Receiving Gifts: Counselors understand the challenges of accepting gifts from the clients and recognize that in some cultures, small gifts are a token of respect and gratitude.

See Text Box 4-1 for APA and AAMFT standards regarding receiving gifts.

TEXT BOX 4-1

American Psychological Association

The APA does not address issues related to receiving or giving gifts.

American Association for Marriage and Family Therapists

AAMFT Standard 3.9 (2015) Gifts: Marriage and family therapists attend to cultural norms when considering whether to accept gifts from or give gifts to clients. Marriage and family therapists consider the potential effects that receiving or giving gifts may have on clients and on the integrity and efficacy of the therapeutic relationship.

Because a counselor will encounter a diverse population of clients, it is paramount to understand that gift giving and receiving is customary in many cultures. Depending on the population a counselor is working with most often, a policy written about gift giving and receiving may benefit the counseling relationship.

Consider Case Illustration 4-4a related to receiving gifts from clients.

CASE ILLUSTRATION 4-4A

Susan is working as a counselor in a nonprofit agency providing counseling to low-income, single-parent, Hispanic women. In December, Ana Elena, who has been attending counseling at the agency for five months, comes to her counseling session bearing a paper bag filled with homemade tamales. Ana Elena presents Susan with the gift and explains that making tamales and giving them to her friends at Christmas is a family tradition. Susan readily accepts the gift and shares with Ana Elena that she will serve the tamales to her family on Christmas Eve. After Ana Elena leaves, Susan is torn whether she should have accepted the tamales as a gift. Susan did not want to offend Ana Elena by refusing the gift, but she also knows Ana Elena has significant financial concerns, and the ingredients and energy required to make the tamales probably increased Ana Elena's financial struggles.

Did Susan act ethically in accepting the tamales from her financially challenged client?

In the previous chapter, the authors discussed ethical decision-making models and the process counselors use in making a decision. In this scenario, Susan had to go through a decision-making process fairly quickly, take many things into consideration, and in the end she made the decision to accept the gift. In making her decision, Susan understood Ana Elena's gift was "a token of respect and gratitude" as mentioned in Standard A.10.f. Therefore, it would most likely be considered an ethical decision that she accepted the tamales. Susan believed to refuse the gift of tamales, which was a token of respect and gratitude from Ana Elena, would negatively impact their counseling relationship. She would also want to be sure to document her decision-making strategy and her rationale for accepting the gift.

Some state licensure or certification boards place a limit on the value of a gift a counselor should accept from a client. This fluctuates across the country, with an average of approximately $50. With any gift, it would be impossible to judge the actual cost incurred by the client, but a good estimate may provide a better ethical result.

Consider Case Illustration 4-4b and another example of an ethical dilemma surrounding the giving and receiving of gifts.

CASE ILLUSTRATION 4-4B

Julio works in a free mental health clinic for Asian refugees. He counsels youth and young adults most often about transition issues in new schools and learning to live in the United States. Because he works with an early adulthood population, he discusses arranged marriages, dating, and career issues related to school graduations. One of his female clients is Ay Quin, who will be getting married soon and has invited him to the wedding ceremony and the reception. The client is Vietnamese and wants to honor Julio by having him be part of the ceremony because he is like family to her. In her culture, Ay Quin would be disgraced if her family knew she was receiving counseling from someone outside her family. So, having Julio be part of the ceremony would make him look more like an advisor or friend instead of a counselor. She stresses that he does not need to pay for anything; she just needs him to be there.

What can Julio do to prepare for this event?

What is the ethical and cultural issue at play?

Does Julio need to participate?

The first question associated with Case Illustration 4-4b inquires as to the best way Julio may be able to prepare for attending the wedding. The best way would be to ask the client what is expected and what are the rules, customs, and traditions in which he would be expected to participate. Information may also be learned by consulting literature or by meeting with the family.

The second question asks about pertinent ethical and cultural issues. The most striking issue is that the client is being put into a difficult spot due to her relationship with Julio. Because her culture does not encourage counseling, the client can mitigate the familial impact by having Julio pose as an advisor or friend. If Julio does not participate in this manner, the client could be shunned by the family, resulting in more psychological trauma.

Whether or not Julio must attend the wedding is a difficult question. On one hand Julio has an obligation to help his client inside the counseling sessions. On the other he has no obligation to help outside the session unless he is advocating for the client. However, in this case, does Julio need to try to change the client's family culture? Sometimes a counselor must choose the battles he/she fights to reduce the harm occurring from impulsive, closed-minded responses. Therefore, it may be in the best interest for Julio to attend the ceremonies but clarify to the client he cannot receive or give gifts. This would include anything he would need to wear. He would need to give back to the family anything he received so as to not be accused of receiving gifts from clients during a traditionally giving ceremony.

Similar to the dilemmas presented in the previous two case illustrations, consider Case Illustration 4-4c, in which the topic of bartering becomes an ethical concern.

CASE ILLUSTRATION 4-4C

Raquel is a licensed professional counselor working as a career counselor at an agency located in a diverse, large metropolitan area in the southwest part of the United States. One of her current clients is Carolina, a 20-year-old woman who has recently moved to the United States from the interior of Mexico. Carolina is a lawful permanent resident, which allows her to legally reside and secure employment within the United States. She is attending counseling at the request of her aunt and uncle, with whom she lives, and is exploring job-seeking skills and local certification programs to better prepare her for employment in her new country.

After several productive counseling sessions, Carolina's aunt and uncle approach Raquel with a concern. They are finding it difficult to continue to pay for Carolina's counseling as she has no insurance and is not covered on their policy. They believe Carolina is benefiting tremendously from the counseling experience and is working hard to achieve the goals she set with Raquel. They, as well as Carolina, want the counseling to continue. Carolina's uncle is a professional massage therapist and offers to provide weekly massages for Raquel, or someone of her choice, in exchange for the counseling. Raquel is aware she has been very stressed for some time and believes taking some time for herself and relaxing with a massage would help her to retain her wellness.

What are the ethical implications if Raquel chooses to barter for counseling services in lieu of traditional monetary payment?

Raquel is aware codes of ethics of mental health service providers caution against bartering; however, she is aware they also *view bartering as a legitimate and ethical option*. In addition, she knows *the code of ethics stresses the importance of the cultural setting within which the bartering relationship takes place*. Raquel believes rejecting all or most bartering arrangements goes against a counselor's professional and ethical commitment to serve clients of diverse economic classes and cultures.

Raquel also is aware that bartering agreements have a potential to create conflicts, exploitation, and misrepresentation of the professional counseling relationship. If she chooses to barter in this case, she must believe the relationship is not exploitative and will need to establish a clear, written contract regarding the agreement.

ACA Standard A.11.a. (2014) Competence Within Termination and Referral: Counselors are knowledgeable about culturally and clinically appropriate referral resources. And suggest these alternatives . . .

Referrals are commonplace in all professional environments. Concomitantly, professional counselors often refer clients to other counselors and for other mental health-related services (e.g., housing assistance, food assistance, psychological testing, etc.). Ethical counselors take culture into consideration when compiling their comprehensive list of referral options and in providing clients with referral resources. Consider Case Illustration 4.5.

CASE ILLUSTRATION 4-5

Barry is a licensed professional counselor in a large metropolitan city with an extremely diverse population and has been in private practice for almost 20 years. He has decided he will be retiring at the end of the month to enjoy spending more time with his family and friends. In preparing for his retirement, Barry knows he must provide referral sources for everyone in his rather large caseload. After all, Barry knows it would be considered unethical (according to Standard A.12. [Abandonment and Client Neglect]) if he were to simply retire and not let his clients know or provide them with referral resources.

What does Barry need to make sure of when providing referrals to his clients?

Barry is acting in an ethical manner by following Standard A.12. (Abandonment and Client Neglect), but he would also want to pay close attention to Standard A.11.a. (Competence Within Termination and Referral). In complying with Standard A.11.a., Barry would want to consider the needs of each of his clients. He is not required to choose specific referral options for each of his clients, but Barry should consider the options he provides. Barry would want to compile a diverse list of counselors with various expertise and therapeutic styles or theories. In doing so, Barry can be assured he is providing his clients with viable options for a better counseling outcome. Even though Barry may give the referrals to his clients, the client may not seek out more counseling through the referral. The ACA Code states, "If clients decline the suggested referrals, counselors discontinue the relationship" (2014, p. 6).

ACA Standard B.1.a. (2014) Multicultural/Diversity Considerations: Counselors maintain awareness and sensitivity regarding cultural meanings of confidentiality and privacy. Counselors respect differing views toward disclosure of information. Counselors hold ongoing discussions with clients as to how, when, and with whom information is shared.

Standard B.1.a. is the first standard of Section B, Confidentiality and Privacy. Similar to many other standards referring to sensitivity and culture, this one reiterates the importance of ongoing conversations with clients regarding privacy and confidentiality. Standard B.1.a. applies to all clients and the need for counselors to be able to put themselves into their clients' shoes and understand the world from the client's perspective. Counselors must understand words (e.g., "confidentiality" and "privacy") have different meanings to different people. Consider Case Illustration 4-6a.

CASE ILLUSTRATION 4-6A

Walter, a counselor who primarily works with adolescent populations, always explains confidentiality to his clients (both parents or guardians and minors) and also explains the limits to confidentiality. He typically says, "If you tell me you're going to hurt yourself, I have an ethical and legal obligation to let your parent or guardian know what is going on. Everything else is confidential." During one counseling session, the adolescent client discusses ways in which he handles stress. He explains that sometimes he takes the end of a paperclip or staple and scratches words into his upper arm. After the discussion, Walter expresses his concern that the client is harming himself and reminds the client that he must tell the client's parent or guardian about the self-harming behavior. The adolescent responds by pleading with the counselor to not share the information and says it is not self-harming behavior; it is just his way of coping. In the end, the client feels betrayed and is hesitant to share any other personal, in-depth information with the counselor, and the counseling relationship is ended.

What happened in this situation that caused the counseling relationship to become ineffective?

What could the counselor have done differently in this situation?

In the example given in Case Illustration 4-6a, the counselor and client have a different understanding about what constitutes "self-harming" behaviors. The counselor, Walter, believes he is fulfilling his ethical obligation by notifying a parent or guardian as required by Standard B.2.a. (Serious and Foreseeable Harm and Legal Requirements). However, the adolescent client does not have the same understanding of "self-harm" and feels betrayed when Walter breaks confidentiality and shares what the client believes to be a "coping skill."

The second question asks what the counselor could have done differently to possibly avoid this awkward situation. Like most situations, there are many "appropriate" ways to respond, and likely there are many things the counselor could have done differently. In Case Illustration 4-6a, it may have been helpful for Walter to discuss his understanding of "hurting oneself" in greater detail during the informed consent process. Instead of simply stating, "If you tell me you're going to hurt yourself, I have an ethical and legal obligation to let your parent or guardian know what is going on," the counselor may have elaborated more on the process he uses to determine whether a behavior is "harmful" and requires parental notification. Consider the following example.

Counselor: *If you let me know you are going to hurt yourself, then I have an ethical and legal responsibility to let someone know about it. The person I typically notify first is your parents or guardians. I know "hurt" is a fairly vague word, and I don't want you to think I am simply going to use it as a way to share every small detail with your parents. If there is ever a time when I feel you might be in danger, I will always discuss it with you first. Together we can figure out the best way to make sure you feel as though your rights to confidentiality are respected and your parents get the information they need to be able to protect you from any potential harm.*

It may have been helpful to have a conversation with the adolescent client regarding his/her concerns once the information is divulged:

Client: *I cope with stress by scratching my arm with a paperclip.*

Counselor: *I hear what you are saying, and as you were talking about scratching your arm, I kept thinking about when we first met, and I mentioned the reasons I would need to let your parents know about what we talk about. I'm worried that you may be hurting yourself, and we may need to let someone else know about it so that you will be safe. What do you think?*

Client: *That's crazy, I'm not hurting myself. I guess I'm scratching my skin, but I'm not going to kill myself. Don't tell my parents about it. They will just freak out and constantly be on my case.*

Counselor: *I understand what you're saying, and I understand that you don't want your parents to freak out over this. Maybe we can find a way to let them know but in a way that is comfortable for you.*

In these examples, the counselor is still able to notify parents or guardians when the issue of self-harm comes up in counseling, but the client would hopefully not feel as though the counselor was betraying him/her. By addressing the differences in meanings words have at the onset, the counselor sets the tone for a collaborative and understanding relationship. The counselor is letting the adolescent know that he/she is a valued and respected member of the counseling relationship.

ACA Standard C.5. (2014) Nondiscrimination: Counselors do not condone or engage in discrimination against prospective or current clients, students, employees, supervisees, or research participants based on age, culture, disability, ethnicity, race, religion or spirituality, gender, gender identity, sexual orientation, marital or partnership status, language preference, socioeconomic status, immigration status, or any basis proscribed by law.

To compare how the APA and AAMFT codes treat discrimination, see Text Box 4-2.

TEXT BOX 4-2

American Psychological Association

APA Standard 3.01 (2010) Unfair Discrimination: In their work-related activities, psychologists do not engage in unfair discrimination based on age, gender, gender identity, race, ethnicity, culture, national origin, religion, sexual orientation, disability, socioeconomic status, or any basis proscribed by law.

(Continued)

(Continued)

American Association for Marriage and Family Therapists

AAMFT Standard 1.1 (2015) Nondiscrimination: Marriage and family therapists provide professional assistance to persons without discrimination on basis of race, age, ethnicity, socioeconomic status, disability, gender, health status, religion, national origin, sexual orientation, gender identity or relationship status.

Consider Case Illustration 4-6b and Hector as he works with a client with whom his own values conflict.

CASE ILLUSTRATION 4-6B

Hector is a professional counselor working in a fairly conservative city in the American Bible Belt. His community is outspoken on assorted political issues, and his state and nationally elected officials tend to be more conservative than the rest of the country. Hector grew up in a family with strong religious beliefs. His family was always doing something at the church, like cooking meals for the elderly, feeding the homeless after the Wednesday and Sunday church services, or volunteering to lead Bible study and Sunday school. Hector has started to see clients pro bono, who come to the church seeking counseling services. The clients come to the counseling center as drop-ins and come from various parts of the city. One of the clients (a 17-year-old) who presents one evening tells Hector he (the client) talked to Hector at a homeless shelter after the client was kicked out of his house. Hector asks why he was kicked out, and the client informs Hector that he told his mom he thought he was gay. Instead of listening to him, the client's mom hit him with her broom and made him leave the house. She locked the doors and would not allow him back in. The client, not knowing what else to do, ended up going to his boyfriend's (a 22-year-old) house and has been staying there for the past week.

What should Hector do as his upbringing and spiritual values include the idea that homosexuality is a sin?

Hector lives in a conservative town, and his values significantly conflict with the concerns presented by his client. The question in Case Illustration 4-6b inquires as to how Hector should move forward with his client. Simply stated, Hector is ethically obligated to avoid imposing his own values and must promote the well-being of his client. There will likely be clients throughout every counselor's career with whom he/she has conflicting values. Professional counselors must be able to put their own values aside and work with clients from diverse backgrounds. In accordance with ethical Standard C.5., professional counselors do not discriminate against individuals.

ACA Standard H.5.d. (2014) Multicultural and Disability Considerations: Counselors who maintain websites provide accessibility to persons with disabilities. They provide translation capabilities for clients who have a different primary language, when feasible. Counselors acknowledge the imperfect nature of such translations and accessibilities.

Later in Chapter 9, the authors will discuss ethical considerations related to technology in more depth. However, this standard (H.5.d.) relates specifically to multicultural issues when using technology. Websites are commonplace and are maintained by the vast majority of counselors. In developing and maintaining websites, it is critical that counselors consider the cultural differences of those people potentially looking to access their websites. Consider the following examples.

CASE ILLUSTRATION 4-7

1. Diego is the owner and manager of a private counseling practice and acts as the clinical supervisor for three other counselors. Diego's practice is located in an upper middle-class area in the southwest part of the country. The community is primarily English speaking, but about 30 to 40 percent of people speak Spanish as the primary language in the household. Diego has hired an outside consultant to develop a webpage to advertise his practice and provide accessibility to current and future clients. On his webpage he lists counselor names and credentials and delineates which counselors are English/Spanish bilingual and which are not. He also includes a personal disclosure statement outlining his views on counseling, theoretical orientation, and other practice specialties. Finally, Diego asks the consultant to include examples of his consent form, release of information, and client rights and responsibilities form, so potential clients can print (if they choose) and bring them to the first session. In consideration of all potential clients and the diverse area in which he is located, Diego lists all forms and information in both English and Spanish.

2. Belinda has just transitioned from working at a community agency to starting her own private counseling practice. One of the first things she wants to do is create a webpage to attract clients. In doing so, Belinda knows she may have individuals from diverse cultures access her page. Among other things, Belinda is careful to make sure the software she uses in developing her webpage is compatible with screen readers. Belinda knows she may have individuals with visual impairments access her webpage, and she wants it to be accessible to all.

In both of these examples the counselors were aware of cultural differences among those who might wish to access their webpages. Additionally, both counselors were careful to address access issues. It may be difficult to ensure webpages are accessible to all persons, but counselors should still strive to meet the needs of as many individuals as possible. A critical component is that counselors have awareness and take actions to provide accessibility when needed. "Awareness" is a term used quite frequently in the ACA

Code of Ethics (2014). Similarly, awareness and counselor self-awareness was discussed more thoroughly in Chapter 2. Standard H.5.d. is yet another example of how counselors must understand the impact their services have on others.

Diversity Considerations in Diagnosis and Assessment

ACA Standard E.5.b. (2014) Cultural Sensitivity: Counselors recognize that culture affects the manner in which clients' problems are defined and experienced. Clients' socioeconomic and cultural experiences are considered when diagnosing mental disorders.

A responsibility of many professional counselors is that of providing or assigning a diagnosis as a way to explain client behaviors. Still, diagnosis is not an exact science. Ford (2006) described diagnosis as a "culturally based value judgment concerning the behavior or beliefs of a client" (p. 155). This standard encourages counselors to consider how culture affects or may influence client behaviors and the way behaviors are explained when assigning a diagnosis. What may be considered appropriate or the norm in one culture may be considered deviant or neurotic in another (Hays, Prosek, & McLeod, 2010; Kress, Eriksen, Rayle, & Ford, 2005). Consider the following questions and how you might explain your reasoning to a client if asked.

EXERCISE 4-1

What is the difference between a child who may be diagnosed as having attention deficit hyperactivity disorder (ADHD) and a child who is described as having "ants in his pants" and a short attention span?

What is the difference between an individual who has bipolar disorder and someone who has many mood swings or ups and downs in his/her life?

What is the difference between someone who is depressed and someone who is having a difficult time right now or doesn't have much energy and has difficulty finding joy in life?

What is the difference between someone who has an adjustment disorder and someone who is having a difficult time with recent changes in his/her life?

The following two standards concern multicultural and diversity issues related to assessments. It is common knowledge that cultural biases exist in some assessment tools. As such, it is critical that professional counselors take culture and context into account when determining which assessments to administer and how to interpret the results.

ACA Standard E.8. (2014) Multicultural Issues and Diversity in Assessment: Counselors select and use with caution assessment techniques normed on populations other than those of the client. Counselors recognize the effects of age, color, culture, disability, ethnic group, gender, race, language preference, religion, spirituality, sexual orientation, and socioeconomic status on test administration and interpretation, and they place test results in proper perspective with other relevant factors.

ACA Standard E.9. (2014) Scoring and Interpretation of Assessments: When counselors report assessment results, they consider the client's personal and cultural background, the level of the client's understanding of the results, and the impact of the results on the client.

See a description of the APA standard for use of assessments in Text Box 4-3.

TEXT BOX 4-3

American Psychological Association

APA Standard 9.02 (2010) Use of Assessments: (a) Psychologists administer, adapt, score, interpret, or use assessment techniques, interviews, tests, or instruments in a manner and for purposes that are appropriate in light of the research on or evidence of the usefulness and proper application of the techniques. (b) Psychologists use assessment instruments whose validity and reliability have been established for use with members of the population tested. When such validity or reliability has not been established, psychologists describe the strengths and limitations of test results and interpretation. (c) Psychologists use assessment methods that are appropriate to an individual's language preference and competence, unless the use of an alternative language is relevant to the assessment issues.

As has been mentioned many times in previous chapters and will continually be highlighted throughout this text, professional counselors must repeatedly consider what is in the best interest of clients. In the case of assessments, counselors may want to consider the following questions:

What is the purpose of the assessment?

What assessment tool(s) will best help fulfill that purpose?

Might the assessment chosen be biased (positively or negatively) toward my client's culture?

In asking these questions, professional counselors will be using caution in selecting an assessment tool and recognizing the effects of culture on test administration and interpretation as required by Standard E.8.

Diversity Considerations in Counselor Education and Supervision

ACA Standard F.11.a. (2014) Faculty Diversity: Counselor educators are committed to recruiting and retaining a diverse faculty.

Diverse faculty members provide diverse experiences and diverse examples for students. It only makes sense that counselor education programs would strive to recruit and retain faculty from diverse cultures to provide the highest-quality education for the students they serve. As was mentioned at the beginning of this chapter, diversity does not simply refer to race or gender. Diversity includes age, gender, socioeconomic status, race, and sexual orientation among many other aspects. In recruiting and retaining counselor educators, there is no specific formula in determining what constitutes a "diverse faculty." There is no checklist to make sure all aspects of diversity are covered for counselor education programs. Similarly, it is impossible to determine individuals' culture simply by judging the color of their skin, sound of their voice, or color of their hair. Like many other aspects of the ACA Code of Ethics, diversity in faculty involves awareness, open discussion, and communication. Awareness is again a critical component of maintaining ethical behavior. Counselor education programs and the faculty within those programs must have self-awareness and evaluate the diversity within the department. Examples of faculty maintaining awareness related to diversity include the following:

A counselor education program in which the faculty is primarily comprised of white males makes a concerted effort to advertise and search for female candidates when a new faculty position is announced.

A counselor education program housed within a primarily Hispanic-serving institution has a fairly balanced faculty in terms of male-to-female ratio and various ethnic backgrounds. However, none of the faculty members are familiar with Hispanic culture or are English/Spanish bilingual. When a new faculty position is open, the search committee gives special consideration to candidates who are English/Spanish bilingual.

A relatively large counselor education program that prides itself on having a diverse faculty realizes the majority of the faculty's expertise is in areas associated with working with adults and elderly populations. As a result, the search committee looks for candidates with backgrounds in working with children and adolescents.

ACA Standard F.11.b. (2014) Student Diversity: Counselor educators actively attempt to recruit and retain a diverse student body. Counselor educators demonstrate commitment to multicultural and diversity competence by recognizing and valuing the diverse cultures and types of abilities that students bring to the training experience. Counselor educators provide appropriate accommodations that enhance and support diverse student well-being and academic performance.

Comparable to the previous standard related to diverse faculty, counselor education programs seek out and recruit diverse students as well. Providing mental health services for a diverse world requires a diverse pool of professional counselors. Not only do counselor educators recruit diverse students, but they also provide appropriate accommodations for all students to ensure students are able to perform at their highest capacity.

ACA Standard F.11.c. (2014) Multicultural and Diversity Competence: Counselor educators actively infuse multicultural and diversity competency in their training and supervision practices. They actively train students to gain awareness, knowledge, and skills in the competencies of multicultural practice.

As stated in the introduction to Section A of the ACA Code of Ethics (2014) and reiterated at the beginning of this chapter, professional counselors continually work and seek out training to understand the diverse cultural backgrounds of the clients they serve. Therefore, counselor education programs begin that process by training and stressing to students the importance of awareness, knowledge, and skills in becoming multiculturally competent. All students are diverse, and each has his/her own culture. Similarly, each student will also have his/her own biases and multicultural blind spots. Counselor educators help bring these into the awareness of the student and thus encourage student growth.

Conclusion

This chapter focused on multiculturalism and diversity. Many aspects of practicing as an ethical professional counselor involve developing and maintaining multicultural competence. Concomitantly, a critical aspect of multicultural competence is self-awareness. Awareness is stressed throughout the ACA Code of Ethics as well as the multicultural competencies developed by Sue, Arredondo and McDavis (1992); e.g., counselor awareness of his/her own cultural values and biases and counselor awareness of the client's worldview). Awareness of client culture, of different communication styles and preferences, of one's own values, of the implications of accepting or denying a gift, and of issues related to access to services are all critical first steps in maintaining an ethical counseling practice. However, awareness is not something that simply happens. Moreover the authors feel as though awareness is often overlooked as a given. Self-awareness is often very difficult because it involves being vulnerable and recognizing one's shortcomings and weaknesses.

Awareness requires reflection and understanding. Once counselors are self-aware, they are able to take action. Therefore, the authors ask you to take time to reflect on your own culture while you consider the following case illustration and answer the discussion questions related to the information you learned in this chapter.

EXERCISE 4-2

You are a counselor in private practice and are working with a 16-year-old girl. She is referred by and brought to counseling sessions each week by her mother and two aunts. Your client's mother and aunts bring her to counseling because they believe that she is "out of control" and extremely disrespectful at home. During sessions, you typically meet with your client while her

(Continued)

(Continued)

mother and aunts wait in the waiting room. After the sessions, your client's mother typically asks you to share if you have any concerns about her daughter and if there is anything important you discussed during session.

Over the first several sessions, you come to learn that your client and her family belong to a radically conservative religious community. Your client explains that her family expects her to communicate only with other individuals who belong to the same religious community. She also states that she is not allowed to go out with any other friends and is never allowed to attend any social functions outside of those sponsored by the church. Your client routinely poses questions to you, such as "Is it wrong for me to want to go and eat pizza with some friends?" and "Why can't I go to the park with my friends to work on homework?" She tells you that she respects her family's beliefs but does not want the same life for herself. She goes on to tell you that she constantly argues with her mother and aunts about the expectations of the church.

At the next session, your client continues to discuss her frustration with her living situation. She confides to you that she has started sneaking out of her house on some nights to go out with some school friends. She claims that she and her friends typically go over to a friend's house and drink wine and just have fun. She claims she enjoys the feeling of being free and how all her problems go away when she is drunk.

As the session begins to come to a close, you remind your client that her mother is going to ask about the things they talked about in the session. Your client begs you not to say anything. She says the punishment will be horrible. She explains that if you tell her mother, the whole church will find out about what she does, and she will be brought in front of the entire church and punished by the church leaders. She claims the punishment is a public shaming and five swats with a wooden switch. Additionally, your client claims that she will never get to see her friends again, and she is sure her mother and aunts will withdraw her from school and all other social outlets.

As you walk back to the waiting room, your client's mother asks what you talked about during the session and if there was anything important she should know about?

How might you respond to the mother's question?

Do you have an ethical obligation to keep the information confidential, or should you share it with your client's parent?

Is there any abuse or neglect involved in this scenario? Do you have an obligation to report information to child or family protective services?

How does culture play into this situation?

Use an ethical decision-making model to determine how you might act.

EXERCISE 4-3

Consider the faculty within the counselor program where you are enrolled. Is there a diverse faculty? What makes the faculty diverse (or causes it to lack diversity)?

Earlier in this chapter, the authors discussed confidentiality and privacy and how words have different meanings in some cultures. The authors gave an example of a misunderstanding regarding clear and foreseeable harm. Think about and share with a classmate other words or phrases that may have different meanings depending on culture. How might those affect confidentiality or privacy and what is shared or not shared?

Part of becoming multiculturally competent is developing self-awareness. Consider your own multicultural competence. What are your strengths in understanding diverse cultures (those that are different than yours)? What aspects of multicultural competence do you struggle with most?

It is common for counselors to feel more comfortable working with some client populations rather than with others. With which populations or issues would you feel most comfortable working?

With which client populations or issues do you feel you would have the most difficulty? Why?

Keystones

- Multicultural competence is necessary for all professional counselors.
- To be multiculturally competent, counselors must first be self-aware.
- Counselors must be aware of their own culture and be accepting of cultural differences in others.
- Ethical counselors are aware of differences in communication and language. Counselors work to provide treatment and information in a way that is understandable to clients.
- Counselors are aware of their own values and choose words and statements carefully so as not to impose their personal values onto clients.
- Giving and receiving gifts have various meanings depending on culture. Counselors consider a client's culture and the meaning behind the gift when deciding whether to accept it.
- Counselor education programs should work to maintain a diverse faculty as well as a diverse student body.

Additional Resources

Cannon, E. P. (2010). Measuring ethical sensitivity to racial and gender intolerance in schools, *Journal of School Counseling, 8*, 1–22.

Day-Vines, N. L., Wood, S. M., Grothaus, T., Craigen, L., Holman, A., Dotson-Blake, K., & Douglass, M. J. (2007). Broaching the subjects of race, ethnicity, and culture during the counseling process, *Journal of Counseling & Development, 85*, 401–409.

Henriksen Jr., R. C., & Trusty, J. (2005). Ethics and values as major factors related to multicultural aspects of counselor preparation. *Counseling and Values, 49*, 180–192.

McLaughlin, J. E. (2002). Reducing diagnostic bias. *Journal of Mental Health Counseling, 24*, 256–270.

Rybak, C. J., Eastin, C. L., & Robbins, I. (2004). Native American healing practices and counseling. *Journal of Humanistic Counseling, Education & Development, 43*, 25–32.

References

American Association for Marriage and Family Therapy. (2015). *Code of ethics.* Retrieved from https://www.aamft.org/iMIS15/AAMFT/Content/legal_ethics/code_of_ethics.aspx

American Counseling Association. (2014). *Code of ethics.* Alexandria, VA: Author.

American Psychological Association. (2010). *American Psychological Association ethical principles of psychologists and code of conduct.* Retrieved from http://www.apa.org/ethics/code/principles.pdf

Arredondo, P., Toporek, M. S., Brown, S., Jones, J., Locke, D. C., Sanchez, J., & Stadler, H. (1996). *Operationalization of the multicultural counseling competencies.* Alexandria, VA: AMCD.

Covey, S. (1989). *The 7 habits of highly effective people.* New York, NY: Free Press.

Ford, G. (2006). *Ethical reasoning for mental health professionals.* Thousand Oaks, CA: Sage.

Hays, D. G., Prosek, E. A., & McLeod, A. L. (2010). A mixed methodological analysis of the role of culture in the clinical decision-making process. *Journal of Counseling & Development, 88*, 114–121. doi:10.1002/j.1556-6678.2010.tb00158.x

Kress, V. E. W., Eriksen, K. P., Rayle, A. D., & Ford, S. J. W. (2005). The *DSM-IV-TR* and culture: Considerations for counselors. *Journal of Counseling & Development, 83*, 97–104. doi:10.1002/j.1556-6678.2005.tb00584.x

Shallcross, L. (2013). Multicultural competence: A continual pursuit. *Counseling Today, 56*(3), 30–43.

Sue, D. W., Arredondo, P., & McDavis, R. J. (1992). Multicultural counseling competencies and standards: A call to the profession. *Journal of Counseling and Development, 70*, 477–486.

5

Clients' Rights and Counselors' Responsibilities

Whenever you find yourself on the side of the majority, it is time to pause and reflect.

—Mark Twain

C hapter 5 focuses on the rights of clients who work with professional counselors and the responsibilities of counselors when working with clients. The chapter will review areas of the code of ethics related to informed consent, record keeping, role changes, and providing competent services. The authors will also discuss morals, values, and beliefs and continue to stress the importance of self-awareness. Throughout the chapter, ethical dilemmas and areas to apply knowledge will focus on challenging students to evaluate their own beliefs about the services they provide. At the conclusion of Chapter 5, readers will specifically be able to accomplish the following:

1. Explain the importance of providing clients with informed consent at the onset of services.

2. Explain ethical expectations regarding what counselors must include in informed consent documentation.

3. Discuss the importance of being thorough in providing all clients with necessary information during the informed consent process.

4. Describe the importance of separating counselor values from the values of the counseling profession.

5. Define ethical requirements related to record keeping, including the maintenance and disposal of records.

6. State the importance of practicing within the bounds of one's competence.

Client Rights

Counselors, like other professionals, take on certain responsibilities as a part of joining the profession. At the same time clients who visit with professional counselors have the right to expect a certain level of care. Consider Case Illustration 5-1 and Roxanne as she visits a counselor for the first time.

CASE ILLUSTRATION 5-1

Roxanne, a 19-year-old, single mother of one, just found out she is three months pregnant with her second child. She was referred to a local counseling agency by her doctor after sharing that she is going through some difficult times with her parents and her current boyfriend. Roxanne has never been to counseling before and is a bit hesitant because she doesn't know what to expect but, as a promise to a friend, has decided to try at least one session.

What would it be like to be in Roxanne's position?

What emotions might she be experiencing as she arrives at her initial session?

What rights does Roxanne have?

Depending on the counselor's own background and experiences, he/she may have varying degrees of knowledge about what Roxanne is actually going through and thus understanding what it might be like to be in her shoes. Regardless of the counselor's own experience and understanding, it is critical for him/her to begin the session with intent on learning about Roxanne's experiences.

Question 2 is a continuation of the first and asks about the emotions Roxanne might be experiencing. Roxanne may be scared, nervous, and anxious or experiencing many other emotions. Even though the counselor may have the best of intentions, he/she is still a complete stranger to Roxanne and someone who must gain Roxanne's trust if he/she hopes to work effectively with her.

In response to Question 3, Roxanne has a right to know what to expect, to know what will be expected of her, and to voluntarily participate or withdraw her participation at any time.

In trying to gain an understanding of how Roxanne, or any client, may feel when accessing counseling for the first time, consider the different emotions you might feel if you were asked to travel to a foreign place, sit down in front of a complete stranger, and share your deepest feelings and concerns with that stranger.

Professional counselors strive to empower clients and encourage them to take control of their own lives, giving them power in the counseling process (Houser & Thoma, 2013). In previous chapters, the authors discussed foundational principles on which many ethical standards are based and, more specifically, the principle of autonomy, which is a client's right to choose and make informed decisions. To make informed decisions, however, clients and students must first have the information needed to make such decisions. Providing the information is the responsibility of the counselor and is most commonly done through the use of informed consent.

Informed Consent

Fisher and Oransky (2008) described informed consent as a process in which the tone is set for a healthy and balanced relationship between counselor and client. The ACA Code of Ethics (2014) primarily describes informed consent in Section A, and the ASCA Code of Ethics (2010) describes it similarly in Standards A.2 and B. Informed consent is a counselor's way of providing the *who, what, when,* and *how* of counseling. You can find details about informed consent for the APA and AAMFT in Text Box 5-1 and Text Box 5-2.

TEXT BOX 5-1

American Psychological Association

The APA's guidelines for obtaining informed consent are broken up into four sections: Section 3.10 (Informed Consent), Section 8.02 (Informed Consent for Research), Section 9.03 (Informed Consent in Assessments), and Section 10.01 (Informed Consent to Therapy). The specifics of each section will be covered in later chapters However, in general, the APA (2010) is similar to the ACA when describing requirements for obtaining informed consent. This is exemplified in Standard 10.01 (Informed Consent to Therapy):

a. *When obtaining informed consent to therapy as required in Standard 3.10 (Informed Consent) psychologists inform clients/patients as early as is feasible in the therapeutic relationship about the nature and anticipated course of therapy, fees, involvement of third parties, and limits of confidentiality and provide sufficient opportunity for the client or patient to ask questions and receive answers.*

(Continued)

(Continued)

b. *When obtaining informed consent for treatment for which generally recognized techniques and procedures have not been established, psychologists inform their clients/patients about the developing nature of the treatment, the potential risks involved, alternative treatments that may be available, and the voluntary nature of their participation.*

c. *When the therapist is a trainee and the legal responsibility for the treatment provided resides with the supervisor, the client or patient, as part of the informed consent procedure, is informed that the therapist is in training and is being supervised and is given the name of the supervisor.*

American Association of Marriage and Family Therapists

The AAMFT provides guidelines related to obtaining informed consent in Standard 1.2 (Informed Consent). Similar to APA ethical guidelines, AAMFT ethical standards concerning the specific type of information provided when obtaining informed consent appear to be less specific and offer more room for interpretation.

AAMFT Standard 1.2 (2015) Informed Consent: Marriage and family therapists obtain appropriate informed consent to therapy or related procedures and use language that is reasonably understandable to clients. When persons, due to age or mental status, are legally incapable of giving informed consent, marriage and family therapists obtain informed permission from a legally authorized person, if such substitute consent is legally permissible. The content of informed consent may vary depending upon the client and treatment plan; however, informed consent generally necessitates that the client: (a) has the capacity to consent; (b) has been adequately informed of significant information concerning treatment processes and procedures; (c) has been adequately informed of potential risks and benefits of treatments for which generally recognized standards do not yet exist; (d) has freely and without undue influence expressed consent; and (e) has provided consent that is appropriately documented.

Who

The "who" is *who* is involved in the counseling process. *Who* are you? What are your credentials? Do you hold a license or certification, and if so, what is it? Do you have any specializations, and what is your experience as a counselor? All of this information is important to share with your clients at the onset of services. As part of making an informed decision about whether or not a counselor has the experiences and qualifications to help them, clients deserve to know some information about their counselor and the counselor's professional background.

The other part of the "who" question is *who* will be involved or *who* will you, the counselor, be meeting with? If you are meeting with an individual, answering that question may be quite simple; however, if you are meeting with a couple, family, or children or adolescents, the answer may be a bit more complicated. The authors believe it is important to go over meeting expectations at the onset of services. Consider Case Illustration 5-2 and some questions the counselor might want to ask as a part of answering the "who" questions in informed consent.

CASE ILLUSTRATION 5-2

Ricardo has an appointment scheduled, and the referral indicates he will be meeting with a 13-year-old male who is experiencing behavior problems at school. At the scheduled time, Ricardo's client, the 13-year-old, arrives with both his mother and father. At the onset of services, while going through the informed consent process, it would be helpful for Ricardo to share some of his own policies with the family as well as understand their expectations.

Does Ricardo prefer to meet with only the 13-year-old alone, or does he feel it would be more productive to meet with everyone together?

Would Ricardo like to meet with the 13-year-old alone for a portion of the session and then meet with the parents for the other portion?

What are the parents' expectations?

What are the 13-year-old's expectations?

All of the questions in Case Illustration 5-2 should be answered at the onset of services. By answering these questions Ricardo, his client, and his client's parents will all be clear on the expectations for counseling and how the counseling process works.

What

The "what" is *what* do counselors include in informed consent? What type of information is necessary? The ACA Code of Ethics (2014) is very helpful in identifying information counselors should include in their informed consent document. Standard A.2.b. (Types of Information Needed) provides a thorough description of required information. The following are topics required to be covered.

The Purpose and Goals of Counseling

What do you do as a counselor? What theoretical approaches and/or specialized techniques do you use in your practice? The authors believe it to be essential for all counselors to be able to articulate what they do as a professional. Review the following interaction between a counselor and client as an example of how a counselor might share the purpose and goals of counseling.

Client: What is counseling all about? What kinds of things do I have to say, and what do you do?

Counselor: I believe counseling is a process. I'm not here to tell you what to do or what not to do or tell you what is right or wrong. I believe you know more about you than I ever will and have it within yourself to make the changes you see fit. Therefore, I'm here to interact with you and learn about you and your concerns and how you would like things to be different. I also believe people make changes based on how they were successful in the past. Therefore, we may spend some time talking about ways that you have been successful in other facets of your life. Finally, I believe many times our thoughts can drive our behaviors. Therefore you might notice me focusing on some of your thought processes at times. I believe by focusing on those, we may be able to determine if some of your thoughts are helping or are hindering you in making it to your end goal. That is a little bit about my beliefs about counseling. I'm wondering if you have any questions about what I said or if that was helpful to you in understanding more about the counseling process.

Benefits Versus Risks of Counseling

Will there be any discomfort to clients as a part of the counseling process? Are there any other risks clients face as a part of meeting with you? Conversely, what are the potential benefits of counseling?

Fees and Billing

What do you charge? Will there be a co-payment? What types of payments do you accept (cash, credit card, or check)? How will billing show up on credit card statements (if you take credit cards)? Do you offer a sliding scale, and if so, what are the requirements to qualify for the sliding scale fees? Do clients pay before or after their sessions?

Confidentiality and Limitations

What does confidentiality mean, and what are the limitations to confidentiality? Who will the counselor share information with and in what situations?

Grievances

If clients are dissatisfied with the services provided, how and to whom can they make a complaint? Among other things in this section, it is critical to include information related to licensure and certification boards and how clients are able to contact them if they have a grievance.

These are a few topic areas that ethically must be included in the informed consent document. A full list of all topics to be included can be found in Standard A.2.b. of the ACA Code of Ethics (2014). However, following the written word of the code of ethics is not always enough. Counselors must be able to understand the meaning and reasoning behind informed consent and deliver the message to clients in a meaningful way. Although counselors may have all the ethically required information (and sometimes more) on their informed consent and go over everything both verbally and in writing, it is the authors' belief that counselors should cater the information they share verbally to the needs of the client (i.e., counselors may emphasize some areas more than others depending on each client's circumstances, past experiences, and mood). Examine Case Illustration 5-3 for three examples of how this might look in practice.

CASE ILLUSTRATION 5-3

Reetu has a new client who is very suspicious about the counseling process and hesitant about what to expect. In this case, it may be helpful for Reetu to speak more in-depth about credentials, licensure, techniques, and confidentiality.

Craig has a new client who is a 16-year-old male who is having anxiety at school. Craig's client is suspicious about counseling because he has heard from friends who have had negative experiences with counselors. The client is worried that everything he says will be told to his parents. In this situation, it may be helpful for Craig to spend extra time talking to both the parents and/or guardians and the 16-year-old about confidentiality and how information will be shared with parents and/or guardians.

Brad has a new client who has questions about insurance billing and what types of payment are acceptable. In this situation, it may be beneficial for Brad to elaborate on billing and payment information.

In Case Illustration 5-3, all three counselors have clients with different concerns. In all three cases, Reetu, Brad, and Craig would still need to cover the consent form in its entirety but may want to spend extra time covering specific parts to ease each client's anxiety.

When

The "when" is *when* is the ideal time to review informed consent with clients? Simply stated, informed consent should be reviewed at the onset of services and then throughout the counseling process periodically (ACA, 2014, A.2.a.).

How

The "how" encompasses many components but starts with *how* counselors interact and set up their relationship with clients. Professional counselors should always be mindful of their primary responsibility "to respect the dignity and to promote the welfare of clients" (ACA, 2014, p. 4). From the first contact with clients to the case closure or last contact, it is not about the counselor; all focus should be directed toward the best interest of the client. It is the counselor's responsibility to understand the client's views, beliefs, and wants and promote those rather than the counselor's own agenda.

Starting the counseling relationship from the position of wanting to understand is crucial, and once the initial tone is set, other "how" questions can be addressed.

How Do Counselors Deliver Informed Consent to Clients and Students?

At the initial meeting between counselor and client, it is the counselor's responsibility to provide the material both in written form and verbally (ACA, 2014). However, informed consent is an ongoing process and should be revisited throughout the counseling process.

How Do Counselors Make Sure Clients Fully Comprehend the Information Provided?

It is the counselors' job to make sure information is delivered in an understandable way to clients, both verbally and in writing. Information must also be both culturally and developmentally appropriate. Therefore, counselors must be able to adjust the material they provide and the way in which they provide it to accommodate the clients they see. Additionally, in situations in which language may be a barrier to understanding services, counselors are responsible for providing adequate services (e.g., interpreter or translator). Consider ACA (2014) Standards A.2.a. and A.2.c.

ACA Standard A.2.a. (2014) Informed Consent: Clients have the freedom to choose whether to enter into or remain in a counseling relationship and need adequate information about the counseling process and the counselor. Counselors have an obligation to review in writing and verbally with clients the rights and responsibilities of both counselors and clients. Informed consent is an ongoing part of the counseling process, and counselors appropriately document discussions of informed consent throughout the counseling relationship.

ACA Standard A.2.c. (2014) Developmental and Cultural Sensitivity: Counselors communicate information in ways that are both developmentally and culturally appropriate. Counselors use clear and understandable language when discussing issues related to informed consent. When clients have difficulty understanding the language that counselors use, counselors provide necessary services to ensure comprehension by clients. In collaboration with clients, counselors consider cultural implications of informed consent procedures and, where possible, counselors adjust their practices accordingly.

How Do Counselors Obtain Consent From Minors or Others Who Are Unable to Give Voluntary Consent?

Minors or individuals under the age of 18 are usually considered unable to give legal consent (Houser & Thoma, 2013). However it is generally considered good practice to include minors in the informed consent process. While minors are unable to give informed consent, they are able to assent to services. By assenting to services, clients are agreeing to participate. Consider ACA (2014) Standard A.2.d.

ACA Standard A.2.d. (2014) Inability to Give Consent: When counseling minors, incapacitated adults, or other persons unable to give voluntary consent, counselors seek the assent of clients to services and include them in decision making as appropriate. Counselors recognize the need to balance the ethical rights of clients to make choices, their capacity to give consent or assent to receive services, and parental or familial legal rights and responsibilities to protect these clients and make decisions on their behalf.

TEXT BOX 5-2

American Psychological Association

APA Standard 3.10 (2010) Informed Consent: (b) For persons who are legally incapable of giving informed consent, psychologists nevertheless (1) provide an appropriate explanation, (2) seek the individual's assent, (3) consider such persons' preferences and best interests, and (4) obtain appropriate permission from a legally authorized person, if such substitute consent is permitted or required by law. When consent by a legally authorized person is not permitted or required by law, psychologists take reasonable steps to protect the individual's rights and welfare.

American Association of Marriage and Family Therapists

Guidelines related to working with minors or those unable to give consent are contained within AAMFT Standard 1.2 (Informed Consent; see Text Box 5-1).

The informed consent process and delivering information to clients is one of the first points of interaction between counselor and client. It sets the tone for counseling and is the beginning of building rapport and trust with clients. The authors believe one of the fundamental errors made by beginning counselors is that the informed consent form turns into a script and is read rather than having a conversation between client and counselor. Part of assuring that clients understand and comprehend services is being able to listen, understand, and respond to their concerns. Informed consent should be a comfortable and relaxed conversation with clients in which the counselor's primary responsibility is to provide clients with information needed to make an informed decision on whether or not they wish to participate in the counseling process.

Counselor Responsibilities

Parallel to the rights of clients are the responsibilities professional counselors assume when becoming a professional counselor. In the following paragraphs the authors discuss counselor responsibilities, including the responsibility to keep and maintain records, to provide competent services, and to avoid imposing one's own morals, values, and beliefs.

Avoiding Imposing Morals, Values, and Beliefs

Being aware of and acknowledging your own morals, values, and beliefs is a vital skill for professional counselors, and it is explicitly stated in the code of ethics that counselors not only be aware of their values but also avoid imposing those values on clients (ACA, 2014). Consider ACA Standard A.4.b.

ACA Standard A.4.b. (2014) Personal Values: Counselors are aware of and avoid imposing their own values, attitudes, beliefs, and behaviors. Counselors respect the diversity of clients, trainees, and research participants and seek training in areas in which they are at risk of imposing their values onto clients, especially when the counselor's values are inconsistent with the client's goals or are discriminatory in nature.

The authors view this as one of the primary responsibilities of all professional counselors, regardless of work setting. In all counseling settings it is not the counselor's job to teach appropriate behaviors or advise clients on the best path to choose in life. Rather, it is the counselor's responsibility to understand the client's values and beliefs and help the client explore them. In Case Illustration 5-4, George is a counselor working with James on some parenting concerns. Consider George's interaction with James, and determine whether you believe George is imposing his values.

CASE ILLUSTRATION 5-4

George is a counselor working at a clinical mental health agency and has about 10 years of experience working with various populations. Today he is working with James, who is a single father of two boys, ages six and nine. James was referred by his sons' school because his sons have had continuous behavior problems, and James expressed to the school counselor and administration that he does not know what to do. George has been meeting with James for a little over a month, and limited progress has been made.

At today's session James voices concerns related to his parenting style. James says he has been talking to friends and other family members, and he thinks he needs to "toughen up his parenting." George responds by acknowledging James's concerns and adds he thinks James should maybe reconsider his stance on refusing to spank his sons as a punishment. "After all," George says, "what you're doing now isn't working, and it's not like spanking is bad. You're not going to hurt them by giving them a little swat every now and then to let them know who is in charge." George smiles a bit and adds "I don't think anyone will report you for abusing your kids if you do it at selected times and don't hit them so hard as to leave a mark."

Is George acting in an unethical manner and imposing his values on James by sharing his own thoughts on discipline techniques?

In Case Illustration 5-4, James has come to counseling to express some concerns about his own parenting skills. George acknowledges James's concerns, but rather than seeking to understand James's values and beliefs more, George suggests to James that he might want to reconsider his stance on certain punishments. In effect, George is telling James about his own values and ways of parenting (i.e., George is imposing his own values related to parenting and discipline.).

While this may seem fairly straight forward in Case Illustration 5-4 with James and George, there are many subtleties in the ways professional counselors interact with clients that may imply right or wrong behaviors. Consider Case Illustration 5-5 in which Jodi, a high school student, discusses some of her job perks with her school counselor.

CASE ILLUSTRATION 5-5

Jodi, a high school student, is talking with her school counselor about her new job:

Jodi: I love my new job at the mall. I shop there all the time anyway, and I get a discount on clothes. Plus, all my friends love it too because I give them my employee discount whenever they come in.

Counselor: Do the managers allow you to do that when they aren't employees?

Jodi: No, but I'm careful about it. I make sure no one is looking, and plus it's only 15 percent, so it's not that big of a deal—not like I'm stealing anything.

Counselor: Well, just be careful. You know it may not seem like stealing to you, but I think your managers would probably feel differently about that. You know, you could probably get fired if you get caught, and the store may even be able to press charges. I'm not trying to tell you what to do. I just want you to be safe and be careful.

(Continued)

> (Continued)
>
> Jodi: Yeah, I know, and wow, you sound a little like my dad with all this breaking-the-law stuff. No worries, I'm super careful about it, and if I do get fired—oh well—it's just a stupid job anyway.
>
> *How do you think the counselor feels about breaking the law and stealing things?*
>
> *Are you able to determine, from this interaction, if the counselor approves or disapproves of Jodi's choice to share her discount with friends?*
>
> *Could this be seen as the counselor imposing his/her own values onto Jodi?*

In Case Illustration 5-5, Jodi's counselor may feel as though she is helping out and trying to keep Jodi safe by trying to get Jodi to look at things from her boss's point of view, but the counselor's values are also showing. In the second statement made by the counselor, it becomes clear the counselor believes Jodi is stealing from the store, and thus Jodi's behaviors are wrong. Even though the counselor does not directly tell Jodi her behaviors are wrong, the counselor's words imply Jodi's actions are wrong or bad.

The second question asks if the reader is able to determine whether the school counselor approves of Jodi's choice to share her discount. Yes, it is quite easy to tell the school counselor does not approve of Jodi's actions. The counselor's words come across as judging and show she does not approve of Jodi's behaviors.

In response to the third question, yes, this could be seen as the counselor imposing his/her values related to stealing or sharing company discounts. While Jodi may not directly complain to her counselor about his/her unethical actions and a complaint may never be made, the counselor's actions may definitely affect the counseling relationship.

Consider a different version of the same situation between Jodi and her school counselor. In Case Illustration 5-6, the same interaction takes place; however, the school counselor is careful to keep his/her own feelings and values out of the conversation.

CASE ILLUSTRATION 5-6

Jodi: I love my new job at the mall. I shop there all the time anyway, and I get a discount on clothes. Plus, all my friends love it too because I give them my employee discount whenever they come in.

Counselor: I can tell by the energy in your voice that you really like this new job, and it seems like there is an added bonus that you get an employee discount. This is something that you get, and then, by the sound of it, the store encourages you to pass your discount along to your friends as well?

Jodi:	No, but I'm careful about it. I make sure no one is looking, and plus, it's only 15 percent, so it's not that big of a deal—not like I'm stealing anything.
Counselor:	OK, so it seems like something they don't really encourage, and I notice you mentioned that you need to be careful about it. I'm wondering about the reasons behind you needing to be careful about it.
Jodi:	Well, I could get fired I guess, but I don't really care if that happens. It's just a stupid job. One of my friends said that I could go to jail, though. That kind of freaks me out, but I don't think I can go to jail because I'm only 16.

How did the counselor respond differently in the second scenario?

Are you able to determine, from the interaction, if the counselor approves or disapproves of Jodi's choice to share her discount with friends?

In Case Illustration 5-6, the counselor kept his/her own beliefs out of the conversation. Rather than asking closed-ended questions, which can often come across as judgmental, the school counselor asked open-ended questions of Jodi to determine Jodi's thoughts related to her actions. Unlike Case illustration 5-5, in Case Illustration 5-6, the reader is not able to determine whether the counselor approves or not.

Case Illustration 5-7, in which Doug, a married father of two, talks to his counselor about a dilemma, provides another similar opportunity to examine the minor nuances of client/counselor interactions.

CASE ILLUSTRATION 5-7

Scenario 1

Doug:	My job is too stressful. I feel like I'm going in circles all of the time, and I don't feel like I belong in my own house. This may sound crazy, but I think I'm just going to run away. I just need some time away and time to think about what to do with my life.
Counselor:	Things are really getting to you lately, and you've gotten to a point where you want to run away from everything. That seems like the best choice right now. I can't stop you, and I'm not going to tell you what to do, but before you make your final decision, let's talk about this some. How do you think it will affect your children? Don't you think they will miss you? And what about your wife? How do you think she will handle it?

(Continued)

(Continued)

Scenario 2

Doug: My job is too stressful. I feel like I'm going in circles all of the time, and I don't feel like I belong in my own house. This may sound crazy, but I think I'm just going to run away. I just need some time away and time to think about what to do with my life.

Counselor: Things are really getting to you lately, and you've gotten to a point where you want to run away from everything. That seems like the best choice right now. Tell me a little more about your decision and what you think about it.

Case Illustration 5-7, similar to Case Illustrations 5-5 and 5-6, provides two examples of counselor/client interactions. In Scenario 1 the counselor may have good intentions and be genuinely concerned about Doug and his family. However, the counselor may also be imposing his/her values and beliefs related to marriage, the role of a father and husband, and communication onto Doug. In the second scenario, the counselor paraphrases the client's concerns and acknowledges feelings similar to the first example. However, in the second example, the counselor continues with an open-ended question asking the client to explain his own thought process and elaborate on his own feelings regarding the decision. In Scenario 2, the counselor takes time to understand the client by asking about Doug's thoughts and ideas about his decision rather than telling Doug what to take into consideration.

Record Keeping

A record is considered any type of physical recording a professional counselor keeps related to his/her practice (Remley & Herlihy, 2014). Records may include myriad types of information, including case notes, voice recordings, contact logs, appointment books, and others.

There are 10 sections of the ACA Code of Ethics (2014) specifically addressing records and record keeping (see Text Box 5-3 and Text Box 5-4 for APA and AAMFT's guidelines for managing records).

ACA Standard A.1.b. (2014) Records and Documentation: Counselors create, safeguard, and maintain documentation necessary for rendering professional services. Regardless of the medium, counselors include sufficient and timely documentation to facilitate the delivery and continuity of services. Counselors take reasonable steps to ensure that documentation accurately reflects client progress and services provided. If amendments are made to records and documentation, counselors take steps to properly note the amendments according to agency or institutional policies.

TEXT BOX 5-3

American Psychological Association

APA Standard 6.01 (2010) Documentation of Professional and Scientific Work and Maintenance of Records: Psychologists create, and to the extent the records are under their control, maintain, disseminate, store, retain, and dispose of records and data relating to their professional and scientific work in order to (1) facilitate provision of services later by them or by other professionals, (2) allow for replication of research design and analyses, (3) meet institutional requirements, (4) ensure accuracy of billing and payments, and (5) ensure compliance with law.

American Association of Marriage and Family Therapists

AAMFT Standard 3.5 (2015) Maintenance of Records: Marriage and family therapists maintain accurate and adequate clinical and financial records in accordance with applicable laws.

Counselors must keep necessary records for rendering services to their clients. Counselors must follow state and local laws, regulations, and agency or institution procedures in keeping records. Finally, counselors must keep sufficient and timely data in their records and must take reasonable efforts to make sure documentation is correct. The depth and detail included in session case notes is left up to each individual counselor, and oftentimes the detail will be determined by the agency or organization for which the counselor works. Depth and detail may also vary depending on the topics discussed during each session. Review Case Illustration 5-8 and the different considerations related to note taking.

CASE ILLUSTRATION 5-8

Mike, a licensed professional counselor, is meeting with Buddy, who is a 15-year-old male experiencing some conflict with his parents. During the session Buddy mentions he has had some recent thoughts of hurting himself. Buddy doesn't have any clear plans and mentions it only as a slight concern because he never thought he would ever even think about doing anything to hurt himself. Mike does a risk assessment with Buddy and determines there is no immediate concern; it was just a passing thought.

Later in the same day Mike meets with Alyson, who is a 15-year-old female experiencing some conflict with her parents. During the session, Alyson talks to Mike about sneaking out of her house recently and going to parties without her parents knowing. She also talks about some recent experimentation with drugs and alcohol.

In Case Illustration 5-8, during the early part of the day when Mike is working with Buddy, Mike will want to be very descriptive in his note taking, documenting Buddy's thoughts of harm and the risk assessment. Doing so will help him remember the details of Buddy's concerns and also will show how Mike did his due diligence in following legal and ethical protocols when a client discusses harm to self. In the second part of Case Illustration 5-8, when Mike meets with Alyson, Mike may want to be less detailed in his note taking. Knowing Alyson is a minor and her parents have access to her file, Mike may choose to be more general in his notes. If Mike were to be very detailed in his notes, and Alyson's parents chose to request access to her file, detailed notes may be harmful to his client.

Counselors should assume their records will be read by others, and oftentimes they are. Notes may be read by clients, their legal guardians, and treatment teams and in legal proceedings and other instances. Being cognizant of the client and the work environment in which he/she works (e.g., workplace policies and procedures) will help counselors best determine the style and types of records to keep.

ACA Standard A.1.c. (2014) Counseling Plans: Counselors and their clients work jointly in devising counseling plans that offer reasonable promise of success and are consistent with the abilities, temperament, development level, and circumstances of clients. Counselors and clients regularly review and revise counseling plans to assess their continued viability and effectiveness, respecting clients' freedom of choice.

Counselors and their clients work together to devise counseling plans (treatment plans) and regularly review and update those plans. Additionally, counseling plans are done in a way respecting the client's freedom of choice. Therefore, clients are encouraged to take an active role in treatment planning. Consider Case Illustration 5-9 and how Lulu and her counselor Jacob work to identify goals for counseling.

CASE ILLUSTRATION 5-9

Lulu was court ordered to counseling as part of a safety plan related to her open case with the Department of Protective and Regulatory Services (Child Protective Services). During the first session, Lulu's counselor, Jacob, reviews her court order with her. The court order encourages Lulu to work on her violent anger outbursts, and she will need to get a job to regain custody of her children. At the end of 60 days, Jacob is expected to provide the court with a summary of Lulu's progress and recommendations to the court. As Jacob is reading the goals the court has encouraged Lulu to work on, Lulu seems disinterested in them and states that she does not have an anger problem and does not need a job. Instead, she wants to talk about how to meet a new boyfriend who is rich and will be able to provide for her and her children.

In this example, what is Jacob's responsibility? Must he address the goals listed in the court order, or should he work with Lulu on the goals she wants?

Is it Jacob's responsibility to change Lulu's mind and make her see she has a problem?

In response to the first question in Case Illustration 5-9, it depends on the relationship Jacob has with the court and/or the Department of Family Services. He may have a responsibility to both parties. However, according the ACA Code of Ethics (2014), Jacob's primary responsibility is to his client. As such, his job is to work with Lulu, so she understands the goals stated on the court order and possible repercussions if those goals are not addressed. In the end it is Jacob and Lulu who must work together to identify treatment goals. They may choose to work on only court-ordered goals, only Lulu's goals, or a mixture of both.

The second question asks if Jacob has an obligation to try and make Lulu understand that she has an anger problem. No, it is not Jacob's responsibility to change her mind. It is Jacob's responsibility to work with Lulu, so she understands the court order and Jacob's obligations to the court (if any) related to the court order.

ACA Standard B.6.b. (2014) Confidentiality of Records and Documentation: Counselors ensure that records and documentation kept in any medium are secure and that only authorized persons have access to them.

TEXT BOX 5-4

American Psychological Association

The APA addresses confidentiality of records in two areas. First, in Standard 6.01 (see Text Box 5-3) and second in Standard 6.02 (2010) Maintenance, Dissemination, and Disposal of Confidential Records of Professional and Scientific Work:

a. *Psychologists maintain confidentiality in creating, storing, accessing, transferring, and disposing of records under their control, whether these are written, automated, or in any other medium.*

b. *If confidential information concerning recipients of psychological services is entered into databases or systems or records available to persons whose access has not been consented to by the recipient, psychologists use coding or other techniques to avoid the inclusion of personal identifiers.*

American Association of Marriage and Family Therapists

AAMFT Standard 2.5 (2015) Protection of Records: Marriage and family therapists store, safeguard, and dispose of client records in ways that maintain confidentiality and in accord with applicable laws and professional standards.

Counselors must make sure records are kept in a secure location and ensure that only authorized individuals have access. The authors encourage counselors to keep records in locked filing cabinets or other areas in which access may be restricted. It may be tempting for some counselors to keep case files in their car (especially if their practice includes making home visits), with the rationale being access to the car is restricted when the car is locked. However, leaving records in a car may leave counselors open to liability if the car is broken into or stolen. Another common concern related to this issue is counselors leaving records unattended in break rooms or other common areas at their place of practice. While this may not seem like cause for great concern, it is important to remember "only authorized persons have access to records" (ACA, 2014, p. 8). By leaving records out, it is possible other counselors or employees without such authorization may be privy to confidential material.

ACA Standard B.6.c. (2014) Permission to Record: Counselors obtain permission from clients prior to recording sessions through electronic or other means.

TEXT BOX 5-5

American Psychological Association

APA Standard 4.03 (2010) Recording: Before recording the voices or images of individuals to whom they provide services, psychologists obtain permission from all such persons or their legal representatives.

American Association of Marriage and Family Therapists

AAMFT Standard 1.12 (2015) Written Consent to Record: Marriage and family therapists obtain written informed consent from clients before recording any images or audio or permitting third-party observation.

Standard B.6.c. (Permission to Record) is likely a point of emphasis in many counselor training programs, especially in those programs requiring students to transcribe or record sessions to turn in for faculty review. Text Box 5-5 lists applicable standards for the APA and AAMFT. See Case Illustration 5-10 as an example of how Standard B.6.c. may apply to a counselor working in private practice.

CASE ILLUSTRATION 5-10

A counselor in private practice schedules clients back-to-back on most days. To see as many clients as possible and to be able to give each client his/her complete attention, the counselor feels it is best to audio record sessions on a handheld digital recorder and then transcribe case notes later on after all her sessions are done for the day. The counselor does her own transcribing and deletes the tapes at the end of each day. It is just her way of keeping track of sessions without the distraction of having to take notes.

Does the counselor need to get permission from each client prior to the sessions?

The answer to the question in Case Illustration 5-10 is yes; the counselor does need to get permission from his/her client prior to recording. ACA Ethical Standard B.6.c. states that counselors must obtain written permission from clients before recording sessions. It does not differentiate based on the reason for the recording.

ACA Standard B.6.d. (2014) Permission to Observe: Counselors obtain permission from clients prior to allowing any person to observe counseling sessions, review session transcripts, or view recordings of sessions with supervisors, faculty, peers, or others within the training environment.

Similar to the previous standard, Standard B.6.d. is very straightforward and directs counselors to obtain written permission prior to observing another counseling session or reviewing a previously taped session with a supervisor, peer, or faculty member. The burden of obtaining permission often falls upon the counselor assigned to a client whose session will be observed. Permission may be obtained at the onset of services (as a part of the informed consent) or another time but must always be obtained prior to allowing others to observe.

ACA Standard B.6.e. (2014) Client Access: Counselors provide reasonable access to records and copies of records when requested by competent clients. Counselors limit the access of clients to their records, or portions of their records, only when there is compelling evidence that such access would cause harm to the client. Counselors document the request of clients and the rationale for withholding some or all of the records in the files of clients. In situations involving multiple clients, counselors provide individual clients with only those parts of records that relate directly to them and do not include confidential information related to any other client.

Counselors must allow clients to access their files and copies of their files if requested. The only exception to this is when counselors feel there is information in a file that may be harmful to the client. In such cases, counselors are required to document the request for information and the reasons for withholding information. See Text Box 5-6 for information about APA and AAMFT standards regarding client access to records.

ACA Standard B.6.f. (2014) Assistance With Records: When clients request access to their records, counselors provide assistance and consultation in interpreting counseling records.

TEXT BOX 5-6

American Psychological Association

The APA does not address patient access to records or assisting patients in understanding records.

American Association of Marriage and Family Therapists

AAMFT Standard 2.3 (2015) Client Access to Records: Marriage and family therapists provide clients with reasonable access to records concerning the clients. When providing coupled, family,

(Continued)

(Continued)

or group treatment, the therapist does not provide access to records without a written authorization from each individual competent to execute a waiver. Marriage and family therapists limit a client's access to their records only in exceptional circumstances when they are concerned, based on compelling evidence, that such access could cause serious harm to the client. The client's request and the rationale for withholding some or all of the record should be documented in the client's file. Marriage and family therapists take steps to protect the confidentiality of other individuals identified in client records.

Although clients are experts in their own lives, they may not be familiar with some of the terminology or forms counselors use when documenting sessions. Therefore, professional counselors must provide assistance to clients when reviewing records. Consider Case Illustration 5-11, and determine whether you believe the counselor's actions would be considered ethical or unethical.

CASE ILLUSTRATION 5-11

Example 1

A client requests access to his/her records. Knowing that he must provide access and assistance, the counselor provides a room where the client can review the records and an instruction manual for interpreting them. The counselor then leaves the room and lets the client know to simply return the file to the front desk when finished.

Example 2

A client requests access to his/her records. Knowing that she must provide access and assistance, the counselor sits down with the client and reads each document in the client's file verbatim.

While an instruction manual may be somewhat helpful, the counselor's assistance efforts in Example 1 would most likely be considered unethical. It is best to sit alongside your client and go through the information personally.

The counselor's efforts in Example 2 would probably be seen as ethical. However, depending on the client, it may come across as antagonistic, tedious, or even belittling.

Both of the examples presented in Case Illustration 5-11 are on opposite ends of the spectrum for "providing assistance" to clients. Ideally, when a client requests to access his/her records (regardless of the setting), counselors will spend some time with the client to make sure his/her needs are met. It may be helpful to use phrases such as these:

How can I help you?

I don't want to be overbearing, but I do want to make sure you understand what you are looking at and the reasons behind this documentation.

Are there specific areas you are interested in reviewing?

ACA Standard B.6.g. (2014) Disclosure or Transfer: Unless exceptions to confidentiality exist, counselors obtain written permission from clients to disclose or transfer records to legitimate third parties. Steps are taken to ensure that receivers of counseling records are sensitive to their confidential nature.

Prior to sharing or transferring any client records, professional counselors must obtain written permission from clients. The only exceptions to this are in cases where exceptions to confidentiality exist (e.g., client is at risk of harming self or others or subpoena requesting documents). Review Case Illustration 5-12, and see how Tammy handles a request from her client's mother to transfer records.

CASE ILLUSTRATION 5-12

Tammy, a licensed professional counselor, has been working with James, a 14-year-old male, for about six months. One afternoon James's mother calls Tammy's office and says James has been acting out at school and home again; she has had enough and has decided to put James in a residential treatment center. James's mother asks Tammy to fax information (case notes and treatment plans) to the intake specialist as soon as possible because the center will not accept James without the documentation. Tammy knows part of the intake paperwork for her office includes a general release of information form she has all new clients sign. However, Tammy typically leaves the top portion of the form blank for situations like these. Wanting to send the requested information off as quickly as possible, Tammy decides to fill in the top portion of the previously signed release form with the residential treatment center's information. She believes this is much more efficient than having James and his mom drive all the way out to her office to sign another form, especially as James's mother gave her permission over the phone.

In Case Illustration 5-12, Tammy is acting in a way she believes is most beneficial to her client and following the request of her client's mother. However, in filling in a previously signed form, she may be acting unethically. Even though permission was given over the phone, Tammy would want to get a new and original form signed by her clients prior to sending any information off to the treatment center.

ACA Standard B.6.h. (2014) Storage and Disposal After Termination: Counselors store records following termination of services to ensure reasonable future access, maintain records in accordance with federal and state laws and statutes such as licensure laws and policies governing records, and dispose of client records and other sensitive materials in a manner that protects client confidentiality. Counselors apply careful discretion and deliberation before destroying records that may be needed by a court of law, such as notes on child abuse, suicide, sexual harassment, or violence.

ACA Standard B.6.i. (2014) Reasonable Precautions: Counselors take reasonable precautions to protect client confidentiality in the event of the counselor's termination of practice, incapacity, or death and appoint a records custodian when identified as appropriate.

Professional counselors are responsible for protecting their client files. Protecting files includes storing them appropriately (even after termination of services) and setting up contingency plans in the event the counselor becomes unable to protect the files him/herself.

Providing Competent Services

Professional ethical codes require counselors to provide competent services to their clientele. According to the ACA Code of Ethics (2014), counselors are required to complete a set number of continuing education hours to maintain competence for licensure; counselors are encouraged to only practice within the boundaries of their competence; counselors are required to monitor their own effectiveness; counselors must only accept jobs for which they are qualified; and counselors only use new techniques after they are properly educated and trained in those techniques. There is a large gray area in determining the difference between what is ethical and unethical in many of these standards.

A question frequently asked is this: How do you know if you are providing competent services? In our years as counselors and counselor educators, we don't believe we have ever heard a counselor say he/she felt he/she was incompetent to work with a particular client or he/she was an incompetent counselor in general. When a complaint is made about a counselor's competence, it is usually done from someone other than the counselor in question. Monitoring one's own competence and effectiveness requires a great deal of humility and self-awareness. It is understanding and knowing there is always something to learn. Self-monitoring involves constant reflection about the interactions you have with clients. As stated in previous chapters, self-monitoring and self-evaluating requires counselors to be humble and vulnerable. Counselors must be open to hearing about strengths and weaknesses. The following are a list of questions recommended to counselors to reflect on when evaluating competency and effectiveness. The questions may be used after every client or as a daily or weekly review of services provided.

Why did I ask one question over another?

What was it that caused me to feel uncomfortable during a session?

What did I do exceptionally well during a session?

What would I do differently if I could redo a session?

Did I act as a professional counselor?

What did I do that was indicative of a professional counselor?

Consider Case Illustration 5-13 and Gary's views on his own competency as a professional counselor.

CASE ILLUSTRATION 5-13

Gary is a veteran counselor with about 10 years of experience. During lunch one day, Greg, a new counselor, talks to Gary about lacking confidence and wondering if he is a "good counselor" providing clients with the help they need. Gary responds by saying, "If you are a good counselor, your clients will come back. If you're not good, they won't." Gary goes on to say, "If clients want advice, you give them advice; if they need someone to complain to, you let them complain; and if they just want a shoulder to cry on, you let them cry on your shoulder. If you don't give them what they want, they won't come back."

In Case Illustration 5-13, Gary's advice may cause clients to "come back" in some instances but does not necessarily mean he is a competent counselor. Gary may not be acting like a professional counselor at all. Competent counselors are skilled and knowledgeable of the core areas identified by the Council for Accreditation of Counseling and Related Educational Programs (CACREP), that is, professional orientation, career development, helping relationships, group work, assessment, and research (CACREP, 2009; Remley & Herlihy, 2014). Moreover, competent counselors are able to effectively use interview and research-based counseling techniques (Remley & Herlihy, 2014). While client attendance may offer some help in determining a counselor's competency, it is certainly not the sole factor.

Case Illustration 5-14 is another example of counselor competence and the importance of practicing within the boundaries of one's own competency. Review Case Illustration 5-14, and see how Krystal may be spreading herself too thin as she works to establish herself as a new licensed professional counselor.

CASE ILLUSTRATION 5-14

Krystal is a newly licensed counselor who has recently taken a job with a local counseling agency. Krystal is a contract counselor. During her orientation, her new boss explains how typically clients will call the main office and speak to a referral specialist. Once all the information is taken, the referral specialist will offer the case to any available counselors. Counselors are then able to choose which cases they wish to take based on their competency and specialty area. Therefore Krystal has the ability to choose her clientele.

Because she is new and trying to start off on the right foot in her new job, Krystal is quick to accept almost every case offered to her. She has clients who range in age from five to 65 years old and have various presenting concerns (i.e., a 14-year-old girl with an eating disorder, a newly married couple who is dealing with an upcoming military deployment, a six-year-old boy whose

(Continued)

(Continued)

father was recently murdered, and a 55-year-old woman who is addicted to pain pills). Krystal knows the only way she will make any money is to take cases, and she doesn't want to turn down too many for fear the referral specialist will stop offering her cases. Krystal has many school loans and a new car to pay for; she can't afford to have any slow weeks without clients.

After several weeks on the job, Krystal meets with her boss for some case consultation. After hearing the wide variety of clients, her supervisor expresses some concern that Krystal may be practicing outside the boundaries of her competence. Krystal disagrees and shares all of her training that qualifies her to work with such a diverse caseload. Krystal states that in addition to her required graduate course work, she took an elective course in grief and loss, one related to addictions, and one on working with military families. Additionally, at her state conference last year, she says she went to some educational sessions related to working with eating disorders. Krystal feels as though she is competent to take any cases dealing with those concerns, even though all of her graduate and postgraduate internship experience was done at a nursing home working with geriatric patients.

Is Krystal practicing within the boundaries of her competence?

What is the threshold for claiming to be "competent" in a certain area? A graduate course? Several graduate courses? Going to a conference? A certificate of achievement from a training?

Question 1 related to Case Illustration 5-14 asks if Krystal is practicing within the boundaries of her competence, and it is difficult to say for sure given the small amount of information given in the case. However, the question should be continually revisited by Krystal as she should continually be assessing her own competence and working toward providing the highest quality of services to her clients. If Krystal ever believes she may need additional training in one area or another, it is her responsibility to seek out such training prior to working with those populations.

The second question inquires as to the threshold for claiming competency in a given area. The authors believe it is more important for counselors to constantly challenge and evaluate their own skills rather than set a bar for competency. It is very difficult to set one standard for every situation because all counselors learn differently and gain varied knowledge from going to conferences, taking graduate courses, or attending trainings. Again, the authors recommend counselors practice self-awareness, openly acknowledge areas of weakness, and address those areas with the help of colleagues and supervisors.

Conclusion

Throughout Chapter 5 the authors discussed clients' rights and counselors' responsibilities. One of the most important rights clients have is the right to understand the counselor process and what they are getting themselves into when entering into a counseling relationship. Clients have the right to informed consent. Concomitantly, a primary duty for counselors is to provide informed consent to their clients. Counselors must also maintain appropriate records and always evaluate their own effectiveness. Take time to complete Exercise 5-1 as a way to apply the knowledge you have learned in this chapter.

EXERCISE 5-1

1. In this chapter, the authors discussed clients' rights and the right to informed consent. Work by yourself or with other classmates to develop an informed consent form you might like to use in your own practice.

2. The 2014 ACA Code of Ethics emphasizes the role of personal values in counseling. Briefly reflect on your own morals, values, and beliefs.

3. With which client populations might it be easier or more difficult for you to work?

4. Personal values are very powerful and ingrained in each and every one of us. How would you know if you were imposing your values onto your client?

5. The latter part of this chapter discussed the importance of counselors practicing within the boundaries of their own competency. Upon your graduation, with which types of client populations would you like to work? Do you feel you will be competent to work with that population? Why, or why not?

Keystones

- Clients have a right to informed consent at the onset of services.
- Counselors are responsible for providing informed consent to clients at the onset of services and also periodically throughout the counseling relationship.
- Informed consent must be delivered both verbally and in writing.
- Counselors are ethically required to work in conjunction with clients to develop treatment plans, and plans must be updated throughout the counseling relationship.
- Counselors must be sure client records are kept secure and not accessible to those who do not have the clients' written permission to review such records.
- Counselors must have written permission to audio or video record counseling sessions.
- Counselors must maintain self-awareness and continually assess their own competency and effectiveness.

Additional Resources

Barnett, J. E., Wise, E. H., Johnson-Greene, D., & Bucky, S. F. (2007). Informed consent: Too much of a good thing or not enough? *Professional Psychology: Research and Practice, 38*, 179–186.

Kuther, T. L. (2003). Medical decision-making and minors: Issues of consent and assent. *Adolescence, 38*(150), 343–58. Retrieved from http://search.proquest.com/docview/195942431?accountid=7122

Laschober, T. C., Eby, L. T. d. T., & Sauer, J. B. (2013). Effective clinical supervision in substance use disorder treatment programs and counselor job performance. *Journal of Mental Health Counseling, 35*(1), 76–94. Retrieved from http://search.proquest.com/docview/1269701242?accountid=7122

Ledyard, P. (1998). Counseling minors: Ethical and legal issues. *Counseling and Values, 42*, 171–177. doi:10.1002/j.2161-007X.1998.tb00423.x

Merlone, L. (2005). Record keeping and the school counselor. *Professional School Counseling, 8*(4), 372–376. Retrieved from http://www.jstor.org/stable/42732633

Mollen, D., Kelly, S. M., & Ridley, C. R. (2011). Therapeutic change: The raison d'être for counseling competence. *The Counseling Psychologist, 39*, 918–927. doi:10.1177/0011000011405221

Sperry, L. (2007). *The ethical and professional practice of counseling and psychotherapy*. New York: Pearson.

Tarvydas, V., Vazquez-Ramos, R., & Estrada-Hernandez, N. (2015). Applied participatory ethics: Bridging the social justice chasm between counselor and client. *Counseling and Values, 60*, 218–233. doi:10.1002/cvj.12015

Welfel, E. R. (2010). *Ethics in counseling & psychotherapy: Standards, research, and emerging issues*. Belmont, CA: Brooks/Cole.

Wiger, D. (2005). *The clinical documentation sourcebook: The complete paperwork resource for your mental health practice* (3rd ed.). Hoboken, NJ: Wiley.

References

American Association for Marriage and Family Therapy. (2015). *Code of ethics*. Retrieved from https://www.aamft.org/iMIS15/AAMFT/Content/legal_ethics/code_of_ethics.aspx

American Counseling Association. (2014). *Code of ethics*. Alexandria, VA: Author.

American Psychological Association. (2010). *American Psychological Association ethical principles of psychologists and code of conduct*. Retrieved from http://www.apa.org/ethics/code/principles.pdf

American School Counselor Association. (2010). *Ethical standards for school counselors*. Alexandria, VA: Author.

Council for Accreditation of Counseling and Related Education Programs. (2009). *CACREP accreditation standards and procedures manual*. Alexandria, VA: Author.

Fisher, C. B., & Oransky, M. (2008). Informed consent to psychotherapy: Protecting the dignity and respecting the autonomy of patients. *Journal of Clinical Psychology: In Session, 64*, 576–588.

Houser, R. A., & Thoma, S. (2013). *Ethics in counseling & therapy: Developing an ethical identity*. Thousand Oaks, CA: Sage.

Remley, T. P., & Herlihy, B. (2014). *Ethical, legal, and professional issues in counseling* (4th ed.). Upper Saddle River, NJ: Pearson.

6

Confidentiality and Privileged Communication

Don't ask yourself what the world needs; ask yourself what makes you come alive. And then go and do that. Because what the world needs is people who have come alive.

—Harold Whitman

Chapter 6 discusses confidentiality, privacy, and privileged communication. All three concepts concern the information counselors share with individuals outside the immediate counselor/client relationship. Confidentiality typically concerns the information clients share with counselors (e.g., the counselor will keep the conversation confidential). The term "privacy" is typically used when discussing the overall counseling relationship (e.g., If I see a client in public, I will usually wait for them to approach me first before I acknowledge I know them. I do this to respect his/her privacy). Last, privileged communication is very similar to confidentiality. However, the term "privileged communication" is typically only used in legal proceedings (e.g., My client asked me to claim privilege on his/her behavior during a divorce proceeding. They did not want me to share confidential information we had discussed during session). All three concepts will be discussed in greater detail. At the conclusion of Chapter 6 readers will specifically be able to do the following:

1. Name the differences between privacy, confidentiality, and privileged communication.

2. Explain the limitations of confidentiality.

3. Discuss the influence counselors' values have on their interpretation of "clear and foreseeable harm" and other limitations to confidentiality.

4. Define limits of confidentiality when working with clients experiencing end-of-life decisions.

5. Explain ethical responsibilities when working with clients who disclose they have a contagious and life-threatening disease.

6. Explain the ethical responsibilities associated with and how to respond to a subpoena.

7. Explain ethical responsibilities related to mandatory reporting.

Confidentiality

Confidentiality is a hallmark of professional counseling. Corey, Corey, and Callanan (2011) describe it as the "central right of a client" (p. 210). Confidentiality ensures what clients say will be held in confidence. Without it, clients may be hesitant to discuss intimate concerns (Ford, 2006). Simply stated, confidentiality means the counselor, both ethically and legally, is not allowed to share information provided by the client. On the contrary, the client is free to share any and all information with whomever they choose (with the exception of group counseling settings, which will be discussed further in Chapter 10). The APA and AAMFT have specific standards regarding confidentiality—see Text Box 6-1.

TEXT BOX 6-1

While the ACA is very specific regarding limits of confidentiality and when counselors are either obligated or have the option of notifying others of confidential information, the APA and AAMFT are less specific in their respective guidelines.

American Psychological Association

The APA discusses limits to confidentiality primarily in two standards, first, in Standard 4.01 (Maintaining Confidentiality); however, rather than giving specific direction, the APA directs psychologists to follow laws or institutional policies. Second, limits to confidentiality are discussed in Standard 4.05.

APA Standard 4.01 (2010) Maintaining Confidentiality: Psychologists have a primary obligation and take reasonable precautions to protect confidential information obtained through or stored in any medium, recognizing that the extent and limits of confidentiality may be regulated by law or established by institutional rules or professional or scientific relationship.

APA Standard 4.05 (2010) Disclosures: (a) Psychologists may disclose confidential information with the appropriate consent of the organizational client, the individual client or patient, or another legally authorized person on behalf of the client or patient unless prohibited by law. (b) Psychologists disclose confidential information without the consent of the individual only as mandated by law or where permitted by law for a valid purpose such as to (1) provide needed professional services; (2) obtain appropriate professional consultations; (3) protect the client, patient, psychologist, or others from harm; or (4) obtain payment for services from a client or patient in which instance disclosure is limited to the minimum that is necessary to achieve the purpose).

American Association of Marriage and Family Therapists

The AAMFT is vague in describing limitations to confidentiality. The only place it is addressed is in Standard 2.1 (Disclosing Limits of Confidentiality). Still, Standard 2.1 does not provide any detail regarding what those limits might be.

AAMFT 2.1 (2015) Disclosing Limits of Confidentiality: Marriage and family therapists disclose to clients and other interested parties at the outset of services the nature of confidentiality and possible limitations of the clients' right to confidentiality. Therapists review with clients the circumstances where confidential information may be requested and where disclosure of confidential information may be legally required. Circumstances may necessitate repeated disclosures.

While confidentiality protects clients from unauthorized disclosures, it is not absolute. In most cases, a counselor must have written consent from his/her client prior to disclosing information to an outside party. However, there are exceptions to confidentiality in which the counselor *may* choose to break or is *required* to break confidentiality and disclose information to outside parties. The following are exceptions to confidentiality.

Duty to Protect

ACA Standard B.2.a. (2014) Serious and Foreseeable Harm and Legal Requirements: The general requirement that counselors keep information confidential does not apply when disclosure is required to protect clients or identified others from serious and foreseeable harm or when legal requirements demand that confidential information must be revealed. Counselors consult with other professionals when in doubt as to the validity of an exception. Additional considerations apply when addressing end-of-life issues.

The requirement to keep information confidential does not apply when disclosure would prevent serious and foreseeable harm to the client or others (ACA, 2014, B.2.a.). This standard, also commonly known as "duty to protect" may come across as fairly straightforward (i.e., if a client reports harming him/herself or the desire to hurt another person, the counselor is required to intervene and notify police, parents, or another outside entity), but like many other standards, there is some gray area and interpretation left up to the counselor. Consider Case Illustration 6-1 and how Rick interprets Standard B.2.a.

CASE ILLUSTRATION 6-1

Rick is a counselor meeting with Jeremiah for the first time today. Jeremiah is a 24-year-old male who claims to need to talk to someone about issues he has been having. During the course of the session, Jeremiah mentions that he believes he has an anger control problem and he would like to work on controlling it. Jeremiah discloses that about three weeks prior to today's session, he became incredibly agitated when he found out his girlfriend was cheating on him. Jeremiah claims to have lost his temper, tying his girlfriend up, cutting her on both her legs and shoulders, and then throwing her in a shallow creek by his house. Jeremiah feels some remorse but still believes she had what was coming to her.

After the session, Rick calls the local police and reports what Jeremiah had told him during session. Rick bases his decision on Section B.2.a. of the ACA Code of Ethics (Serious and Foreseeable Harm). Rick's rationale for breaching confidentiality is that he feels Jeremiah is a danger to society. If he assaulted someone like this once, he will do it again. He says, "A tiger can't change his stripes."

Did Rick act in an ethical manner and interpret Standard B.2.a. appropriately?

In Case Illustration 6-1, there may be arguments to be made for either keeping information confidential or breaking confidentiality and reporting to an outside authority. Depending on the counselor's morals, values, beliefs, and previous life experiences, he/she may come to different conclusions as to what constitutes serious and foreseeable harm and thus what his/her next step should be. In Case Illustration 6-1, Rick's actions most likely would be considered unethical. Standard B.2.a. requires counselors to break confidentiality for "clear" and "foreseeable" harm. The behavior Rick reported to the police was one that happened in the past, not one which will clearly happen in the future. Rick has strong beliefs about the possibility of Jeremiah hurting someone in the future; however, Jeremiah did not indicate in any way that he was going to hurt another person or whom he would hurt.

Continuing with Case Illustration 6-1, a closer look at Rick reveals personal values including a strong belief against violence of any kind. Additionally, two years previously, while jogging he was assaulted by a man who had a history of violent behaviors. Those beliefs and experiences may have likely influenced his interpretation of serious and foreseeable harm. On the contrary, if Rick had a close family member with a violent temper or history of criminal behaviors and that family member was making positive changes in his/her life, or Rick did not have the experience of being assaulted, he may interpret serious and foreseeable harm differently.

In previous chapters the authors discussed the importance of counselor self-awareness and knowing and taking responsibility for one's own personal values. In the following scenarios, decide whether you believe a counselor should break confidentiality and notify a third party (i.e., a duty to protect the client).

CASE ILLUSTRATION 6-2

A 19-year-old male client discloses to his clinical mental health counselor that he goes out on weekends to attend parties and drink with friends. While he claims to not drink "too much," he does admit to drinking to the point of passing out on several occasions.

A 14-year-old male student discloses to his school counselor that he has shoplifted clothing and shoes from a local department store on numerous occasions and even shows off the new shoes he is wearing, claiming to have stolen them the previous weekend.

A 35-year-old female client discloses to her clinical mental health counselor that she is tired of living with HIV and is going to discontinue taking any and all medications.

A 17-year-old female client discloses to her clinical mental health counselor that she is sexually active with multiple partners. She further explains that she is actively trying to get pregnant and refuses to use any type of contraception.

A 15-year-old female student discloses to her school counselor that she routinely makes cuts on her upper arm to alleviate stress and anxiety.

An 11-year-old male shares with his clinical mental health counselor that he sometimes sneaks out of his house in the middle of the night to ride his bicycle around the neighborhood where he lives. He says he likes to look at the moon and stars.

Do any of the above scenarios qualify as "clear and foreseeable harm," requiring the counselor to break confidentiality and disclose information to an outside party?

Consider morals, values, beliefs, and life experiences and how they might influence a counselor's interpretation.

The first question of Case Illustration 6-2 asks if any of the scenarios qualify as "clear and foreseeable harm." All of these examples again involve gray areas in which counselors must interpret the meaning of "clear and foreseeable harm." Depending on the counselor's values and life experiences, he/she may interpret the standard in different ways. It is the author's opinion that none of the situations presented in Case Illustration 6-2 (given only the information provided in the case illustration) substantiate breaking confidentiality and notifying an outside party. In a real session, the counselor would want to explore each of the situations more and determine if additional information presented would reach the threshold of "clear and foreseeable harm" and require a disclosure.

The second question asks how morals, values, and beliefs may affect a counselor's interpretation of Standard B.2.a. Consider the first example, in which a 19-year-old client reports drinking heavily. A counselor may have strong beliefs about the importance of following the law and being 21 before having the maturity to handle alcohol. Another counselor may have had a friend or family member recently injured or killed in an alcohol-related incident. In both cases, those counselors may tend to have stronger beliefs about the danger associated with excessive drinking. A counselor who considers him/herself a "social drinker" and drinks excessively on weekends with friends may be less likely to have the same views about the dangers of excessive drinking.

Another scenario presented in Case Illustration 6-2 presents a 14-year-old boy who steals clothing from department stores. The boy even shows off his stolen shoes from a recent "shopping trip." Some counselors may have stronger beliefs and views about the dangers associated with theft than others. For example, one counselor may determine clear and foreseeable harm exists (and a duty to inform the client's parents) because the 14-year-old is certain to eventually get caught and have to answer for his crimes and the punishment and a criminal history would "harm" his chances for pursuing a successful career. On the contrary, a different counselor would see the behaviors as clearly against the law but not make the same conclusions about breaking the law constituting "clear and foreseeable harm."

The examples given in Case Illustration 6-2 exemplify the importance of using an ethical decision-making model when determining whether to break confidentiality and disclose information. Also discussed in Chapter 3 was the importance of process and being thorough when using a decision-making model. Related to the situations in Case Illustration 6-2, counselors must be careful to be thorough in understanding their own values related to alcohol use or binge drinking, multiple relationships, risky sexual behaviors, self-injurious behaviors, shoplifting, and so on. Again, as discussed in previous chapters, counselors must be self-aware and separate their own values and beliefs from the values of the counseling profession.

Duty to Warn

Duty to warn is also associated with Standard B.2.a. (Serious and Foreseeable Harm and Legal Requirements). In the previous paragraphs, the authors primarily discussed counselors' obligations when clients were themselves in clear and foreseeable harm. The second part of Standard B.2.a. requires counselors to protect "identified others from clear and foreseeable harm" as well. When clients make threats to harm others, counselors have a duty to break confidentiality and notify proper individuals or authorities (i.e., law enforcement). In such cases where there is an identified victim, counselors may not only have a duty to notify law enforcement but also the intended victim (*Tarasoff v. Regents of University of California*, 1976). However, this duty to warn does not exist in all states. In some states (Texas and Ohio), duty to warn is either not recognized, or the law requires counselors to respond to threats in different ways. Consider Case Illustration 6-3 as an example of duty to warn.

CASE ILLUSTRATION 6-3

A licensed professional counselor, Joan, is working with Diane, who is a 39-year-old female who originally sought a counselor to work through some relationship problems she has been having. At today's session, Diane comes in and is extremely agitated. She spends the first half of the session talking about her recent breakup with her boyfriend and how betrayed she feels because her boyfriend "dumped her to hook up with her back-stabbing best friend." Diane continues to talk about the betrayal she feels from both her boyfriend and her friend, whom she has known for more than 10 years. Toward the end of the session, Diane begins to disclose her plan to "take out" both her friend and her now ex-boyfriend. Diane says she has a gun and knows where her friend lives. Diana plans to wait in the parking lot of her friend's apartment and shoot both her friend and her ex-boyfriend this Sunday when they return home from a weekend trip.

What are Joan's ethical and legal obligations in this situation?

In response to the question in Case Illustration 6-3, Joan has an ethical obligation to notify the proper authorities about Diane's plans according to Standard B.2.a. In fulfilling her obligation, Joan would likely want to call her local police department and explain who she was and Diane's plans. After making the report, Joan would want to be certain to document her actions thoroughly. Joan's legal obligations would depend upon the state in which she lives. If Joan lived in Texas, she would not be legally required to contact the intended victims. In fact, if Joan lived in Texas, she would be breaking the law if she were to notify the intended victims. On the contrary, if Joan lived in California, she would be legally required to notify both intended victims if she had the ability to do so. Professional counselors are encouraged to know and have working knowledge and understanding of their specific state laws regarding duty to warn.

End-of-Life Decisions

ACA Standard B.2.b. (2014) Confidentiality Regarding End-of-Life Decisions: Counselors who provide services to terminally ill individuals who are considering hastening their own deaths have the option to maintain confidentiality, depending on the applicable laws and the specific circumstances of the situation and after seeking consultation or supervision from appropriate professional and legal parties.

"Counselors who provide services to terminally ill individuals who are considering hastening their own deaths have the option to maintain confidentiality" (ACA, 2014, p. 7). Standard B.2.b. continues by directing counselors to base their decision (whether to break confidentiality) on state and federal laws, consultation with other professionals, and the circumstances of the situation. Keeping this in mind, consider Case Illustration 6-4.

CASE ILLUSTRATION 6-4

George, a 23-year-old male, has been seeing his counselor Karen since being diagnosed with terminal cancer. George and Karen have a strong relationship, and George feels as though Karen is one of the few people in his life who will listen to his concerns rather than tell him what he should or should not do. Karen takes her job as a professional counselor very seriously and, since meeting George, has spent a significant amount of time researching cancer and available treatment options. Recently, Karen has stumbled on some new research showing great promise in treating George's specific type of cancer. Karen thinks it may be helpful to George but is hesitant to share it with him because she doesn't want to come across as "giving advice" or "imposing her own agenda." Karen also knows George has been through many clinical trials since his diagnosis and has commented several times about his lack of interest in trying any more of them.

At today's session, George mentions he has some pretty important things to discuss. He discloses that over the last couple of weeks his pain has become more and more unbearable. George says he has done a great deal of thinking and praying and has reached a decision to end all this pain and speed up his inevitable death. He then goes on to describe his plans to overdose on his sleeping pills this weekend when he gets home from visiting with some friends and family. He doesn't want to tell his parents or friends because he doesn't want them to worry about it or try to change his mind. George talks in detail about his journey in making the decision to hasten his own death. It is clear to Karen that George has put a great deal of thought into his decision.

As the session comes to a close, George expresses his extreme gratitude to Karen for all her help and support. After George leaves, Karen reflects on her session with George and wonders about her ethical and legal obligations. She wonders if she has any obligation to report George's plans to end his life.

Does Karen have an ethical responsibility to break confidentiality and share George's plans?

If so, with whom should she share the information?

In Case Illustration 6-4, Karen has a client who openly shares his plans to end his own life. Karen's client, George, is adamant about overdosing on sleeping pills when he returns from a trip to visit with his family and friends. Knowing this information, Karen must determine how to act and whether she will break confidentiality and share the information with a third party. In the absence of any specific laws in her state, Karen is left with the option of whether she will break confidentiality and notify an outside party of George's plans. After consulting a legal expert and consulting with colleagues, Karen would also want to consult the ACA Code of Ethics (2014) and review Standard B.2.b. related to end-of-life decisions. In doing so, Karen would see she has the option to break or maintain confidentiality (i.e., counselors who provide services to terminally ill individuals who are considering hastening their own deaths have the option to maintain confidentiality).

In deciding how to act, Karen would want to be sure to separate her own values and beliefs and determine what might be in George's best interest. For example, depending on Karen's own views about death, dying, and assisted suicide, she may feel more strongly about one action or another. Karen would need to consider all possible options and the benefits and consequences of each choice. In situations such as the one presented in Case Illustration 6-4, counselors may be tempted to make judgments about what is "right" and what is "wrong" based on the counselor's own morals, values, and beliefs. For example, Karen might have thoughts or make statements such as these:

Taking sleeping pills and killing yourself is wrong.

It's not right for George to kill himself; his family will be devastated.

You just can't do that; it's just not right.

The counselor's job is not to determine what is right or wrong. It is the counselor's job to listen and understand the client and to promote his/her autonomy and welfare. However Karen decides, she must ultimately choose how to act, implement her choice, and document the process.

Contagious, Life-Threatening Diseases

ACA Standard B.2.c. (2014) Contagious, Life-Threatening Diseases: When clients disclose that they have a disease commonly known to be both communicable and life threatening, counselors may be justified in disclosing information to identifiable third parties, if the parties are known to be at serious and foreseeable risk of contracting the disease. Prior to making a disclosure, counselors assess the intent of clients to inform the third parties about their disease or to engage in any behaviors that may be harmful to an identifiable third party. Counselors adhere to relevant state laws concerning disclosure about disease status.

Similar to the standards discussed previously, when working with clients who have a contagious, life-threatening disease, counselors are left with a choice to either keep information confidential or share with identifiable third parties. Before making the determination, professional counselors are also encouraged to assess whether the client intends to tell the identified third party on his/her own. Professional counselors are also directed to follow all pertinent state laws. Consider Case Illustration 6-5 related to Standard B.2.c.

CASE ILLUSTRATION 6-5

Client: Since I received my test results a few weeks ago and found out I'm HIV+, I have been living life to the fullest and partying every night.

Counselor: What do you mean "living life to the fullest"?

(Continued)

(Continued)

Client: Going out, partying, drinking, just doing whatever with whoever.

Counselor: Are you being careful? I mean, you don't want to give this to anyone else, do you?

Client: To be honest, I don't even care. The person who gave it to me didn't care enough about me to say something, so why should I care about anyone else?

Counselor: Don't you think it's the right thing to do? If you don't want to tell them yourself, maybe we could talk to them together?

Client: No.

Counselor: Well then give me a list of their names so that I can let them know. You can't do this to people.

Did the counselor act in an ethical manner?

Case Illustration 6-5 involves a client and counselor who clearly have different values and beliefs about a person's obligation to share his/her medical history with those with whom they are sexually active. Based on the short interaction, the counselor would most likely be seen as acting in an unethical manner. The counselor clearly has some strong values related to sexually transmitted diseases and is imposing those values onto his/her client by badgering and pleading with the client to produce a list of names of the people with whom he/she was sexually active. Standard B.2.c. states counselors "may be justified in disclosing information to identifiable third parties," assuming there is an identified third party. Standard B.2.c. does not give permission for counselors to persuade, coax, or guilt clients into providing contact information of identifiable third parties. Case illustration 6-5 is another example of how counselor values may be imposed onto clients.

Case Illustration 6-5 involves a client who is known to be HIV+ and is hesitant to reveal information that would allow the counselor to disclose the diagnosis to an at-risk third party. Professional counselors may also encounter situations where there is risk-taking behavior but no confirmed diagnosis or disclosure of a diagnosis. Consider Case Illustration 6-6, also related to Standard B.2.c. (Contagious Life-Threatening Diseases).

CASE ILLUSTRATION 6-6

Connie and Linda have been meeting with a couple's counselor for about six months to work on some of their communication issues. They have been thinking about adopting a child for some time and want to make sure they have all their issues worked out before bringing a child into their family. Last week, Connie approached her couple's counselor about getting some individual counseling to work on her own issues a little more. Connie's couple's counselor referred her to Paul. During the first session with Paul, Connie revealed she has been incredibly anxious lately. She wants Paul to help her find some coping strategies to handle her anxiety and maybe even a referral to a psychiatrist for medication. As Paul discusses the situation further, Connie discloses that she has cheated on her partner Linda several times over the past three years and is worried Linda may find out and leave her. Complicating things more, one of Connie and Linda's mutual friends, and someone Connie had a brief affair with, posted on a social media outlet that she was recently diagnosed as HIV+. Even though the friend has contacted Connie to encourage her to get tested, Connie has no interest and believes that if she gets tested, it will only let out the secret she cheated on Linda. Connie says, "Those affairs are in the past and need to stay in the past. If Linda ever found out about them, she would leave me, which would absolutely destroy my life."

After finishing the session with Connie, Paul finds himself to be concerned for Connie's partner (Linda) and her health. After reflecting on the session for a few minutes he reviews his ACA Code of Ethics, reads Standard B.2.c. related to contagious and life-threatening diseases, and determines it important to notify Linda about the possible danger as he feels Connie will not tell Linda herself. Specifically, Paul rationalizes his decision based on one part of Standard B.2.c. (i.e., Counselors may be justified in disclosing information to identifiable third parties, if the parties are known to be at serious and foreseeable risk of contracting the disease. Prior to making a disclosure, counselors assess the intent of clients to inform the third parties about their disease or to engage in any behaviors that may be harmful to an identifiable third party).

Is Paul acting ethically by notifying Linda of the potential danger?

In Case Illustration 6-6, Connie is currently in a committed relationship and may pursue adopting a child in the near future. She has cheated on her partner several times over the past few years and has recently been made aware one of her past affairs is HIV+. The section of the ACA Code of Ethics most relevant here (B.2.c.) states that counselors may be justified in disclosing information when the client discloses that they have a disease. In this situation, Connie has not disclosed she has a contagious, life-threatening disease. However, she has disclosed that she has been sexually active with someone who has tested positive for such a disease. Complicating the situation, Connie refuses to get tested herself for fear of losing the relationship with her partner.

The question in Case Illustration 6-6 asks whether Paul acted ethically by notifying Linda about his client's possible disease. The answer is no; he did not act in an ethical manner. Paul read Ethical Standard B.2.c. and picked out the section supporting the action he wanted to take rather than considering the entire standard. In doing so, Paul showed a lack of self-awareness and understanding of his own values. If Paul were more self-aware, he would have understood his strong beliefs related to this situation and been cautious to avoid allowing his own values to guide his decision. Paul overlooked the fact Connie did not disclose she had a contagious, life threatening disease. Thus, Paul had no ethical backing to break confidentiality.

Court-Ordered Disclosures

ACA Standard B.2.d. (2014) Court-Ordered Disclosure: When ordered by a court to release confidential or privileged information without a client's permission, counselors seek to obtain written, informed consent from the client or take steps to prohibit the disclosure or have it limited as narrowly as possible because of potential harm to the client or counseling relationship.

The majority of professional counselors will be subpoenaed at some point in their career. Case Illustration 6-7 presents a situation in which Tommy, a professional counselor, is served with a subpoena. Review the example, and consider how you might act if you were in the same situation.

CASE ILLUSTRATION 6-7

Tommy, a professional counselor with more than 10 years of experience, was surprised when a peace officer showed up at his office today to deliver a subpoena. The subpoena directed Tommy to appear in court on a specific day to testify on issues related to one of his current clients and provide copies of all case notes related to the topic.

What should Tommy do?

Should Tommy tell his client about the subpoena?

Does Tommy need written permission from his client to share information?

Question 1 in Case Illustration 6-7 asks what Tommy should do about the subpoena. When this occurs, the authors suggest first contacting an attorney or legal advisor. If counselors don't have a private legal consultant, several professional counseling associations offer free legal care and advice to their membership. Contacting an attorney may be beneficial in a number of ways (i.e. determining the legitimacy of the subpoena, advisement as to the steps to take in responding to the subpoena, and what to expect throughout the process). It may also be helpful for counselors to be aware of state statutes related to confidentiality and privilege. Nonetheless, as discussed in Chapter 3, professional counselors are expected to be experts in mental health and counseling, not law.

The second question asks if Tommy should talk to his client about the subpoena. Yes, as a professional counselor, your primary responsibility is to your client. Always include the client in the process. Even if your client is not in favor of you disclosing information or sharing your documents, it is beneficial to the counseling relationship to discuss the matter and your ethical and legal responsibilities as a professional counselor.

Finally, the third question inquires about consent to release information and whether Tommy needs his client's permission to share information—yes and no. Getting a client's written consent is always the ideal; however, sometimes it is not absolutely necessary. In the case of a subpoena, you may be asked to share information even if your client does not sign a written consent. Contacting an attorney or other legal professional is a counselor's best option in understanding the specific legal requirements when issued a subpoena.

Sharing Information With Subordinates, Interdisciplinary Teams, and Third-Party Payers

ACA Standard B.3.a. (2014) Subordinates: Counselors make every effort to ensure that privacy and confidentiality of clients are maintained by subordinates, including employees, supervisees, students, clerical assistants, and volunteers.

Oftentimes professional counselors hold supervisory positions in private practice, agency, school, hospital, or other settings. In such cases, counselors are responsible for their subordinates and making sure they uphold client confidentiality. Consider Case Illustration 6-8 in which the counselor, Jacey, must deal with a mistake made by of one of her subordinates.

CASE ILLUSTRATION 6-8

Jacey, an experienced counselor, owns her own practice and has an office assistant she has hired to help with answering phones, filing, and insurance billing. Today, Jacey's assistant leaves early because she is not feeling well. So she won't fall behind on her work, the office assistant decides to take some client files and other billing materials home with her, even though it is against agency policy. In her rush to get out the door and in her car, the office assistant accidentally drops a treatment plan and some other case notes in the parking lot. Later in the same day, Jacey finds out about the dropped documents because her afternoon client brings them in and says she thinks someone dropped them.

Who is responsible for the dropped documents and breach of confidentiality?

Can Jacey be held accountable, even though she wasn't the one who made the mistake?

In Case Illustration 6-8, Jacey's administrative assistant makes an unfortunate mistake as she is rushing out to her car. The administrative assistant is the one who dropped the documents, but both the assistant and Jacey are responsible for the breach of confidentiality. If there were to be a complaint made about the breach of confidentiality, Jacey would be the one who would ultimately be held responsible. Ultimately the counselor is the responsible party and is the one who will be held accountable for any unethical behaviors.

ACA Standard B.3.b. (2014) Interdisciplinary Teams: When services provided to the client involve participation by an interdisciplinary or treatment team, the client will be informed of the team's existence and composition, information being shared, and the purposes of sharing such information.

Interdisciplinary teams are common in many settings in which counselors work (e.g., behaviors hospitals, community clinics, residential settings, etc.). When professional counselors provide services as part of an interdisciplinary team, they are responsible for informing the client of the existence of the team, the information to be shared, and the purpose of sharing information (ACA, 2014, B.3.b.). See Case Illustration 6-9 as an example of how Bill incorporates the requirements of ACA Standard B.3.b. into his daily work with his client Mr. Brown.

CASE ILLUSTRATION 6-9

Bill is a professional counselor and works at an inpatient hospital primarily with adults who are dealing with serious addictions. Today he is going to meet with Mr. Brown for the first time. In addition to going over informed consent, Bill includes some additional information related to the treatment team at the facility. As he walks into the room, Bill introduces himself and says, "Hi, Mr. Brown. My name is Bill, and I wanted to come by and meet with you today and see how I might be able to be helpful to you. I'm a professional counselor here at the hospital and work with several other people (whom you might have already met). The job of this treatment team is to make sure we provide the best services for you while you're here at the facility. In addition to me, the other members of your treatment team include a psychiatrist, social worker, and physician. Because I am only one part of your whole treatment team, there is some information about our sessions I will share with the other members. The information I commonly share includes your treatment plan, goals for treatment, and other observations such as your general mood and temperament. The main reason for sharing information among the team is so we can all be up-to-date related to your condition. Additionally, it may also be beneficial to you as you will not have to repeat yourself every time a different member of the team meets with you. Do have any questions about this?"

In Case Illustration 6-9, Bill fulfills the requirements of ACA Standard B.3.b. by letting his client know about the treatment team on which he works. Bill informs his client about other members of the treatment team, the purpose of sharing information, and the types of information he generally shares with the team. Additionally, Bill asks his client for any questions. In doing so, Bill is engaging his client in the process and being transparent about the services he provides.

ACA Standard B.3.d. (2014) Third-Party Payers: Counselors disclose information to third-party payers only when clients have authorized such disclosure.

When working with insurance agencies or other third-party payers, counselors are required to obtain the client's permission prior to disclosing any confidential information.

Considerations

In all case illustrations presented throughout the first part of this chapter, professional counselors are either required or have the option to disclose confidential information. When the decision is made to break absolute confidentiality and share information, counselors must then decide *what* they will share and *how* they are going to share it. For the most part, professional counselors will be either sending or sharing documents or having personal conversations with those to whom they are disclosing information. Whatever the situation, "counselors take precautions to ensure the confidentiality of all information transmitted through the use of any medium" (ACA, 2014, p. 7). If professional counselors choose to have a personal conversation, they are sure to discuss confidential information "only in settings in which they can reasonably ensure client privacy" (ACA, 2014, p. 7). Finally, when disclosing information, "only essential information is revealed" (ACA, 2014, p. 14). Consider Case Illustration 6-10 in which two graduate students, Zach and William, use their break time to consult over cases.

CASE ILLUSTRATION 6-10

Zach and William are counseling graduate students currently working at the University Counseling Center during their internship semester. Because they both have a break in scheduling from 12 to 2 p.m. every afternoon, the two friends typically walk over to the student center to have lunch. They also use their lunchtime to consult on cases. Even though there are many people around in the lunch area, the two believe it is safe to talk as they only use client first names and "nobody is paying attention to them anyway."

Upon returning to the clinic one afternoon, they are both asked to meet with their supervisor to discuss some concerns voiced by a client. During the meeting Zach and William's supervisor indicates a long-time client voiced some concerns about student counselors talking about clients in the cafeteria area. The supervisor further explained how the client who voiced the concerns typically has lunch at the university cafeteria each week prior to walking over to the clinic for his session. The client was very upset when he heard the two counselors sitting and talking about clients in such an open area.

Did Zach and William act in an unethical manner?

In Case Illustration 6-10, Zach and William spend time during their lunch break consulting about cases and feel as though they are safe talking about their clients because they only use first names and they believe no one is paying attention to them anyway. Zach and William would most likely be seen as acting unethically according to ACA Standard B.3.c. (Confidential Settings). Counselors are to discuss confidential information only when there is some assurance of confidentiality (ACA, 2014). Even though the two only used first names, it was clear to others in the area (and especially to the client who heard them) that they were talking about clients.

Confidentiality Versus Privacy

Confidentiality and privacy may sound like similar constructs but, in fact, have some distinct differences. Confidentiality is the obligation of professional counselors to respect the privacy of clients and the information they provide. On the contrary, privacy is the client's right to keep the counseling relationship a secret. Professional counselors should monitor their behaviors in and out of the office setting to ensure they do not invade their clients' privacy (Corey, Corey, & Callanan, 2011). Privacy involves not only the communications between counselor and client, but also the storage and disposal of records.

Storage and Disposal of Records

ACA Standard B.6.h. (2014) Storage and Disposal After Termination: Counselors store records following termination of services to ensure reasonable future access, maintain records in accordance with federal and state laws and statutes such as licensure laws and policies governing records, and dispose of client records and other sensitive materials in a manner that protects client confidentiality. Counselors apply careful discretion and deliberation before destroying records that may be needed by a court of law, such as notes on child abuse, suicide, sexual harassment, or violence.

According to Standard B.6.h. counselors must abide by all "federal and state laws governing records, and dispose of client records and other sensitive materials in a manner that protects client confidentiality" (ACA, 2014, p. 8). Doing so usually involves shredding materials (either by hand or by using a service) rather than simply throwing them in a trash dumpster.

Waiting Rooms

Waiting rooms often pose a problem when thinking about client privacy. In school and agency settings, there may be multiple counselors working from the same office and only one waiting room. At any time there may be multiple individuals waiting for their appointments in the same waiting room and therefore no assurance of absolute privacy (e.g., Two neighbors may both have appointments at the same counseling agency at the same time and on the same day unbeknownst to each other. If they see each other in the same waiting room, the privacy of each person's counseling involvement is broken). Counselors working as independent practitioners or in private practice may have more control in protecting client privacy.

Either way, the authors recommend spacing client appointments appropriately to allot time so clients leaving session do not interact with clients arriving for sessions, thus protecting the privacy of clients' counseling involvement.

Credit Card Billing

Credit cards offer a convenient alternative to paying with cash or checks, but counselors who accept credit cards must pay special attentional to protecting their clients' privacy. Consider Case Illustration 6-11 in which Jake uses his parents' credit card to pay for his counseling sessions.

CASE ILLUSTRATION 6-11

Jake, a 19-year-old male, arrives at his counseling session today and is upset at his counselor. He accuses his counselor of being negligent in protecting the privacy of his counseling involvement. Jake claims earlier in the week his parents confronted him and asked why he felt the need to see a counselor. When Jake asked how they knew, his parents said they were reviewing their credit card bill and noticed a charge from Mike's Counseling Agency. In response to Jake, the counselor informed Jake that if he doesn't want his parents to know about his counseling, then he shouldn't use their credit card. Instead he should pay in cash or use another method of payment.

What could Mike have done to avoid this situation with Jake?

Case Illustration 6-11 provides an example of the importance of being thorough during the informed consent process. The counselor, Mike, could have avoided this uncomfortable encounter if he were more thorough during his informed consent. For example, when Mike reviewed his policy regarding payment of fees, he might have quickly reviewed how his agency's billing might appear on credit card bills. Doing so would have given Jake necessary information to make an informed decision about how he would like to pay for services. By responding the way he did in Case Illustration 6-11, Mike is likely hurting the rapport he has built with Jake and ultimately negatively affecting the counseling relationship.

Phone Calls

Phone calls between professional counselors and clients are necessary for a number of reasons (e.g., scheduling and confirming appointment times); however, to avoid unintentionally invading clients' privacy, there is certain information the authors recommend reviewing during the informed consent process.

In the event the counselor needs to contact the client by phone, which is the preferred phone number to use?

If there is no answer when the counselor calls the client and the counselor is given the option to leave a message, would the client prefer the counselor leave a message or not?

If the client would like the counselor to leave a message, given the option, how would the client like the counselor to identify him/herself in the message?

Public Encounters

Depending on where professional counselors live and work, they may be more or less likely to encounter clients outside of session (i.e., counselors working in smaller communities may be more likely to encounter clients in their daily activities than those living in larger communities). Similar to the previous section concerning phone calls, it is critical counselors monitor their behaviors so as not to unintentionally invade a client's privacy. Consider Case Illustration 6-12 and how Robin responds when she encounters one of her clients at the gym.

CASE ILLUSTRATION 6-12

Robin, a professional counselor, owns her own practice and typically schedules all her appointments after lunch and in the early evenings because she enjoys going to the gym to exercise in the mornings. Robin has been a member of her gym for quite some time and has many friends (both professional and personal) who work out at the same gym. Today, while on the treadmill, Robin notices one of her clients is there at the gym at the same time. Robin feels a bit awkward and wonders if she should go over and say hi to her client or if she should try to avoid her client noticing her, leave, and change her workout schedule.

What should Robin do in this situation? (Go say hi to her client? Act like she doesn't see her? Leave immediately? Something else?)

What are the possible consequences of Robin's actions?

How could Robin have avoided this awkward situation?

In response to the first question in Case Illustration 6-12, there is not a clear-cut answer as to what Robin should do. However, in deciding what she might do, Robin would certainly want to use an ethical decision-making model and determine what might be in the best interest of the client.

In response to Question 2 there may be many consequences of Robin's choice of how to handle the situation, some of which may positively affect her relationship with her client and some which may negatively affect the relationship. For example, if Robin goes over to say hi and her action is unwelcome from her client, then it may negatively affect the counseling relationship. Conversely, if Robin decides to not say hi and avoid her client, the client may feel a bit rejected, thus negatively affecting the counseling relationship. Regardless of her response to either quickly leave or go over and quietly say hello to her client, it is unlikely Robin would face any type of ethical complaint from a licensure board. If Robin's actions are viewed negatively by her client, the most likely consequence would be a damaged relationship.

This potentially awkward situation could be avoided if Robin were to add situations like these to the informed consent process. For example, while discussing confidentiality Robin could say to her clients, "Given that this is a relatively small community, there is potential for us to encounter each other outside of the office setting. If we do end up meeting someplace outside of a counseling session, what would be most comfortable for you? I don't want you to feel as though I am being rude and ignoring you if I don't come over to say 'Hi.' However, I also don't want to invade your privacy if you would prefer I don't say 'Hi' or acknowledge I know you in public. What would be best for you?" By having the conversation at the onset of services, Robin would be able to know her client's wishes and thus avoid the situation of having to guess as to what would be the best course of action.

Mandatory Reporting (Protecting Children and Vulnerable Adults)

When professional counselors suspect a child or vulnerable adult is being abused or neglected, they are ethically and legally mandated to report their suspicions to the proper authorities (ACA, 2014; Child Abuse Prevention and Treatment Act, 1974). The previous statements may be seen as common knowledge to most graduate students (especially those pursuing a counseling degree). In situations in which the abuse is clearly identifiable, the authors believe counselors are more confident in their reporting. However, in situations in which the abuse is not as clear, counselors may question their actions more. Consider Case Illustration 6-13 in which Bailey, a school counselor, must determine whether to make a report.

CASE ILLUSTRATION 6-13

Bailey is a school counselor at a local middle school. Today he is meeting with Justin, a sixth grader, after Justin's teacher referred him to the counselor's office. As Justin walks in, Bailey notices Justin has a significant limp and is heavily favoring his left leg. Bailey also notices Justin has a bandage around one of his arms. Justin hands Bailey a referral slip that says only "Justin doesn't seem like himself today. Can you talk to him and see what's going on?" Justin is hesitant to talk but does open up a bit and says he has been falling behind on his homework, and so things have been difficult at home. When asked about his bandage and limp, Justin discloses information about how his parents are really into working out, and when he or his little sister fall behind on school work, their punishment is to do "exercise stuff." Justin further explains how when he or his sister make lower than an A on an assignment, they are made to run, do push-ups, sit-ups, and pull-ups during their two-hour homework time. Justin says it has been happening a lot recently because his schoolwork has been getting much more difficult. He claims to not be as worried about himself but does mention his little sister (age 10) gets sick sometimes while doing her exercises. When Bailey asks Justin what he thinks of the exercises, Justin claims he knows his parents just want the best for him and his sister, but the exercises are hard, and he is noticing how his shoulders and feet hurt much more lately, especially now as it is getting closer to summer and the temperature is getting up into the 90s.

Is this abuse?

Does Bailey need to report this behavior?

The short answer to question one of Case Illustration 6-13 is that we don't know. Bailey is a school counselor and not a family services investigator or law enforcement officer. Therefore it is not Bailey's responsibility to know for sure if Justin's injuries are the result of abuse.

The response to the second question associated with Case Illustration 6-13 is yes. If Bailey has any suspicion Justin's injuries are in any way associated with abuse, then he is required to report the behaviors to the proper authorities. It is not Bailey's responsibility to determine if this is abuse or not; it is Bailey's responsibility to report if he has any suspicion at all. Once he makes the report, it is the responsibility of those to whom he makes the report to investigate and determine the degree of concern.

Conclusion

In Chapter 6 the authors discussed issues related to confidentiality, privacy, and privileged communication. In short, Chapter 6 was about when and how professional counselors share information about the counseling relationship with those outside the counseling relationship. In some instances counselors are directed or obligated to break confidentiality (i.e., in situations where there is suspected abuse or neglect of a child or if there is clear and foreseeable harm to a client or identifiable other). In other situations counselors are given the option to break confidentiality (i.e., when a client discloses he/she has contagious, life-threatening disease or when a terminally ill client discloses they plan to hasten their own death). As in all situations, counselors must maintain self-awareness, understanding their own morals, values, and beliefs and how those beliefs affect their interpretation of ethical standards. When counselors begin imposing their own values, believing they know what is "right" and "wrong" for clients, they are no longer acting as a counselor.

Having read Chapter 6 and understanding counselors' ethical responsibilities related to confidentiality, privacy, and privileged communication, the authors invite you to review Exercise 6-1 and answer the associated questions.

EXERCISE 6-1

Dr. Jacobs is a primary care physician and a well-known family practice physician in his community. He is a private pay client and originally scheduled a counseling appointment with you to address his chronic use and abuse of illicit and prescription drugs. During his first few counseling sessions, Dr. Jacobs described his recent medical history and his use of painkillers, which he uses to deal with chronic pain. His use of painkillers eventually progressed into using more illicit drugs (cocaine and methamphetamines), and now he is concerned his drug habits may be getting excessive and out of control. He goes on to tell you his drug use has never caused him any trouble at work, and he has never been arrested for being under the influence. Dr. Jacobs is adamant he is "careful" and is a "responsible drug user." His main concern is he wants to work on "taming" his drug use to make sure it does not ever interfere with his ability to treat his own patients. Dr. Jacobs believes his drug use has not progressed to a dangerous level yet and wants to work on managing his stress and pain in other ways.

At today's session, you notice Dr. Jacobs acting out of the ordinary and displaying some unusual behavior. When you confront him about his behavior and ask if he is under the influence, he admits to taking a few pills earlier in the day but nothing over his "usual dose." Dr. Jacobs tells you not to worry; he is not wasted and has even been careful to get someone else to drive him around today because he doesn't feel he can safely drive.

At the end of the session, while walking out to the waiting room, you are surprised to see Dr. Hame, another well-respected family practice physician and a colleague of Dr. Jacobs, who is there to drive Dr. Jacobs back to their office. While you are rescheduling your next appointment and collecting payment from Dr. Jacobs, you overhear the two doctors talking about the remainder of the day. Dr. Jacob tells his colleague he only has two more appointments in the afternoon and some paperwork to complete. As the two walk out, you hear Dr. Jacobs say, "My two patients this afternoon aren't anything serious. I should be able to make it through just fine."

What would you do in this situation?

Use an ethical decision-making model to determine how you might act.

Identify the problem.

Review relevant ethical codes and laws.

Understand your own morals, values, and beliefs and how they might influence your interpretation of the code of ethics and laws.

Identify possible courses of action.

Identify benefits and consequences of possible courses of action.

Consult with others.

Decide on a course of action and implement.

Do you have an ethical responsibility to report Dr. Jacobs's behaviors and drug use?

If you do have a responsibility to report the behaviors, to whom should the report be made? The police? The medical board? Dr. Jacobs's employer?

Keystones

- Confidentiality protects clients from unauthorized disclosures but is not absolute.
- Counselors' own morals, values, beliefs, and life experiences will likely influence their understanding of what constitutes "clear and foreseeable harm."
- If counselors determine clear and foreseeable harm exists, they have an obligation to report the future harm to the appropriate authorities.

- When a client discloses plans to harm an identifiable third party, the counselor may have an obligation to warn the intended victim (depending on state law).
- When working with terminally ill clients who plan to hasten their own death, counselors have the option to break confidentiality and disclose the information to appropriate authorities.
- When working with clients who disclose they have a contagious and life-threatening disease, counselors have the option to break confidentiality to notify appropriate parties.
- When counselors are served with a subpoena and asked to share client documents, it is always best to contact an attorney or legal expert to receive advice on how to act.
- When working with treatment or interdisciplinary teams, counselors must inform clients about the purpose of the team and what types of information will be shared with other members of the team.
- Counselors are ethically permitted to share confidential information with their subordinates and are responsible for educating subordinates of the importance of confidentiality.
- To avoid potentially awkward public encounters with clients, counselors should review client preferences for handling such situations during the informed consent process.
- Counselors are legally and ethically required to report suspected child abuse.

Additional Resources

Bradley, L. J., Hendricks, B., & Douglas, R. (2011). Postmortem confidentiality: An ethical issue. *The Family Journal, 19*(4), 417–420.

Burkemper, E. M. (2002). Family therapists' ethical decision-making processes in two duty-to-warn situations. *Journal of Marital and Family Therapy, 28*(2), 203–211.

Coduti, W. A., & Luse, M. M. (2015). Rural ethics and mental health: An overview for rehabilitation counselors. *Journal of Applied Rehabilitation Counseling, 46*(1), 40–47. Retrieved from http://search.proquest.com/docview/1672889667?accountid=7122

Costa, L., & Altekruse, M. (1994). Duty-to-warn guidelines for mental health counselors. *Journal of Counseling and Development, 72*(4), 346. Retrieved from http://search.proquest.com/docview/219121988?accountid=7122

Del Mauro, J. M., & Jackson Williams, D. (2013). Children and adolescents' attitudes toward seeking help from professional mental health providers. *International Journal for the Advancement of Counselling, 35*(2), 120–138.

Kress, V. E., Hoffman, R. M., Adamson, N., & Eriksen, K. (2013). Informed consent, confidentiality, and diagnosing ethical guidelines for counselor practice. *Journal of Mental Health Counseling, 35*(1), 15–28.

McCurdy, K. G., & McCurdy, K. C. (2003). Confidentiality issues when minor children disclose family secrets in family counseling. *The Family Journal, 11*(4), 393–398.

Moyer, M., & Sullivan, J. (2008). Student health risk behavior: When do school counselors break confidentiality? *Professional School Counseling, 11*(4), 236–245.

O'Connell, W. P. (2012). Secondary school administrators' attitudes toward confidentiality in school counseling. *National Association of Secondary School Principals. NASSP Bulletin, 96*(4), 350–363. Retrieved from http://search.proquest.com/docview/1287938884?accountid=7122

Ponton, R. F., & Duba, J. D. (2009). The ACA code of ethics: Articulating counseling's professional covenant. *Journal of Counseling and Development, 87,* 117–121.

Scriggins, L. P. (2002). Legal ethics, confidentiality, and the organizational client. *The Business Lawyer, 58*(1), 123–141. Retrieved from http://www.jstor.org/stable/40688119

Sullivan, J. R., & Moyer, M. S. (2008). Factors influencing the decision to break confidentiality with adolescent students: A survey of school counselors. *Journal of School Counseling, 6*(24), 236–245.

References

American Association for Marriage and Family Therapy. (2015). *Code of ethics.* Retrieved from https://www.aamft.org/iMIS15/AAMFT/Content/legal_ethics/code_of_ethics.aspx

American Counseling Association. (2014). *Code of ethics.* Alexandria, VA: Author.

American Psychological Association. (2010). *American Psychological Association ethical principles of psychologists and code of conduct.* Retrieved from http://www.apa.org/ethics/code/principles.pdf

Child Abuse Prevention and Treatment Act of 1974, 42 USC §§5101–5106.

Corey, G., Corey, M. S., & Callanan, P. (2011). *Issues and ethics in the helping professions* (8th ed.). Belmont, CA: Brooks/Cole, Cengage Learning.

Ford, G. G. (2006). *Ethical reasoning for mental health professionals.* Thousand Oaks, CA: Sage.

Tarasoff v. Board of Regents of the University of California, 17 Cal. 3d 425, 551 (1976).

7

Ethics in Theory, Practice, and Professional Relationships

I am always more interested in what I am about to do than what I have already done.

—Rachel Carson

Chapter 7 reviews the ethics of practice and the daily activities of being a professional counselor. The authors discuss everything from relationships with other professionals to being an employer and being an employee. All related areas of the code of ethics will be discussed in detail; however, emphasis will be put on how the code can be applied to real-world activities. There are many gray areas in the ethical code, and readers will again be challenged to evaluate not only their decisions on many ethical dilemmas but also how they go about making a decision on how to act. This chapter will focus primarily on ethics surrounding theory, practice, and maintaining professional relationships. At the conclusion of Chapter 7, readers will specifically be able to accomplish the following:

1. Explain the ethical and practical importance of integrating theory into practice.

2. Define ethical considerations related to diagnosis.

3. Discuss the importance of forming positive relationships with others and respecting different theoretical approaches to counseling.

4. Discuss the importance of providing a safe and nondiscriminatory work environment for employees.

5. Define ethical considerations related to advertising one's counseling practice.

6. Explain ethical requirements in setting and collecting fees.

7. Name counselor's ethical obligations when determining when to refer clients to other professionals.

8. State the importance of representing one's credentials appropriately.

Theory and Techniques

Choosing a theory or theories with which to work and establishing effective techniques are critical developmental steps for almost all counselors. Counseling programs seeking accreditation from CACREP are required to include counseling theories in their core course work; even graduate programs not seeking CACREP accreditation infuse theory into much of their course work (CACREP, 2009). Theory guides practice (Corey, Corey, & Callanan, 2011). The ACA Code of Ethics (2014) discusses theory in a couple of areas. First, in the introduction of Section C, "Counselors have a responsibility to the public to engage in counseling practices based on rigorous research methodologies" (ACA, 2014, p. 8), and also in Standard C.2.b., "While developing skills in new specialty areas, counselors take steps to ensure the competence of their work and protect others from possible harm (ACA, 2014, p. 8). Above and beyond following a specific theory or theories, the authors strongly believe ethical counselors should take great care in understanding the tenets of the theory or theories they choose. Each theory is based on the beliefs, personality, and understandings of the theory's originator (Corey, Corey, & Callanan, 2011), and an ethical counselor works to adjust theory to his/her own personality and style. Consider Case Illustration 7-1 in which Mark and James both integrate theory into their practice.

CASE ILLUSTRATION 7-1

Scenario 1

Mark, a counselor in training, has been asked by his instructor to demonstrate his mastery of a "chosen" theory. Mark must audio tape one of his counseling sessions and share the tape with his instructor and supervisor. Although he is a little nervous about his assignment, Mark knows he really likes Solution Focused Brief Therapy (SFBT) due to his interest in working in a school setting. He says he also likes SFBT because "he is good at figuring out solutions for his clients." Plus, he is familiar with Scaling and the Miracle Question. A brief portion of Mark's session follows.

Mark: How are you doing today?
Client: Alright.

(Continued)

(Continued)

Mark: Let me start out with finding out what you want to work on. I'm going to ask you a Miracle Question. If you woke up tomorrow morning and a miracle occurred because you were at counseling today, what would that miracle be?

Client: Umm, I guess I would feel better and not feel so trapped in my house.

Mark: OK, so you want to feel better. On a scale of 1 to 10, how good do you feel right now?

Client: About a 4.

Mark: OK, so you don't feel very good right now. I think we can find a solution to help you feel better. You said you feel trapped. Have you tried getting out of your house more? What about going and doing things with friends?

Scenario 2

James, a counselor in training, has also been asked by his instructor to demonstrate his mastery of a "chosen" theory. Similar to Mark, James must also audio tape one of his counseling sessions and share the tape with his instructor and supervisor. James is also most comfortable in using SFBT due to his interest in working in a school setting. Additionally, in James's own life, he believes in looking for small changes to facilitate larger changes. He feels as though individuals are best able to make positive changes if they look for what is going right in life and build on the positives to achieve goals. James also likes the Miracle Question. He sees it as a way to help clients identify small, specific goals to work on in treatment. Additionally, James feels as though Scaling questions really help him get a sense of where his clients are at with various emotions.

James: How are you doing today?

Client: Alright.

James: Alright, so what brings you in today? How can I be helpful?

Client: Umm, I guess I just want to feel better. I feel so trapped sometimes.

James: OK, so you want to feel better. What do you mean by better?

Client: I don't know. I just would be better.

James: OK, so let me ask you, on a scale of 1 to 10, how confident are you that coming to counseling will be helpful to you?

Client: About a 4.

James: Describe what you mean by a 4.

Client: I've been to counseling before, and it wasn't very helpful. I'm not optimistic this will be any better. But I'm here and willing to give it a shot.

James: So you haven't had much success with counseling in the past, and you're not convinced this is going to help, but you thought you would give it one more chance.

> **Client:** Sure.
>
> **James:** So let me ask you a question. If you woke up tomorrow and something had happened overnight that made you "feel better," how would you know you were feeling better?
>
> **Client:** I'm not sure. Maybe I would just have more energy to go out and do yard work?
>
> **James:** You would do more yard work. So if you got up in the mornings and went out to do yard work, then you would be feeling better? Maybe we could talk more about some strategies to help you with your energy to get out and do yard work; doing so may snowball into helping you have more energy overall.

In Case Illustration 7-1, and specifically Scenario 1, Mark uses SFBT techniques but lacks a thorough understanding of the theory and how to use the techniques effectively. Mark has likely read his counseling theories book and understands the basic terminology associated with SFBT but lacks the in-depth understanding necessary to effectively integrate SFBT techniques into his sessions. Mark seems to use the Miracle Question and Scaling sporadically, without knowing the purpose of either technique. On the contrary, James understands the underlying purpose of the SFBT techniques and uses them effectively in his session. James not only understands the terminology associated with SFBT; he also has a more in-depth understanding of the theory as a whole. Whereas Mark seems to use generic, "cookie-cutter" terms associated with SFBT without rhyme or reason, James is more strategic in his approach.

Being an ethical counselor involves more than simply using the words and techniques of a given theory. It involves understanding the purpose behind the technique, knowing the theory's view of the client/counselor relationship, and adapting the theory to one's own personality. In thinking about your own theory and gaining an in-depth understanding of that theory, the authors encourage you to consider the following questions.

Which theory or theories do you gravitate toward most?

What are the major tenets of those theories?

What are your own personal beliefs about how people make changes in their lives?

Do you see any similarities between your own personal beliefs about change and the theories you gravitate toward?

Diagnosis

ACA Standard E.5.a. (2014) Proper Diagnosis: Counselors take special care to provide proper diagnosis of mental disorders. Assessment techniques (including personal interviews) used to determine client care (e.g., locus of treatment, type of treatment, recommended follow-up) are carefully selected and appropriately used.

Diagnosis is a powerful tool and should not be taken lightly. Counselors are careful to provide proper diagnosis and consider various assessment strategies to determine the best course of care for clients.

ACA Standard E.5.b. (2014) Cultural Sensitivity: Counselors recognize that culture affects the manner in which clients and problems are defined and experienced. Clients' socioeconomic and cultural experiences are considered when diagnosing mental disorders.

Similar to the requirements of Standard E.5.a., Standard E.5.b. requires counselors to use extreme caution when providing a diagnosis. As previously stated in Chapter 4, professional counselors consider culture when making a diagnosis and understand how culture impacts life experiences and how problems are defined.

ACA Standard E.5.c. (2014) Historical and Social Prejudices in the Diagnosis of Pathology: Counselors recognize historical and social prejudices in the misdiagnosis and pathologizing of certain individuals and groups and strive to become aware of and address such biases in themselves or others.

Counselors are cognizant of social prejudices that accompany the diagnosis or misdiagnosis of certain populations and address their own biases.

ACA Standard E.5.d. (2014) Refraining From Diagnosis: Counselors may refrain from making and/or reporting a diagnosis if they believe that it would cause harm to the client or others. Counselors carefully consider both the positive and negative implications of a diagnosis.

Diagnosis provides a definition for treatment; it delivers standard terminology for describing a client's presenting concern (Welfel & Patterson, 2004). However, diagnosis is not a must for professional counselors. The ACA Code of Ethics (2014) permits counselors to refrain from diagnosis. Although it may be considered ethical to refrain from diagnosis, counselors working with managed care companies will most likely need to provide a diagnosis to receive third-party payment for services. Even with these guidelines, diagnosis continues to be subjective in nature. See Text Box 7-1 for information about handling diagnoses in the APA and AAMFT. Review Case Illustration 7-2 related to diagnosis, and consider how you might act if you were in Floyd's situation.

CASE ILLUSTRATION 7-2

Floyd is a licensed professional counselor and a certified school counselor. He is single and has sole custody of his two children. Due to the recent downturn in the economy, Floyd has been having trouble making ends meet and has decided to take on a second job (part time) in addition to his regular job as a school counselor. Floyd has started working at a local counseling agency. Although the extra money isn't going to make his family rich, Floyd is now able to catch up on all his bills and won't be forced to sell his house and downsize.

Today, Floyd's clinical supervisor meets with him to review his cases and consult. His supervisor expresses some concern because Floyd uses "V-codes" quite often when making diagnoses. Floyd defends his diagnosis and explains he feels strongly that the V-codes are most appropriate considering his clients' presenting problems and the treatment needed. His supervisor expresses her understanding but explains to Floyd how many insurance companies do not view V-codes as acceptable diagnoses and therefore will not reimburse when they are used. The supervisor goes on to explain that because Floyd is paid based on the clients he sees, he will not be paid if the insurance companies do not pay for the diagnoses he provides. She further encourages Floyd to switch his diagnoses and says, "Just change it to an adjustment disorder or something else that isn't bad. Your clients won't care; they probably don't even know the difference between the two. At least you will get paid." Floyd's supervisor then reiterates that the decision is up to him, but no one will know or care if he makes the change.

In Case Illustration 7-2, Floyd has an ethical and possibly even a moral dilemma. When counselors find themselves involved in an ethical dilemma, it is always important to engage in an ethical decision-making process. What follows is an example of how Floyd may use an ethical decision-making process to help him decide how to act.

Identify the Problem

Floyd is struggling financially to the point where he has taken on a part-time counseling job to help make ends meet. Floyd has been told by his clinical supervisor that he may not be paid for his counseling because many insurance companies do not accept V-codes (which Floyd has used in many of his current cases) as acceptable diagnoses. Floyd was encouraged by his clinical supervisor to change his diagnoses to get paid.

Review Relevant Ethical Codes and Laws

ACA (2014) E.5.a. (Proper Diagnosis) says counselors take special care in making a proper diagnosis.

ACA (2014) I.2.d. (Organizational Conflicts) states that if demands of an organization conflict with the ACA Code of Ethics, counselors talk to their supervisors about the concern and express their dedication to following the code of ethics.

Understand Your Own Morals, Values, and Beliefs and How They Might Influence Your Interpretation of the Code of Ethics and Laws

Floyd feels very strongly about maintaining his professionalism and rarely (if ever) cuts corners related to his work as a professional counselor. He takes great care in understanding his clients and tends to lean toward underdiagnosing rather than "labeling" one of his clients with something more severe. If it were up to Floyd, he wouldn't diagnose at all, but he knows he must provide something when working with managed care.

Identify Possible Courses of Action

Floyd could immediately go to all of his case files and switch all of his diagnoses from a V-code to an adjustment disorder or something else. Floyd could refuse to switch his diagnoses and keep them the way they are. Floyd could refuse to switch his diagnoses (similar to the previous choice) and also express concern to his supervisor about how she encouraged him to change his diagnoses.

Identify Benefits and
Consequences of Possible Courses of Action

If Floyd chooses to switch his diagnoses, he will have the benefit of getting paid for the time and energy he is putting into this new job. However, in doing so, Floyd may have to bend on his own morals and values. Floyd may also be acting in an unethical manner based on Standard E.5.a. If Floyd chooses not to makes changes to his diagnoses, then he will most likely not be paid for any of the services he is providing. Consequently, he will be working the hours at his part-time job but won't see any benefits and will still have trouble making ends meet with his financial situation. However, he will maintain his morals, values, and professionalism. If Floyd chooses to discuss his concerns with his supervisor, he will likely have all the same consequences listed previously but may also suffer some consequences related to his employment (depending on how his supervisor responds to him voicing his concerns).

Consult With Others

Floyd could consult with colleagues and would also want to consult with his state board for licensure.

Decide on a Course of Action and Implement

In the end, Floyd decides to hold firm to his choice to use V-codes. He also chooses to discontinue his work at the agency and seek part-time employment in other areas. Floyd made the decision to quit primarily due to his strong sense of professional responsibility and not wanting to compromise his morals by changing his diagnoses simply to get a paycheck.

> **TEXT BOX 7-1**
>
> **American Psychological Association**
>
> The APA addresses ethics related to diagnosis in only one standard, 9.01 (Bases for Assessments). In Standard 9.01 psychologists are instructed to "base the opinions contained in their recommendations, reports, and diagnostic or evaluative statements, including forensic testimony, on information and techniques sufficient to substantiate their findings" (APA, 2010, p. 12).
>
> **American Association for Marriage and Family Therapists**
>
> The AAMFT does not address issues related to diagnosis in their ethical standards.

Professional Relationships

Professional counselors seldom work in a vacuum. In fact, the majority of professional counselors work with other professionals on a daily basis (e.g., consultation, referrals, and professional development activities). Therefore, building strong, positive working relationships with others is a necessity to provide quality services (Remley & Herlihy, 2014). Section D of the ACA Code of Ethics (2014) offers additional guidelines for counselors. The following are summaries of ethical guidelines covered in Section D and a brief explanation of each.

ACA Standard D.1.a. (2014) Different Approaches: Counselors are respectful of approaches that are grounded in theory and/or have an empirical or scientific foundation but may differ from their own. Counselors acknowledge the expertise of other professional groups and are respectful of their practices.

As discussed previously, there are numerous and diverse theories, techniques, and approaches to counseling. Likewise, the clientele with which counselors work gravitate toward many different approaches and styles. Counselors should be respectful of approaches that are different from their own (i.e., there are many ways to be a professional counselor).

ACA Standard D.1.b. (2014) Forming Relationships: Counselors work to develop and strengthen relationships with colleagues from other disciplines to best serve clients.

Simply stated, build relationships with others. Part of being a successful, ethical counselor is knowing how to provide and find the best services for clients. Meet and build relationships with other professional counselors, psychologists, psychiatrists, social workers, and so on. You never know when you will need the help of others. Building positive working relationships with professionals from other disciplines not only benefits clients but is also beneficial to counselors in terms of building referral sources.

ACA Standard D.1.c. (2014) Interdisciplinary Teamwork: Counselors who are members of interdisciplinary teams delivering multifaceted services to clients remain focused on how to best serve clients. They participate in and contribute to decisions that affect the well-being of clients by drawing on the perspectives, values, and experiences of the counseling profession and those of colleagues from other disciplines.

If counselors work as part of an interdisciplinary team, they remain focused on how to best serve clients. Counselors participate and fulfill their obligations as team members (i.e., be a good team member, and do your part as a professional counselor).

ACA Standard D.1.d. (2014) Establishing Professional and Ethical Obligations: Counselors who are members of interdisciplinary teams work together with team members to clarify professional and ethical obligations of the team as a whole and of its individual members. When a team decision raises ethical concerns, counselors first attempt to resolve the concern within the team. If they cannot reach resolution among team members, counselors pursue other avenues to address their concerns consistent with client well-being.

When working with an interdisciplinary team, counselors are careful to share their professional and ethical obligations. If there is a conflict, counselors first try to resolve the issue with the team members. If the first attempt is not successful, counselors then pursue other efforts to ensure the well-being of the client. In all situations, the well-being of the client is the end goal. See how the APA addresses professional cooperation in Text Box 7-2.

TEXT BOX 7-2

American Psychological Association

APA Standard 3.09 (2010) Cooperation With Other Professionals: When indicated and professionally appropriate, psychologists cooperate with other professionals to serve their clients and patients effectively and appropriately.

American Association for Marriage and Family Therapists

The AAMFT does not address issues related to working with other professions in their ethical standards.

ACA Standard D.1.e. (2014) Confidentiality: When counselors are required by law, institutional policy, or extraordinary circumstances to serve in more than one role in judicial or administrative proceedings, they clarify role expectations and the parameters of confidentiality with their colleagues.

Similar to the requirement to clarify roles with clients, counselors must clarify their role and constraints of confidentiality with interdisciplinary teams or other colleagues.

ACA Standard D.1.f. (2014) Personnel Selection and Assignment: When counselors are in a position requiring personnel selection and/or assigning of responsibilities to others, they select competent staff and assign responsibilities compatible with their skills and experiences.

When counselors are in a position in which they are responsible for hiring new personnel, they are careful to choose competent staff.

ACA Standard D.1.g. (2014) Employer Policies: The acceptance of employment in an agency or institution implies that counselors are in agreement with its general policies and principles. Counselors strive to reach agreement with employers regarding acceptable standards of client care and professional conduct that allow for changes in institutional policy conducive to the growth and development of clients.

When counselors accept a job at an agency, they are basically saying that they agree with the policies and procedures of the agency.

ACA Standard D.1.h. (2014) Negative Conditions: Counselors alert their employers of inappropriate policies and practices. They attempt to effect changes in such policies or procedures through constructive action within the organization. When such policies are potentially disruptive or damaging to clients or may limit the effectiveness of services provided, and change cannot be affected, counselors take appropriate further action. Such action may include referral to appropriate certification, accreditation, or state licensure organizations, or voluntary termination of employment.

If an agency policy does not seem ethical, professional counselors alert the employer of the violation and try to work out a better course of action. If counselors are not able to come to a mutually agreeable decision with employers, they take action to either notify appropriate certification or licensure boards or voluntarily resign from their position.

ACA Standard D.1.i. (2014) Protection From Punitive Action: Counselors do not harass a colleague or employee or dismiss an employee who has acted in a responsible and ethical manner to expose inappropriate employer policies or practices.

Professional counselors do not harass or fire employees if those employees are acting ethically showing the agency's wrongdoings.

Advertising

When considering advertising, professional counselors are given some flexibility in the ways in which they may advertise and promote services (Ford, 2006). There are several ethical standards that provide specific direction to counselors. (See Text Box 7-3 for details about credentials and advertising described in the APA and AAMFT.)

ACA Standard C.3.a. (2014) Accurate Advertising: When advertising or otherwise representing their services to the public, counselors identify their credentials in an accurate manner that is not false, misleading, deceptive, or fraudulent.

Professional counselors must be accurate and ensure information presented to the public is true and not misleading. Standard C.3.a. is exemplified in Case Illustration 7-3. Consider the examples given and whether they might be considered "true" and "non-misleading."

CASE ILLUSTRATION 7-3

Lifelong Happiness Couples & Family Counseling Center

Perfect Solutions Family Therapy. We guarantee a solution!

Friendship Counseling Agency

The first example in Case Illustration 7-3 would be considered misleading due to the use of the term "lifelong happiness." The term implies that families seeking services will enjoy lifelong happiness. The second example, similar to the first, is misleading. Rather than implying happiness, the counseling agency in Example 2 guarantees a solution will be reached. Therefore the agency gives clients false hope that there will be a solution to problems. In the third example the name implies the counselor/client relationship is similar to that of a friendship. Example 3 is also misleading and gives clients a distorted view of appropriate boundaries.

ACA Standard C.3.c. (2014) Statements by Others: When feasible, counselors make reasonable efforts to ensure that statements made by others about them or about the counseling profession are accurate.

Standard C.3.c. reminds professional counselors that the counselor is responsible for making sure others' statements are true and accurate about said professional counselor. Consider Case illustration 7-4 and how Rachel is introduced to the families with which she works.

CASE ILLUSTRATION 7-4

Rachel is a master's-level, licensed professional counselor. She has a contract with her local courthouse to provide counseling to truant students as part of each student's court order. While the counseling is not mandatory, the judge highly encourages all families seen in his courtroom to take advantage of the counseling as an alternative to community service or paying a fine. Because of the judge's encouragement, many families take advantage of Rachel's counseling services.

During today's court docket, Rachel sits in the courtroom and hears the judge explaining the counseling services she provides. She hears the judge say to some parents, "I highly encourage you sign up and take advantage of the services Ms. Rachel provides. She is a psychologist and works with families and kids. She really knows how to manipulate their brains, so your kids will start going to school again and do what you want them to do."

What should Rachel do?

According to Standard C.3.c., Rachel's responsibilities include not only speaking to the families referred to her, but she must also speak to the judge making the referrals. Rachel should talk to her new clients and the judge about her credentials (she is a master's-level licensed professional counselor and not a psychologist) and the description of the services she provides (she may want to clarify the services she provides and clear up the misconception she "manipulates brains").

In addition to the two standards listed previous, the ACA Code of Ethics (2014) directs professional counselors to avoid soliciting testimonials from current or past clients.

ACA Standard C.3.b. (2014) Testimonials: Counselors who use testimonials do not solicit them from current clients, former clients, or any other persons who may be vulnerable to undue influence. Counselors discuss with clients the implications of and obtain permission for the use of any testimonial.

Counselors also refrain from using their places of employment to recruit clients, supervisees, or consultees for their own private practice.

ACA Standard C.3.d. (2014) Recruiting Through Employment: Counselors do not use their places of employment or institutional affiliation to recruit clients, supervisors, or consultees for their private practice.

Finally, by the nature of the profession, counselors are in a position of power and have great influence over many, if not all, of the clients with whom they meet.

ACA Standard C.3.e. (2014) Products and Training Advertisements: Counselors who develop products related to their profession or conduct workshops or training events ensure that the advertisements concerning these products or events are accurate and disclose adequate information for consumers to make informed choices.

If professional counselors have developed products or present workshops, they are careful to ensure all advertising related to those products or workshops is done accurately and not delivered in a deceptive manner.

ACA Standard C.3.f. (2014) Promoting to Those Served: Counselors do not use counseling, teaching, training, or supervisory relationships to promote their products or training events in a manner that is deceptive or would exert undue influence on individuals who may be vulnerable. However, counselor educators may adopt textbooks they have authored for instructional purposes.

In Case Illustration 7-5, Kerri and Terry have developed a few products that they sell at their newly opened private practice. Consider Case Illustration 7-5 as an example of how Ethical Standards C.3.e. and C.3.f. may look in practice.

CASE ILLUSTRATION 7-5

Kerri and Terry are friends who have opened a private practice together. They are both licensed professional counselors and have named their practice Counseling and Stuff. Due to their knowledge about the financial strains accompanying starting a private practice and the difficulty of

(Continued)

(Continued)

establishing oneself over the first couple years, the two counselors have decided to offer other products in addition to counseling. Kerri and Terry have worked very hard and are both trained in stress and anxiety reduction strategies. They sell their relaxation tapes for $10 each at their office to any clients who may wish to have some of the songs and music Kerri and Terry use during sessions. Additionally, they have aromatherapy soaps and candles for sale and displayed in the lobby, which vary in price from $5 to $25.

Are Kerri and Terry acting ethically by deciding to sell some items in their counseling office? Why, or why not?

At first look, Kerri and Terry seem to be acting ethically in their practices. However, the limited information provided in Case Illustration 7-5 does not include anything related to how Kerri and Terry advertise or market their tapes or aromatherapy items. According to Ethical Standard C.3.e., Kerri and Terry must be sure to advertise the products accurately and provide clients with enough information to make an informed choice. Kerri and Terry must also avoid applying undue pressure to clients when marketing their products. The following examples are provided to highlight differences in how Kerri and Terry might interact with clients.

Scenario 1

Client: I noticed you have some candles and soaps out in the lobby. Do you make those yourself?

Kerri: Yes, they are 100 percent natural.

Client: How helpful are they?

Kerri: We wouldn't have them out there if we didn't think they were effective. I highly encourage you to pick out one or two for yourself. I guarantee you will be able to manage your stress and anxiety much better at home if you have one. We burn the same candles here, and if you have one at your home, smelling the same smells will really help you remember to implement the strategies we talked about today.

Scenario 2

Client: I noticed you have some candles and soaps out in the lobby. Do you make those yourself?

Kerri: Yes, they are 100 percent natural.

Client: How helpful are they?

Kerri: That is a great question, and I think it depends. There is certainly nothing magical about them. We have had some individuals swear by them and believe them to be excellent. On the contrary, there are certainly many others who believe them to be ineffective. I believe it is just personal preference. We have them available but certainly don't want to make any false claims about their effectiveness.

In Scenario 1, Kerri "highly encourages" the client purchase items and implies buying items will increase the effectiveness of treatment, thus possibly acting unethically according to Standard C.3.f. (ACA, 2014). On the contrary, in Scenario 2, Kerri is open and honest about the effectiveness of the products on display. Kerri reports other clients have had mixed feelings about the products and does not put any undue pressure on the client to make a purchase.

TEXT BOX 7-3

American Psychological Association

The APA discusses advertising and presenting one's credentials accurately in Section 5 (Advertising and Other Public Statements). A list of all pertinent standards follows.

APA Standard 5.01 (2010) Avoidance of False or Deceptive Statements: (a) Public statements include but are not limited to paid or unpaid advertising, product endorsements, grant applications, licensing applications, other credentialing applications, brochures, printed matter, directory listings, personal resumes or curricula vitae, or comments for use in legal proceedings, lectures and public oral presentations, and published materials. Psychologists do not knowingly make public statements that are false, deceptive, or fraudulent concerning their research, practice, or other work activities or those of the persons or organizations with which they are affiliated. (b) Psychologists do not make false, deceptive, or fraudulent statements concerning (1) their training, experience, or competence; (2) their academic degrees; (3) their credentials; (4) their institutional or association affiliations; (5) their services; (6) the scientific or clinical basis for, or results of degree of success of, their services; (7) their fees; or (8) their publications or research findings. (c) Psychologists claim degrees as credentials for their health services only if those degrees (1) were earned from a regionally accredited educational institution or (2) were the basis for psychology licensure by the state in which they practice.

APA Standard 5.05 (2010) Testimonials: Psychologists do not solicit testimonials from current therapy clients or patients or other persons who because of their particular circumstances are vulnerable to undue influence.

APA Standard 5.06 (2010) In-Person Solicitation: Psychologists do not engage, directly or through agents, in uninvited in-person solicitation of business from actual or potential therapy clients or patients or other persons who because of their particular circumstance are vulnerable to undue influence. However, this prohibition does not preclude (1) attempting to implement

(Continued)

(Continued)

appropriate collateral contacts for the purpose of benefiting an already engaged therapy client or patient or (2) providing disaster or community outreach services.

American Association for Marriage and Family Therapists

The AAMFT addresses advertising in Section 9. See below for specific standards related to advertising.

AAMFT Standard 9.1 (2015) Accurate Professional Representation: Marriage and family therapists accurately represent their competencies, education, training, and experience relevant to their practice of marriage and family therapy in accordance with applicable laws.

AAMFT Standard 9.2 (2015) Promotional Materials: Marriage and family therapists ensure that advertisements and publications in any media are true, accurate, and in accordance with applicable law.

AAMFT Standard 9.5 (2015) Educational Credentials: Marriage and family therapists claim degrees for their clinical services only if those degrees demonstrate training and education in marriage and family therapy or related fields.

AAMFT Standard 9.7 (2015) Specialization: Marriage and family therapists represent themselves as providing specialized services only after taking reasonable steps to ensure the competence of their work and to protect clients, supervisees, and others from harm.

AAMFT Standard 9.8 (2015) Correction of Misinformation: Marriage and family therapists correct, wherever possible, false, misleading, or inaccurate information and representations made by others concerning the therapist's qualifications, services, or products.

Fees and Billing

Cottone and Tarvydas (2007) recommend counselors be "cautious and fair" in setting their fees (p. 140). Remley and Herlihy (2014) add that fees should be set in a way that is not discriminatory to any. Finally, once fees are set, they should not be changed unless services are discontinued and then started again. Oftentimes fee structures and billing methods are included in the informed consent process and thus are a contract between client and counselor (see Chapter 5 for more information). Ethical guidelines are set forth in Standard A.10.c. See Text Box 7-4 for fee and billing guidelines in the APA and AAMFT.

ACA Standard A.10.c. (2014) Establishing Fees: In establishing fees for professional counseling services, counselors consider the financial status of clients and locality. If a counselor's usual fees create undue hardship for the client, the counselor may adjust fees, when legally permissible, or assist the client in locating comparable, affordable services.

In adjusting fees, professional counselors may consider a sliding scale fee structure. Sliding scale fees offer benefits such as making services available to those who might otherwise not be able to afford counseling but also may bring about some unforeseen and unintended ethical concerns. Similar to previous chapters in which counselors have been encouraged to practice self-awareness, the authors again recommend that the professional counselor reflect on the type and quality of services provided to sliding scale-paying clients versus those paying full price. What follows are a few questions to consider.

Do you provide lower-quality services to clients who may be paying sliding scale fees as compared to those paying full price (e.g., come to session less prepared, less present during session, more easily distracted)?

Do you schedule sliding scale clients at less convenient times, or are you less flexible in scheduling or rescheduling with sliding scale clients?

How might you monitor your behaviors to ensure you provide high-quality services to all clients, regardless of their payment method?

TEXT BOX 7-4

American Psychological Association

APA Standard 6.04 (2010) Fees and Financial Arrangements: (a) As early as is feasible in a professional or scientific relationship, psychologists and recipients of psychological services, reach an agreement specifying compensation and billing arrangements. (b) Psychologists' fee practices are consistent with law. (c) Psychologists do not misrepresent their fees. (d) If limitations to services can be anticipated because of limitations in financing, this is discussed with the recipient of services as early as is feasible. (e) If the recipient of services does not pay for services as agreed, and if psychologists intend to use collection agencies or legal measures to collect the fees, psychologists first inform the person that such measures will be taken and provide that person an opportunity to make prompt payment.

American Association of Marriage and Family Therapists

Guidelines related to setting and collecting fees are covered in Section 8 of the AAMFT Code of Ethics (Financial Arrangements). Specific standards follow.

AAMFT Standard 8.1 (2015) Financial Integrity: Marriage and family therapists do not offer or accept kickbacks, rebates, bonuses, or other remuneration for referrals. Fee-for-service arrangements are not prohibited.

AAMFT Standard 8.2 (2015) Disclosure of Financial Policies: Prior to entering into the therapeutic or supervisory relationship, marriage and family therapists clearly disclose and explain to clients and supervisees: (a) all financial arrangements and fees related to professional services, including charges for cancelled or missed appointments; (b) the use of collection agencies or legal measures for nonpayment; and (c) the procedure for obtaining from the client, to the

(Continued)

(Continued)

extent allowed by law, if payment is denied by the third-party payer. Once sessions have begun, therapists provide reasonable notice of any changes in fees or other charges.

AAMFT Standard 8.4 (2015) Truthful Representation of Services: Marriage and family therapists represent facts truthfully to clients, third-party payers, and supervisees regarding services rendered.

Referrals

The 2014 ACA Code of Ethics is very clear about counselor referrals and when it is appropriate for counselors to refer. See Text box 7-5 for related information from the APA and AAMFT.

ACA Standard A.11.a. (2014) Competence Within Termination and Referral: If counselors lack the competence to be of professional assistance to clients, they avoid entering or continuing counseling relationships. Counselors are knowledgeable about culturally and clinically appropriate referral resources and suggest these alternatives. If clients decline the suggested referrals, counselors discontinue the relationship.

ACA Standard A.11.b. (2014) Values Within Termination and Referral: Counselors refrain from referring prospective and current clients based solely on the counselor's personally held values, attitudes, beliefs, and behaviors. Counselors respect the diversity of clients and seek training in areas in which they are at risk of imposing their values onto clients, especially when the counselor's values are inconsistent with the client's goals or are discriminatory in nature.

TEXT BOX 7-5

American Psychological Association

The APA discusses terminating therapeutic relationships with clients but does not include "values" in the standard. Please see the following for specific standards.

APA Standard 10.10 (2010) Terminating Therapy: (a) Psychologists terminate therapy when it becomes reasonably clear that the client or patient no longer needs the service, is not likely to benefit, or is being harmed by continued service. (b) Psychologists may terminate therapy when threatened or otherwise endangered by the client or patient or another person with whom the client or patient has a relationship. (c) Except where precluded by the actions of clients or patients or third-party payers, prior to termination psychologists provide pretermination counseling and suggest alternative service providers as appropriate.

American Association for Marriage and Family Therapists

The AAMFT also provides its members guidance related to referrals; however, it does not include any discussion of therapist values within the standard. Please see the following.

AAMFT Standard 1.10 (2015) Referrals: Marriage and family therapists respectfully assist persons in obtaining appropriate therapeutic services if the therapist is unable or unwilling to provide professional help.

Review Case Illustration 7-6 as an example of how both Standards A.11.a. and A.11.b. might apply to a real situation. In Case Illustration 7-6, Kayla struggles with one of her clients and chooses to refer the client out based on her interpretation of the code of ethics and wanting to do the "right" thing.

CASE ILLUSTRATION 7-6

Kayla has just received her licensure and has started providing contract counseling for a local agency. Being a new counselor and still having the contents of her ethics class fresh in her mind, Kayla is very careful about choosing her cases and does not want to practice outside the boundaries of her competence. She knows taking on too many clients would be unethical and might possibly indirectly harm one or more of her clients. After meeting with a new client, Jesse, for a few sessions, Kayla begins to realize that Jesse has some very strong, conservative religious beliefs. Kayla, being an atheist herself, struggles with some of the statements Jesse makes during sessions. It has even gotten to the point on a few occasions where Kayla can sense herself wanting to confront Jesse on some of his beliefs. Reflecting on her sessions, Kayla feels as though she is not the best counselor for Jesse because they have such drastically different religious beliefs and decides her best course of action is to refer Jesse to another counselor. She backs up her decision with Standard A.11.a. of the ACA Code of Ethics (2014): "If counselors lack the competence to be of professional assistance to clients, they avoid entering or continuing counseling relationships..."

Is Kayla acting in an ethical manner by referring Jesse to another counselor based solely on his strong religious beliefs? Why, or why not?

In Case Illustration 7-6, Kayla references Standard A.11.a. (Competence Within Termination and Referral). However, Kayla failed to read further in the code of ethics to Standard A.11.b. (Values Within Termination and Referral). The latter standard specifically directs professional counselors to "refrain from referring prospective and current clients based solely on the counselors' personally held values, attitudes, beliefs, and behaviors" (ACA, 2014, p. 6). In Case Illustration 7-6, Kayla's values and religious beliefs are interfering with her ability to work with Jesse. In letting her values interfere, Kayla is neglecting Standard A.4.b. requiring counselors to be aware of and avoid imposing their own values, attitudes, beliefs, and behaviors (ACA, 2014).

Another often overlooked component of Standard A.11.b. is in its first sentence (i.e., counselors refrain from prospective and current clients . . .). To exemplify this component of Ethical Standard A.11.b., examine Case Illustration 7-7 in which Kayla and Jesse's interaction is reworded, consisting only of an intake phone call.

CASE ILLUSTRATION 7-7

Kayla has just received her licensure and has started providing contract counseling for a local agency. Being a new counselor and still having the contents of her ethics class fresh in her mind, Kayla is very careful about choosing her cases and does not want to practice outside the boundaries of her competence. She knows taking on too many clients would be unethical and might possibly indirectly harm one or more of her clients. Today Kayla receives a call from a prospective new client, Jesse. As part of her normal intake procedures, Kayla asks Jesse for some basic contact information including phone number, address, date of birth, insurance number. Additionally, Kayla asks Jesse about his reason for seeking out counseling services. In response Jesse describes his current conflict with his parents and family about his recent life-style change. Jesse talks briefly about a new church he has joined and some of the practices of his new congregation. Kayla begins to realize Jesse has some strong, conservative religious beliefs. Kayla, being an atheist herself, struggles with many of the statements Jesse makes during the phone call. Kayla can sense herself wanting to confront Jesse on his beliefs. While talking with Jesse over the phone, Kayla feels as though she is not the best counselor for him because they have such drastically different religious beliefs and decides her best course of action is to refer Jesse to another counselor. She backs up her decision with Standard A.11.a. of the ACA Code of Ethics (2014): "If counselors lack the competence to be of professional assistance to clients, they avoid entering or continuing counseling relationships . . . " Therefore, at the end of the call, Kayla shares her thoughts about referring Jesse to another counseling agency due to her incompetence and feeling as though she would not be able to understand his current struggles. She then provides Jesse with a list of four other counseling agencies, including two places specializing in "Christian counseling."

Did Kayla act in an ethical manner in referring Jesse to another counselor?

The primary difference between Case Illustration 7-6 and 7-7 is that in the latter, Jesse is a prospective client and has not yet signed a consent form or met with Kayla for a formal counseling session. However, Kayla is still acting in an unethical manner by referring Jesse to another counseling agency due to a value conflict. According to ethical Standard A.11.b., professional counselors may not refer a client or prospective client based on values. The moment Jesse reached out to Kayla for counseling, he became a prospective client.

Review Case Illustration 7-8, and determine which situations may be appropriate for referral and which may be inappropriate.

CASE ILLUSTRATION 7-8

Example 1

Tony, a licensed professional counselor with minimal experience, is quite shy in his personal life and becomes very nervous around women. He has determined his nervousness and anxiety do not affect his professional practice except in rare situations. He traditionally accepts both male and female clients. When meeting with female clients, he can usually tell after the first session if he will become too nervous or anxious to work with them effectively. If he does find himself becoming overly nervous, he simply refers those clients out to another therapist and bases his decision on his incompetence.

Example 2

Tanya works as a professional counselor in a private practice. She has 10 years of experience and likes to describe the population she works with as "those with normal, everyday concerns." After meeting with a new client, she realized the client participates in non-suicidal self-injury (NSSI) and has some past history with disordered eating. Tanya had one class in her graduate studies related to eating disorders but nothing additional. She feels incompetent to work with this client and therefor refers out.

Example 3

Logan is a professional counselor, and his new client originally reported seeking services for intimacy issues. However, after several sessions Logan's client confided in him the intimacy issues with her husband are mainly due to her lack of interest in her husband. Instead, she finds herself fantasizing about young boys. The client assures Logan she knows this is morally wrong and would never act on her fantasies; she simply wants help to address her thoughts. Logan consults with his supervisor and divulges that he is truly disgusted by his client's fantasies. Logan wants to refer his client out to someone else. During the consultation, Logan's supervisor questions him about imposing his values. Logan acknowledges his supervisor's concerns but then claims he has no training in working with child molesters or sexual deviants and feels as though he is incompetent to work with this client.

Example 4

Sachin is a professional counselor working in an agency setting. He has met with his client for several weeks related to self-esteem issues. Today his client has brought his partner with him to session and asks if Sachin would be willing to work with both of them as a couple. Sachin

(Continued)

> (Continued)
>
> feels a bit uncomfortable because he has never done couples counseling before. He shares his lack of experience with his client and says he would feel irresponsible and unethical if he were to meet with them as a couple as he lacks the knowledge and experience. Sachin offers to provide the couple with a referral to someone with more experience in couples counseling and also offers to keep meeting with his client individually if his client wishes to do so.
>
> *In which of these examples might the counselor be acting ethically, and in which might they be acting in an unethical manner?*

The first example provided in Case Illustration 7-8 involves Tony, who becomes very shy and nervous around certain women. When Tony senses himself becoming overly shy around a client, he refers the client out as a way to prevent his shyness from interfering with his clinical effectiveness. While Tony's self-awareness and ability to recognize his own nervousness is commendable, his actions would likely be considered unethical. Tony's shyness and nervousness are issues he must learn to overcome.

The second example concerns Tanya's work with clients who participate in NSSI. Tanya is acting ethically in referring her client who participates in self-injurious behaviors. Tanya has limited training in working with her client's specific issues. NSSI is a clinical concern rather than a value.

In Example 3 Logan is likely acting in an unethical manner. His comment about not having "experience working with child molesters or sexual deviants" reveals his strong feelings about his client's thoughts. Logan is unable to put his own morals, values, and beliefs aside and lacks unconditional positive regard for his client. Instead he is judging his client's thoughts. Logan's judgmental attitude is a value conflict rather than a clinical competency issue.

In the fourth example Sachin is likely acting ethically by offering to refer his client and client's partner to another counselor. If Sachin is inexperienced in providing couples counseling, it would be unethical for him to provide couples counseling.

Credentials

There are numerous licensures, certifications, and titles professional counselors hold. Additionally, there are many terms used to describe mental health workers (e.g., therapist, counselor, psychotherapist, mental health counselor, shrink, psychoanalyst, etc.). Counselors in training often ask what they are able to call themselves and which terms are acceptable to use. According to the ACA Code of Ethics (2014) there is not one specific term to use. The primary requirement is that professional counselors are honest and forthcoming about their licensure, education background, and professional membership.

ACA Standard C.4.a. (2014) Accurate Representation: Counselors claim or imply only professional qualifications actually completed and correct any known misrepresentations of their qualifications by others. Counselors truthfully represent the qualifications of their professional colleagues. Counselors clearly distinguish between paid and volunteer work experience and accurately describe their continuing education and specialized training.

Review Case Illustration 7-9 related to Ethical Standard C.4.a., and see how Dawn handles a potentially awkward situation.

CASE ILLUSTRATION 7-9

Dawn is a master's-level professional counselor, holds a license, and typically works with a wide range of clients at her private practice. Knowing Dawn is a counselor and is highly thought of in her faith community, Dawn's pastor has asked her to speak about effective communication strategies at a couple's retreat the church has scheduled. At the retreat, the pastor introduces Dawn as a "marriage and family therapist" and an "expert in helping couples communicate with each other."

What should Dawn do?

In Case Illustration 7-9, it is Dawn's responsibility to correct the pastor's introduction and correctly identify her licensure and qualifications. Throughout counselors' careers they will have interactions with individuals with varying degrees of understanding of the mental health professions and professional counseling. According to Standard C.4.a. professional counselors have a duty to educate others about the counseling profession. When counselors are misrepresented it is the counselor's responsibility to correct the misrepresentation.

ACA Standard C.4.b. (2014) Credentials: Counselors claim only licenses or certifications that are current and in good standing.

Ethical Standard C.4.b. is very similar to Standard C.4.a. Both relate to counselors accurately representing credentials. However, Standard C.4.b. is more specific by prohibiting counselors from claiming licensures or certifications not kept current and in good standing. In Case Illustration 7-10, Emily makes a questionable decision when applying for a new position.

CASE ILLUSTRATION 7-10

Emily is a doctoral-level counselor and has been a counselor supervisor in the past; however, due to her current job responsibilities, she has not kept her supervisory status with her state licensure board current. Today, Emily's administrative supervisor has notified her of a new

(Continued)

(Continued)

position opening as a counselor supervisor. The administrator, not knowing Emily has let her supervisory status lapse, encourages Emily to submit her application. Emily agrees and submits her application and résumé, claiming to be a state-approved counselor supervisor. Emily's rationale is that she has the education and experience requirements to renew her supervisory status. She will submit the necessary paperwork and be officially credentialed as a supervisor and be fully credentialed again before anyone ever knows she let it lapse.

Did Emily act ethically?

In Case Illustration 7-10, Emily did not act ethically. Instead, Emily should have mentioned to her administrative supervisor that her supervisory credential was not current and she would need to update her status prior to applying. Emily was not transparent about her credentials and therefore was not in compliance with the ACA Code of Ethics (2014).

ACA Standard C.4.c. (2014) Educational Degrees: Counselors clearly differentiate between earned and honorary degrees.

ACA Standard C.4.d. (2014) Implying Doctoral-Level Competence: Counselors clearly state their highest earned degree in counseling or a closely related field. Counselors do not imply doctoral-level competence when possessing a master's degree in counseling or related field.

Ethical Standards C.4.c. and C.4.d. are quite similar to previous standards discussed. The primary difference being Standards C.4.c. and C.4.d. require counselors to be fully transparent about educational degrees instead of credentialing. Review Case Illustration 7-11 to see how these two standards may apply to actual situations.

CASE ILLUSTRATION 7-11

Mike is a master's-level professional counselor and works primarily with adolescents and young adults. Today, Mike is working with a new client and meeting with both the parent and child for the intake session. During the intake session, Mike continually hears his client's parent refer to him as Dr. Mike (e.g., This is Dr. Mike. I want you to talk to him and tell him what you have been feeling. We're going to come and visit Dr. Mike every week, and he will be someone you can trust and talk to about your problems).

What should Mike do?

In Case Illustration 7-11, it is critical Mike reiterate to the client (and parent) that he is not a doctoral-level practitioner. However, it is also important Mike keep in mind how he may want to word his clarification so as to avoid having it turn into a potentially awkward situation where he is correcting the parent in front of the child.

ACA Standard C.4.e. (2014) Accreditation Status: Counselors accurately represent the accreditation status of their degree program and college or university.

When applying for employment or listing their educational degree in other situations, counselors are honest and forthright about the accreditation status of their educational institution (e.g., CACREP-accredited program or non-CACREP-accredited program).

ACA Standard C.4.f. (2014) Professional Memberships: Counselors clearly differenti-ate between current, active memberships and former memberships in associations. Members of ACA must clearly differentiate between professional membership, which implies the possession of at least a master's degree in counseling, and regular membership, which is open to individuals whose interests and activities are consistent with those of ACA but are not qualified for professional membership.

Simply stated, professional counselors and others who are members of professional organizations are honest about their membership status and their affiliations to profes-sional organizations.

Conclusion

Counseling is a profession and therefore counselors must have knowledge and skills to behave professionally throughout every aspect of their daily activities. Chapter 7 reviews counselors' ethical responsibilities related to being a professional. Chapter 7 also includes areas specifically emphasized in the 2014 ACA Code of Ethics, for example, values and counselor transparency regarding credentialing and educational background. An emphasis on values can be seen in ethical standards related to making referrals. Similarly, transparency in educational training and credentialing is addressed in multiple standards. Throughout Chapter 7 the authors discussed the importance of being compe-tent in providing services, setting appropriate and consistent fee structures, making appropriate referrals, and representing oneself accurately, among other topics. Using your knowledge gained in Chapter 7, please address the ethical dilemma and discussion questions presented in Exercise 7-1.

EXERCISE 7-1

Rick is a master's student and is one semester away from graduating with his master's degree in clinical mental health counseling. While in school, Rick has been able to find a full-time job closely related to his professional interest, and although it doesn't pay much, the job is accom-modating to his school schedule. Rick feels lucky to be able work at the local courthouse where he was hired by a justice of the peace as a "truancy case manager." He works with the judge to help truant students get back into school and be successful. Rick likes his job and generally

(Continued)

(Continued)

gets along with everyone. Recently, Rick has been asked to work with another of the judge's colleagues (Dr. S.) who facilitates "parenting groups" for the parents of truants who come into the courtroom. As part of their court order, the judge typically directs the truants and their parents to attend two to three parenting groups. The judge introduces the truants and parents to Dr. S., who the judge describes as "an expert in understanding family relationships."

Over the course of the next few weeks, Rick goes to the parenting groups and is able to talk more with Dr. S. Rick sees his interactions with Dr. S. as a way to learn from someone who has been in the counseling field and who has expertise in the area Rick wishes to work.

However, Rick is a bit surprised when he asks Dr. S. about his background and learns Dr. S. is a retired podiatrist. Dr. S. says, "When I retired from my practice as a podiatrist, I became interested in helping families, and this is a perfect way for me to give back to the community. Rick is also a bit concerned when he learns about the curriculum and corresponding games Dr. S. has created and uses as the primary focus of the parenting groups. Dr. S. recommends all parents purchase one or more of the games ($10 each) used during the groups and reminds parents about how using the games and curriculum even after the groups have concluded will be viewed favorably by the judge and will likely result in leniency on the judge's behalf.

Feeling as though he is caught in a dilemma, Rick schedules a time to talk with his supervisor. Rick explains the situation but also discusses his fear of losing his job. Rick describes the judge and Dr. S. as being very good friends, and Rick does not want to be viewed as "not a team player." Rick also knows the judge created this position specifically for Rick as a favor, and saying something may cause him to lose his job.

What do you believe Rick should do in this situation?

What are the potential pros and cons of Rick's decision (however he chooses to act)?

Use an ethical decision-making model to determine how you might act if you were in Rick's situation.

Keystones

- To provide competent counseling services, counselors must have an in-depth understanding of their chosen theory.
- Culture affects how clients understand problems and therefore must be considered in diagnosis.
- Counselors are able to refrain from diagnosis when it may cause harm to clients.
- Counselors must respect different approaches to counseling when they are grounded in theory.
- Ethical counselors form relationships with professionals from other disciplines to better serve clients.

- When counselors participate on interdisciplinary teams, they are focused on providing quality services to clients and are transparent with team members about ethical obligations.
- When counselors accept employment they are accepting the policies and principles of their employers.
- Counselors do not participate in or condone harassment of colleagues for acting in an ethical manner.
- When advertising, counselors are truthful and avoid deception.
- Counselors are prohibited from referring current or prospective clients based on value conflicts.
- Counselors are truthful and transparent about credentials and educational training.

Additional Resources

Atinga, R. A., Abekah-Nkrumah, G., & Domfeh, K. A. (2011). Managing healthcare quality in Ghana: A necessity of patient satisfaction. *International Journal of Health Care Quality Assurance, 24*(7) 548–563.

Bennett-Levy, J. (2006). Therapist skills: A cognitive model of their acquisition and refinement. *Behavioural and Cognitive Psychotherapy, 34*, 57–78. doi:10.1017/S1352465805002420.

Chung, R. C. Y., Bemak, F., Ortiz, D. P., & Sandoval-Perez, P. A. (2008). Promoting the mental health of immigrants: A multicultural/social justice perspective. *Journal of Counseling & Development, 86*, 310–317. doi:10.1002/j.1556-6678.2008.tb00514.x

Colburn, A. A. N. (2013). Endless possibilities: Diversifying service options in private practice. *Journal of Mental Health Counseling, 35*(3), 198–210. Retrieved from http://search.proquest.com/docview/1404761162?accountid=7122

Eriksen, K., & Kress, V. E. (2006). The DSM and the professional counseling identity: Bridging the gap. *Journal of Mental Health Counseling, 28*(3), 202–217. Retrieved from http://search.proquest.com/docview/198712395?accountid=7122

Glosoff, H. L., Corey, G., & Herlihy, B. (2006). Avoiding detrimental multiple relationships. In B. Herlihy & G. Corey (Eds.), *ACA ethical standards casebook* (6th ed., pp. 209–215). Alexandria, VA: American Counseling Association.

Gonyea, J. L. J., Wright, D. W., & Earl-Kulkosky, T. (2014). Navigating dual relationships in rural communities. *Journal of Marital and Family Therapy, 40*(1), 125–136. doi:http://dx.doi.org/10.1111/j.1752-0606.2012.00335.x

Ivey, A. E., & Ivey, M. B. (1998). Reframing *DSM-IV*: Positive strategies from developmental counseling and therapy. *Journal of Counseling & Development, 76*, 334–350. doi:10.1002/j.1556-6676.1998.tb02550.x

Kress, V. E., & Shoffner, M. F. (2007). Focus groups: A practical and applied research approach for counselors. *Journal of Counseling & Development, 85*, 189–195. doi:10.1002/j.1556-6678.2007.tb00462.x

Stumbo, N. J., & Carter, M. J. (1999). National therapeutic recreation curriculum study. Part A. Accreditation, curriculum and internship characteristics. *Therapeutic Recreation Journal First, 33*(1), 46–60.

Ward v. Wilbanks, No. 10-2100, Doc. 006110869854 (6th Cir. Court of Appeals, Feb. 11, 2011). Retrieved from http://www.counseling.org/resources/pdfs/EMUamicusbrief.pdf

Wilcoxon, S. A., Magnuson, S., & Norem, K. (2008). Institutional values of managed mental health care: Efficiency or oppression? *Journal of Multicultural Counseling and Development, 36,* 143–154.

References

American Association for Marriage and Family Therapy. (2015). *Code of ethics.* Retrieved from https://www.aamft.org/iMIS15/AAMFT/Content/legal_ethics/code_of_ethics.aspx

American Counseling Association. (2014). *Code of ethics.* Alexandria, VA: Author.

American Psychological Association. (2010). *American Psychological Association ethical principles of psychologists and code of conduct.* Retrieved from http://www.apa.org/ethics/code/principles .pdf

Corey, G., Corey, M. S., & Callanan, P. (2011). *Issues and ethics in the helping professions* (8th ed.). Belmont, CA: Brooks/Cole Cengage Learning.

Cottone, R. R., & Tarvydas, V. M. (2007). *Counseling ethics and decision making* (3rd ed.). Upper Saddle River, NJ: Pearson Merrill Prentice-Hall.

Council for Accreditation of Counseling and Related Educational Programs. (2009). *CACREP: The 2009 standards* [*statement*]. Alexandria, VA: Author.

Ford, G. G. (2006). *Ethical reasoning for mental health professionals.* Thousand Oaks, CA: Sage.

Remley, T. P., & Herlihy, B. (2014). *Ethical, legal, and professional issues in counseling* (4th ed.). Upper Saddle River, NJ: Pearson.

Welfel, E. R., & Patterson, L. E. (2004). *The counseling process* (6th ed.). Pacific Grove, CA: Brooks/ Cole.

8

Appropriate Boundaries and Multiple Relationships

There's always room for improvement; it's the biggest room in the house.

—Louise Heath Lebor

Boundaries and multiple relationships can be one of the more difficult areas for students to understand. Students often tend to make very gray areas into black and white or right and wrong. Every student knows not to have sex with his/her clients, but what about seeing clients in public and unforeseen social interactions? Chapter 8 will discuss issues such as the one aforementioned, when counselors find themselves sexually attracted to clients and when clients may be attracted to you as a counselor. Finally, the authors will cover giving and receiving of gifts. Again, this tends to be an area that is easy to talk about but more difficult when actually putting the behaviors into action. Throughout Chapter 8 ethical dilemmas and case illustrations will focus on students understanding how they react to these situations and how their reactions may affect the counseling relationship with clients. At the conclusion of Chapter 8, readers will specifically be able to do the following:

1. Discuss the importance of maintaining appropriate and consistent boundaries with clients.

2. Discuss the importance of documenting all boundary extensions with clients.

3. Explain how to handle sexual attraction both toward a client and from a client.

4. Name ethical standards related to relationships with former clients.

5. List ethical requirements related to counseling friends and family members.

6. Define ethical obligations concerning the giving and receiving of gifts.

7. Define ethical standards related to bartering with clients.

Maintaining Boundaries With Clients

Boundaries and maintaining the delicate balance between appropriate and inappropriate relationships with clients was identified in *Counseling Today* as one of the five most common ethical concerns (Meyers, 2014). Due to the nature of the profession, counselors are routinely involved in intimate conversations. Correspondingly, counselors are typically trained to be empathetic listeners who take great care in being attentive to their clients' trepidations. It is no wonder professional relationships may have a propensity to wander past what may be considered ethical or appropriate and become unethical or inappropriate. Boundary crossings and violations happen in the most subtle ways and are difficult to recognize, and many professionals do not even agree on what may be considered appropriate or inappropriate (Remley & Herlihy, 2014). Therefore counselor self-awareness is essential to prevent inappropriate and possibly harmful relationships from developing. Consider Case Illustration 8-1 and how Arturo tries to "promote the well-being" of his client Reid.

CASE ILLUSTRATION 8-1

Arturo, a 56-year-old professional counselor, works for a nonprofit counseling agency and primarily works with low-income families who are unable to afford other mental health services. Arturo has been working with Reid, a 23-year-old male who sought out counseling services to help him manage the stress and anxiety that started after he enrolled in college. Arturo learns Reid's parents kicked him out of the house when he was 18 after learning Reid's girlfriend was pregnant. For the past five years, Reid has struggled to provide for his girlfriend and daughter by working long hours at minimum-wage jobs. Reid decided to enroll in college as a way to further his education and land a higher-paying job. Although Reid is excited about college, he feels extreme stress due to the financial burden his schooling places on his family. Arturo and Reid have built a very strong relationship, and Arturo enjoys working with Reid since Reid reminds Arturo a little of himself. Arturo feels a special obligation to Reid because Arturo knows he would not be in the place he is today without the help of others when he was struggling.

Reid arrives about 30 minutes late for session today, is out of breath, and seems overly frustrated. After a brief discussion, Arturo learns Reid's car, which has had many mechanical failures lately, ran out of gas on the way to session. Reid is frustrated because of having to walk in the heat but also because he has a final exam for school right after his counseling session and fears he will fail because he probably won't be able to get there on time. Additionally, Reid is overwhelmed by the financial stressors his car is causing lately and his end-of-month bills. Reid expresses concern that he won't be able to buy food for his family until he gets paid in two days.

Knowing this is his last session of the day, Arturo tells Reid, "Come on, I will take you to your test, and we can have the rest of our session in the car." Reid is somewhat hesitant, but trusts Arturo, and is relieved he will get to his final exam. Arturo stops by a gas station, buys gas, and then drives Reid to his car to fill it up. Arturo then pulls $100 from his wallet and gives it to Reid. He says, "Take this, so you don't have to worry about food for the next couple days. I want you to do well on your final, and you don't need to be worrying about feeding your family." When Reid tries to refuse, Arturo convinces him to take it, saying, "Consider this just a gift from a friend. We all need friends to help us out every so often."

Did Arturo act in an ethical manner by helping his client in such a way?

In Case Illustration 8-1, Arturo sees some of himself in his client, Reid, and wants to help. Arturo feels a responsibility to pay it forward because others helped him in the past when he was struggling. Furthermore, Arturo knows Reid is struggling financially and wants to help him be successful and further his education. As a result, Arturo gives Reid a ride to his car, buys him gas, and even gives him cash out of his own wallet to help pay for food until the end of the month. In determining the ethicality of Arturo's actions, the ACA Code of Ethics (2014) offers some guidance, although there are no standards specifically addressing Arturo's situation. In response to the question posed in Case Illustration 8-1, Arturo's actions would most likely be seen as inappropriate primarily due to the manner in which Arturo acted and not necessarily his actions. The most appropriate ethical standards related to Case Illustration 8-1 are the following.

ACA Standard A.6.b. (2014) Extending Counseling Boundaries: Counselors consider the risks and benefits of extending current counseling relationships beyond conventional parameters. Examples include attending a client's formal ceremony (e.g., a wedding or commitment ceremony or graduation), purchasing a service or product provided by a client (excepting unrestricted bartering), and visiting a client's ill family member in the hospital. In extending these boundaries, counselors take appropriate professional precautions such as informed consent, consultation, supervision, and documentation to ensure that judgment is not impaired and no harm occurs.

ACA Standard A.6.c. (2014) Documenting Boundary Extensions: If counselors extend boundaries as described in A.6.a. and A.6.b., they must officially document, prior to the interaction (when feasible), the rationale for such an interaction, the potential benefit, and anticipated consequences for the client or former client and other individuals significantly involved with the client or former client. When unintentional harm occurs to the client or former client, or to an individual significantly involved with the client or former client, the counselor must show evidence of an attempt to remedy such harm.

Both these standards express the importance of documenting the counselor's decision-making process and actions taken.

In Case Illustration 8-1, Arturo did not have the luxury of an extended time period to make his decision (if he is going to act). Therefore, Arturo was forced to move through an ethical decision-making process rather quickly (as discussed in Chapter 3) and be sure to address certain questions. For example, Arturo would have wanted to reflect on the following questions:

Is his judgment impaired due the countertransference he has with Reid?

What is the motivation for helping Reid?

What would it be like for Reid to have his counselor buy him gas and give him money?

Is the $100 a gift or a loan?

What are the potential consequences of giving Reid a ride to his car? Buying him gas? Giving him cash to help pay his bills?

In addition to asking these questions of himself, Arturo would want to have a discussion with Reid (before taking any action) to include Reid in the decision-making process. See the following example as a possible conversation between Arturo and Reid.

Arturo: *Reid, as you're talking about all of this going on, I'm feeling an urge to want to help you out. I'm wondering what you would think about us finishing this session in the car. I can take you to get some gas and then to your car, so you can get to your final exam on time.*

Reid: *(Reid would either express appreciation and willingness or would express discomfort and unwillingness.)*

Arturo: *Reid, I know you are struggling with bills this month, and I can't help long term, but think I may be able to help you out today. Would it be alright with you if I gave you a few dollars to help out with food for the rest of the month? This would be a gift (or loan).*

Reid: *(Reid would agree or disagree.)*

In situations like Arturo's and others, where there is no direct guidance from the code of ethics or law, a decision-making process is critical in determining how to act in the best interest of the client.

Social Relationships With Clients

In previous versions of the ACA Code of Ethics, terms such as "dual relationships" (ACA, 1995) and "potentially beneficial interactions" (ACA, 2005) were used when discussing social relationships between counselors and clients. In its most current form, the ACA Code of Ethics uses "extending counseling boundaries" when discussing interactions between counselors and clients outside of the professional relationship. The APA and AAMFT use terms like "multiple relationships." See Text Box 8-1 for more information. When professional counselors are faced with a situation potentially extending counseling boundaries, they are required to first "consider the risks and benefits of extending current counseling relationships beyond conventional parameters" and "take appropriate professional precautions such as informed consent, consultation, supervision, and documentation to ensure that judgment is not impaired and no harm occurs" (ACA, 2014, p. 5). If professional counselors choose to act and extend the boundaries of the relationship, after considering all the potential risks and benefits, they must document their decision (i.e., rationale for extending boundaries, potential benefits, and potential consequences) (ACA, 2014).

As with all ethical dilemmas, there is a continuum, and some situations may be easier to navigate than others (e.g., going out to a have drinks with a client after session would likely be viewed as inappropriate by most professional counselors). However, in situations where there is not as clear of an answer, the question remains: How do counselors know if extending the boundaries of the counseling relationship is appropriate?

The simple answer is that it depends. As noted, the ACA Code of Ethics requires professional counselors to consider the benefits, consequences, and the rationale for acting. Once those factors are considered, it is the counselor's responsibility (along with the client) to make a decision on the best course of action. Consider Case Illustration 8-2 in which Dawn struggles with whether to buy Girl Scout cookies from her students.

CASE ILLUSTRATION 8-2

The Case of Dawn

Dawn is a school counselor working at an elementary school. Each spring, several of the students in her school ask her to purchase Girl Scout cookies to support their troop. Dawn always wonders if it is appropriate for her to purchase cookies from her students or if it is considered an inappropriate boundary extension. Dawn, like most everyone else, looks forward to buying Girl Scout cookies each year and would ideally like to support the students at her school. Nevertheless, she has always declined buying any from her students due to her concern about the appropriateness of her actions.

Would it be ethical for Dawn to order Girl Scout cookies from her students?

In Case Illustration 8-2, Dawn may seem like she is being overconcerned or overcautious about her decision to buy cookies or not. However, there may be some unanticipated ethical concerns if she does not fully consider her actions. Before making her decision, Dawn would want to follow the ACA Code of Ethics and consider her rationale, any potential benefits, and potential consequences of her decision. Review the following example.

Rationale

It's important for Dawn to understand why she may or may not want to buy cookies from these students. Dawn must understand her motivation.

Why does she want to buy cookies from her students at school?

Is the student asking her one of her "favorites" in the school?

Does Dawn have current or past experience with the Girl Scouts and feel strongly about supporting the program?

Potential Benefits

What, if any, are the potential benefits to Dawn buying Girl Scout cookies?

How might buying cookies potentially benefit this student (e.g., Is this a student who has a history of extreme shyness? Will buying these cookies possibly encourage the student to be more assertive and outgoing?)?

Potential Consequences

What, if any, are the potential consequences?

How might buying cookies have negative effects?

In addition to thinking about these questions, it's critical for Dawn to document her reasons. Additionally, the authors encourage counselors to explore other questions. If Dawn is going to buy cookies from one student, is she willing to buy fund-raising items from every student who comes and asks her to support his/her program? In Chapter 1 the authors discussed the principle of justice or being fair and consistent with all clients. If Dawn does not support fundraising efforts of all students, is she acting with justice in mind?

Case Illustration 8-3 offers another example of the need for counselors to consider various factors when determining the ethicality of extending counseling boundaries. Consider how Mickey responds to his clients' invitation to attend their recommitment ceremony.

CASE ILLUSTRATION 8-3

The Case of Mickey

Mickey is a couple's counselor and has been working with the Smiths for several months. The Smiths have made tremendous progress and attribute much of it to their sessions with Mickey. As a result they have asked Mickey if he would honor them by attending their recommitment

> ceremony at which the couple will renew their vows to each other. The ceremony will be a small gathering (15–30 people) of those who have played significant roles in the Smiths' lives.
>
> *Would it be an appropriate boundary extension for Mickey to attend the ceremony?*

Case Illustration 8-3 again examines the ethicality of extending counseling boundaries, and in this scenario Mickey must determine whether he should attend the recommitment ceremony of his clients. When counselors are invited to social events, they have the choice to attend or not attend. In many cases the event may be one in which the counselor is excited about or looking forward to attending. In other cases, the invitation may be to an event that the counselor would not like to attend, depending on the counselor's own interests and hobbies. Whichever the case, counselors must engage in an ethical decision-making process. Related to Case Illustration 8-3, Mickey must consider the potential benefits and consequences of attending the ceremony. He must also consider the potential benefits and consequences of declining the invitation (e.g., if he declines, how might it affect the relationship he has with his clients). Whichever route Mickey chooses, it is important for him to have a thorough discussion with his client(s) prior to taking any action.

Smiths: Mickey, over the past few months, we have made many changes in our relationship, and we are going to celebrate our progress with a recommitment ceremony renewing our vows to each other. Because you have been such a great inspiration and big part of our success, we would like you to be there to celebrate with us. Will you please come and celebrate with us?

Mickey: I really appreciate your asking, and I would love to attend, but before I say yes or no, I believe it's important we talk about it a bit more.

Smiths: Sure, what would you like to talk about?

Mickey: Well, going back to our first session when we went over confidentiality, I let you know that I always want to respect your privacy. Going to this party, how might the privacy of your counseling possibly be broken? Additionally, I imagine in interacting with other people at the ceremony, some might ask how I know the two of you. How would you like me to identify myself if I am asked?

After making his decision, Mickey would want to be sure to document his ethical decision-making process. Case Illustrations 8-2 and 8-3 examined extending counseling boundaries in situations where the counselor was invited to purchase cookies and attend a recommitment ceremony. In both situations the counselor was able to choose if he/she wanted to extend counseling boundaries. In some occasions counselors happen to interact with clients outside the traditional relationship without choosing to do so. Consider Case Illustration 8-4 and how Anthony handles an interaction with his client while working out at the gym.

CASE ILLUSTRATION 8-4

Antonio, a professional counselor, works with a wide variety of clients. In his time away from the office, Antonio enjoys activities with his family and exercising at the community gym. He lifts weights as a way to relieve stress and also enjoys the friendships he has developed with others at the gym. Because he is typically there five or six times a week, Antonio also knows the staff and employees at the gym quite well. While working out one day, Antonio noticed a familiar face as he moved from one machine to another. Shelby, one of Antonio's newer clients noticed Antonio and walked over to him to say hi. She was excited to see him and shook his hand, expressing her excitement in seeing a familiar face at the gym. Antonio said hi but was limited in his conversation. He felt a bit awkward seeing one of his clients in public and was not sure how to handle the interaction. Therefore he let Shelby know he was in a bit of a hurry and did not have much time to talk. Antonio cut his workout short and went home as a way to get out of the awkward situation.

At her next session, Shelby again mentioned how great it was to see Antonio at the gym. She also began to question Antonio more about his exercise habits and the times he typically works out. She said it's always nice to work out when there is a friendly face in the room. Shelby also pointed out there are often many open offices at the gym and inquires as to whether they may be able to reserve one and have her counseling sessions there. Because Antonio did not want to create another awkward situation and because he is very comfortable with the employees at the gym and the space overall, Antonio agrees to Shelby's proposal. Antonio calls the gym each week to reserve a vacant office for him and Shelby to meet. After their session is over, both go out, complete their workouts, and then continue on with their days.

Did Antonio act in an ethical manner?

In Case Illustration 8-4, Antonio is approached by one of his clients while working out at the gym. The client then inquires as to whether counseling sessions can be held at the gym on a weekly basis as both individuals are there anyway (i.e., a convenient way to save both of them time and travel). At first glance, many counselors might have a strong negative reaction, believing Antonio to be highly unethical for even considering the idea. Still, it is always critical to engage in an ethical decision-making process to determine the ethicality of actions. According to Ethical Standards A.6.b. and A.6.c., Antonio would need to consult with others to determine if his judgment was impaired, consider all potential benefits and consequences of meeting at the gym, and document his entire decision-making process. Although meeting at the gym may not be every counselor's preferred way to conduct sessions, it may be ethical in this situation.

TEXT BOX 8-1

American Psychological Association

The APA uses the term "multiple relationships" to address relationships outside of the therapeutic relationship between psychologists and clients. "Multiple relationships" are described in Standard 3.05.

APA Standard 3.05 (2010) Multiple Relationships: (a) A multiple relationship occurs when a psychologist is in a professional role with a person and (1) at the same time is in another role with the same person, (2) at the same time is in a relationship with a person closely associated with or related to the person with whom the psychologist has the professional relationship, or (3) promises to enter into another relationship in the future with the person or a person closely associated with or related to the person.

A psychologist refrains from entering into a multiple relationship if the multiple relationship could reasonably be expected to impair the psychologist's objectivity, competence, or effectiveness in performing his or her functions as a psychologist or otherwise risks exploitation or harm to the person with whom the professional relationship exists.

Multiple relationships that would not reasonably be expected to cause impairment or risk exploitation or harm are not unethical.

(b) If a psychologist finds that, due to unforeseen factors, a potentially harmful multiple relationship has arisen, the psychologist takes reasonable steps to resolve it with due regard for the best interests of the affected person and maximal compliance with the ethics code.

(c) When psychologists are required by law, institutional policy, or extraordinary circumstances to serve in more than one role in judicial or administrative proceedings, at the outset they clarify role expectations and the extent of confidentiality and thereafter as changes occur.

American Association for Marriage and Family Therapists

The AAMFT uses similar terminology to that of the APA and describes "multiple relationships" in Standard 1.3.

AAMFT Standard 1.3 (2015) Multiple Relationships: Marriage and family therapists are aware of their influential positions with respect to clients, and they avoid exploiting the trust and dependency of such persons. Therapists, therefore, make every effort to avoid conditions and multiple relationships with clients that could impair professional judgment or increase the risk of exploitation. Such relationships include, but are not limited to, business or close personal relationships with a client or the client's immediate family. When the risk of impairment or exploitation exists due to conditions or multiple roles, therapists document the appropriate precautions taken.

Sexual Attraction to Clients

There is no doubt a counselor will find a client sexually attractive at some point during his/her career, and according to Pope, Keith-Spiegel, and Tabachnick (1986), sexual feelings occur in both male and female therapists. Considering the nature of the counseling relationship, there is no wonder attractions occur. The authors argue that people generally tend to be attracted to those who meet the following criteria:

They find them to be physically attractive → *There will be clients who find their counselors physically attractive.*

They are good listeners → *Counselors are trained to be good listeners.*

They pay attention → *Counselors are trained to be attentive to their clients.*

They care for them → *Counselors are trained to be empathetic to clients.*

Similar to clients being attracted to counselors, the opposite is also true. Professional counselors will find themselves attracted to some clients. Counselors are human. As such, they have ups and downs in their own relationships; they have a need to feel wanted and feel important. Comparable to their clients, counselors may be attracted to clients due to the following reasons:

They find them to be physically attractive → *There will be clients counselors find physically attractive.*

They make them feel important → *Clients often look up to counselors as experts.*

They share similar interests → *Counselors will have clients with whom they have similar hobbies or interests.*

They feel as though they connect with them → *Counselors will have clients they feel a certain connection with (e.g., those who have a similar past or have endured similar hardships or life situations).*

Understanding these attractions may and often do occur, the ACA Code of Ethics (2014) and most state laws are very clear (as are the APA and AAMFT—see Text Box 8-2 and Text Box 8-3).

ACA Standard A.5.a. (2014) Sexual and/or Romantic Relationships Prohibited: Sexual and/or romantic counselor/client interactions or relationships with current clients, their romantic partners, or their family members are prohibited. This prohibition applies to both in-person and electronic interactions or relationships.

Simply stated, professional counselors are ethically and legally prohibited from having sexual or romantic relationships with clients.

Similar to ACA Standard A.5.a. (Sexual and/or Romantic Relationships Prohibited), there are other standards that address sexual and romantic relationships with clients and past clients.

ACA Standard A.5.b. (2014) Previous Sexual and/or Romantic Relationship: Counselors are prohibited from engaging in counseling relationships with persons with whom they have had a previous sexual and/or romantic relationship.

TEXT BOX 8-2

Sexual relationships with current clients and engaging in therapeutic relationships with individuals with whom one has had previous sexual or intimate relationships is prohibited by both the APA and AAMFT.

American Psychological Association

APA Standard 10.05 (2010) Sexual Intimacies With Current Therapy Clients or Patients: Psychologists do not engage in sexual intimacies with current therapy clients or patients.

APA Standard 10.07 (2010) Therapy With Former Sexual Partners: Psychologists do not accept as therapy clients or patients persons with whom they have engaged in sexual intimacies.

American Association for Marriage and Family Therapists

AAMFT Standard 1.4 (2015) Sexual Intimacy With Current Clients and Others: Sexual intimacy with current clients or with known members of the client's family system is prohibited.

Counselors are prohibited from counseling those with whom they have previously been sexually or romantically involved. Consider Case Illustration 8-5 and how Sasha handles a request for counseling from someone with whom she was in a previous relationship.

CASE ILLUSTRATION 8-5

Sasha is a professional counselor who dated Shane approximately six years ago. The couple broke up as both seemed to lose interest in each other and have not talked much since they ended their relationship. Shane, going through a recent traumatic event, called Sasha's office today to set up an intake appointment.

What would be the best course of action for Sasha in this situation?

In Case Illustration 8-5, it is Sasha's responsibility to listen and acknowledge Shane's request for services. It is also Sasha's responsibility to explain to Shane that it would be considered unethical for her to engage in a counseling relationship with Shane due to their past history (i.e., "Shane, I understand your wanting counseling considering all you have been through lately, and I'm honored you thought of me. However, it would be unethical of me to enter into a counseling relationship with you considering our past history."). Additionally, Sasha would want to provide Shane with some referrals to best help him receive the help he is seeking (i.e., "Shane, although I'm not able to be your counselor, these are few other counselors in the area who may be able to provide what you are looking for.").

ACA Standard A.5.c. (2014) Sexual and/or Romantic Relationships With Former Clients: Sexual and/or romantic counselor/client interactions or relationships with former clients, their romantic partners, or their family members are prohibited for a period of five years following the last professional contact. This prohibition applies to both in-person and electronic interactions or relationships. Counselors, before engaging in sexual and/or romantic interactions or relationships with former clients, their romantic partners, or their family members, demonstrate forethought and document (in written form) whether the interaction or relationship can be viewed as exploitive in any way and/or whether there is still potential to harm the former client; in cases of potential exploitation and/or harm, the counselor avoids entering into such an interaction or relationship.

TEXT BOX 8-3

Each professional association addresses sexual intimacies with former clients in different ways. The ACA requires counselors to avoid such relationships for a minimum of five years, the APA shortens the waiting period to two years, and the AAMFT prohibits relationships with former clients completely.

American Psychological Association

APA Standard 10.08 (2010) Sexual Intimacies With Former Therapy Clients or Patients: (a) Psychologists do not engage in sexual intimacies with former clients or patients for at least two years after cessation or termination of therapy.

(b) Psychologists do not engage in sexual intimacies with former clients or patients even after a two-year interval except in the most unusual circumstances. Psychologists who engage in such activity after the two years following cessation or termination of therapy and of having no sexual contact with the former client or patient bear the burden of demonstrating that there has been no exploitation, in light of all relevant factors, including (1) the amount of time that has passed since therapy terminated; (2) the nature, duration, and intensity of the therapy; (3) the circumstances of termination; (4) the client's personal history; (5) the client's current mental status; (6) the likelihood of adverse impact on the client; and (7) any statement or actions made by the therapist during the course of therapy suggesting or inviting the possibility of a post-termination sexual or romantic relationship with the client.

American Association for Marriage and Family Therapists

AAMFT Standard 1.5 (2015) Sexual Intimacy With Former Clients and Others: Sexual intimacy with former clients or with known members of the client's family system is prohibited.

Sexual and/or romantic relationships with former clients, their family members, or their family members' romantic partners is prohibited for a period of five years following the last contact. However, before becoming involved with past clients, counselors engage in (and document) a thorough and thoughtful decision-making process. This process should examine how the involvement may be exploitive and whether the relationship has the potential to cause harm to the former client. If the relationship may be seen as exploitive or may cause harm, then it is the counselor's responsibility to avoid entering into the relationship. Review Manny's actions in Case Illustration 8-6 as he is careful to wait the minimal five years before pursuing a romantic relationship with his past client.

CASE ILLUSTRATION 8-6

Manny is a single recent graduate who is working on his licensure and certification hours at a local career counseling agency. At his apartment complex's holiday party, he recognizes one of his past clients (Adriana), who he had not known lived in his building. Adriana also notices Manny and approaches him to speak briefly about how much his services had been helpful. Manny thanks her and says he is glad he could help. The conversation is short, and Manny ends up leaving to visit with some other friends. Over the next few months, Manny sees Adriana on various occasions during his regular routines (i.e., checking mail, visiting the apartment pool, etc.). As a consequence Manny and Adriana's interactions become more frequent, and a natural, mutual attraction seems to take place. Manny understands his ethical obligation (nothing romantic or sexual for at least five years) and has consulted with several friends (outside of the counseling field). As a result, he decides to continue seeing Adriana but only as friends. Manny knows it has been almost four years since their last professional contact, so he will be "just friends" with Adriana until five years and then maybe try moving into a more official relationship with her. He rationalizes his decision based on the fact that Adriana was his client while he was doing his internship for his graduate degree (it isn't like he was a licensed counselor), and he remembers that she had very minimal concerns and was only a client of his for three sessions. Manny is hesitant to discuss the whole ethics thing with Adriana. He doesn't think it is a big deal and doesn't want to scare her off. Whenever the topic comes up, he just says he has been hurt in past relationships and wants to take things really slow for now.

What, if any, part of ACA Standard A.5.c. is Manny in compliance with?

What, if any, part of ACA Standard A.5.c. is Manny not in compliance with?

Manny's behaviors are questionable in Case Illustration 8-6. He is in compliance with the written words of the ACA Code of Ethics (2014). He has not entered into a romantic or sexual relationship with Adriana until the five-year requirement has passed. Nonetheless, on page three of the ACA Code of Ethics (2014), counselors are directed to act in a manner consistent with the "spirit as well as the letter" of ethical standards. While Manny is in compliance with the letter, he is not in compliance with the "the spirit" of the standard. Manny is not transparent and honest with Adriana and would most likely be guilty of not showing forethought prior to entering into the relationship.

ACA Standard A.5.d. (2014) Friends or Family Members: Counselors are prohibited from engaging in counseling relationships with friends or family members with whom they have an inability to remain objective.

As discussed many times previously, the ACA Code of Ethics (2014) gives some direction but leaves the ultimate decision up to the counselor and puts the responsibility on the counselor to make a thoughtful decision. Related to Standard A.5.d., most would likely agree that it would be unethical for a professional counselor to provide counseling to his/her sister, father, or best friend. However, determining the ethical appropriateness of counseling friends or family members becomes much more difficult in other (less clear-cut) situations. Consider Case Illustration 8-7, where Myra is contacted by a college roommate.

CASE ILLUSTRATION 8-7

Myra is a professional counselor living in a relatively small rural community approximately 50 miles from a larger metropolitan area. She is one of only a few professional counselors in her community and the only one who specializes in working with substance abuse. One day Myra's friend Kasey (they were good friends and roommates in college and now have kept in touch sporadically via social media) calls Myra to talk about her sister, Renee, who is struggling with alcohol. Kasey asks Myra if she would be willing to work with Renee and help her with her alcohol struggles. Myra understands the ACA Code of Ethics Standard A.5.d. but rationalizes that Renee is more of an acquaintance than a friend. She has not talked to Renee in over a year, and when she has seen Renee in the past, it has always been at Kasey's family functions. Additionally, Myra is very aware she is the only substance abuse counselor within approximately 50 miles. If she were to refuse to meet with Renee, Renee would face a considerable barrier in getting the help she needs.

Would it be ethical for Myra to engage in a counseling relationship with Renee?

In Case Illustration 8-7, it may be tempting for Myra (or any other counselor) to simply say "yes" or "no" to Kasey's request without giving the situation much thought. One might choose to provide services to Renee because Kasey was a close friend in the past but not as much now. Also, Myra does not really know Renee and would easily be able to stay objective. Another counselor may believe providing services to Renee would be unethical because the ACA Code of Ethics says that "counselors are prohibited from engaging in counseling relationships with friends or family members." Even though Myra has not seen or talked to Renee in a year, she is still the sister of a close friend. Case Illustration 8-7 requires Myra to use an ethical decision-making process to determine whether to accept the referral from Kasey. There is no clear guidance given by laws or ethical codes for Myra to apply in a prescription-type manner. She must apply relevant codes of ethics, examine her own morals, values, and beliefs, consider all possible choices and consequences, and eventually make a decision on how to act. However Myra chooses, it is crucial for her to document her decision-making process in case her decision is ever challenged.

ACA Standard A.5.e. (2014) Personal Virtual Relationships With Current Clients: Counselors are prohibited from engaging in a personal virtual relationship with individuals with whom they have a current counseling relationship (e.g., though social and other media).

Similar to Standard A.5.a., professional counselors must avoid engaging in personal virtual relationships with those whom they currently have a counseling relationship. This standard is new to the 2014 ACA Code of Ethics and covers all venues of social and other media (i.e., counselors should avoid connecting with their clients via their personal Facebook, LinkedIn, or other social media accounts).

Receiving Gifts

ACA Standard A.10.f. (2014) Receiving Gifts: Counselors understand the challenges of accepting gifts from clients and recognize that in some cultures, small gifts are a token of respect and gratitude. When determining whether to accept a gift from clients, counselors take into account the therapeutic relationship, the monetary value of the gift, the client's motivation for giving the gift, and the counselor's motivation for wanting to accept or decline the gift.

See Text Box 8-4 for gift guidelines from the AAMFT.

TEXT BOX 8-4

American Psychological Association

The APA does not address giving or receiving gifts in their code of ethics.

American Association for Marriage and Family Therapists

AAMFT Standard 3.9 (2015) Gifts: Marriage and family therapists attend to cultural norms when considering whether to accept gifts from or give gifts to clients. Marriage and family therapists consider the potential effects that receiving or giving gifts may have on clients and on the integrity and efficacy of the therapeutic relationship.

Regardless of their work setting, most counselors will encounter a client or two presenting them with a gift. Gifts may vary in size, value, and substance. For some counselors, it may cause feelings of discomfort or uneasiness as to whether it is appropriate (ethical) to accept a gift from a client (Anderson, 2011). Standard A.10.f. requires professional counselors to go through several steps in the process of determining whether to accept a gift from a client.

Counselors Understand the Challenges of Accepting Gifts

Professional counselors understand there is not a prescriptive universal right or wrong to accepting gifts. There are many things to take into account when determining the ethicality of accepting or declining a gift.

Counselors Recognize in Some Cultures Small Gifts Are a Token of Respect and Gratitude

Professional counselors understand clients come from various backgrounds and cultures. Therefore counselors take into account the culture of the client when determining whether to accept a gift. This requirement is also reiterated in Chapter 4, where the authors discuss ethics related to multiculturalism and diversity.

Counselors Take Into Account the Therapeutic Relationship

How might accepting or refusing the gift affect the therapeutic relationship? If the counselor refuses the gift, does it come across as offensive to the client? If the counselor accepts the gift, does the client feel as though he/she will (or is entitled to) get better or more preferential treatment if he/she continues to bring gifts?

Counselors Take Into Account the Monetary Value of the Gift

Approximately how much does the gift cost? Some authors (Anderson, 2011; Brendel, et al., 2007) suggest an appropriate price range of $10 to $20, and states may have various laws specifically allowing for either less or more expensive gifts. For example, Texas law prohibits counselors from accepting a gift costing more than $50. Nevertheless, some clients may feel the need to give more elaborate and costly gifts as a way to say thank you (i.e., concert tickets, jewelry, gift cards, cash, etc.). In such cases, it is generally considered poor practice to accept large, elaborate gifts as it may put the counselor at risk for losing objectivity. Other clients may give homemade gifts (i.e., baked goods or personal artwork, etc.). In these instances the authors recommend counselors avoid accepting gifts individually. Instead, counselors may want to accept the gift on behalf of the office and share it with the entire office setting. For example, if a client brings a box of homemade brownies as a gift, the counselor would want to acknowledge the hard work put into making the brownies, accept them on behalf of the office, and share them with everyone.

Counselors Take Into Account the
Client's Motivation in Giving the Gift

What is the meaning behind the gift? Is your client trying to manipulate your objectivity, or is this a genuine token of appreciation?

Counselors Take Into Account Their
Own Motivation for Accepting the Gift

Yet again, self-awareness is key in this situation. Why is the counselor wanting to accept (or deny) the gift? Review the scenarios presented in Case Illustration 8-8, and determine whether or not you believe it would be appropriate for the counselor to accept the gift.

CASE ILLUSTRATION 8-8

Scenario 1

A client who is in counseling for issues related to drug and alcohol abuse brings her counselor a $15 bottle of whiskey as a thank-you gift at her last session.

Scenario 2

An adolescent boy brings his counselor a picture he drew at school.

Scenario 3

A couple who is being seen for marriage counseling brings their counselor a plate of homemade cookies at the first intake session.

Scenario 4

A high school student brings his school counselor a Starbucks gift basket as a holiday gift. The basket includes some coffee, a coffee mug, and a $50 gift card to Starbucks.

Scenario 5

A woman brings her counselor a bookmark inscribed with "thank you for all that you do" to her counselor.

In Scenario 1 a client brings a bottle of whiskey to her counselor as a gift. Although the gift is under the $20 suggested price range, at first glance this would most likely be seen as inappropriate due of the nature of the gift. However, as suggested previously, a discussion with the client may unveil more information about the motivation behind the gift, changing this from an inappropriate to possibly an appropriate gift. For example, during a discussion about the gift, this client may elaborate on the importance alcohol has played in her life. Knowing she could not stay sober if the alcohol was still in her home, she may be giving each of her unopened bottles to significant people in her life or those who have made a significant impact on her recovery. The client may see her counselor as a significant force in her recovery, and by giving a bottle of her alcohol to the counselor, she is being open and honest about her recovery.

Scenario 2 involves a boy who brings a self-drawn picture to his counselor. In most all situations, this would be seen as appropriate.

Scenario 3 involves a couple bringing cookies to their counselor at the first session. While most likely appropriate in all situations, the counselor would want to be sure to discuss gifts with his/her clients, assuring them that bringing a gift (cookies) is not necessary and certainly not expected by the counselor. Concomitantly, it is recommended (if the counselor does accept the cookies) that he/she accept them on behalf of the entire office and make them available to everyone rather than accepting them personally (e.g., Thank you so much. I will put these in the break room, so the whole office can enjoy them.).

Scenario 4 may become a common occurrence for anyone training to become a professional school counselor. Across the United States it is common for students to bring their teachers and administrators gifts at various times throughout the school year. Working in a school setting, professional school counselors may find themselves in potentially awkward situations when students present them with a gift. The situation presented in scenario 4, while likely very tempting, may be seen as inappropriate or unethical if the school counselor were to simply accept the gift without discussing it more with the student. Similar to many situations discussed previously, the process is most important. Consider the following two interactions:

Student:	*Hi Mr. M. Have a great summer. Since this is the last day of school, I wanted to give you this basket and tell you thank you for all your help this year. You really helped me a lot.*
School Counselor:	*Wow, this is very kind of you, and how did you know I love coffee? I can definitely use this.*
Student:	*You were an incredible help to me this year, and it's my small way of letting you know how much I appreciate all you do. It's just a mug, some coffee, and a gift card. I got it for you because every time I see you, you're drinking coffee.*
School Counselor:	*Wow, amazing! Thank you! I will use this mug every day, and this fancy coffee is much better than the generic stuff they give us in the teacher's lounge. I will be sure to keep this in my drawer here, so nobody finds it and uses it up. Wow! A $50 gift card—this will be very useful to me over the summer. I think I go to Starbucks almost every day.*
Student:	*I'm glad you like it. Have a great summer.*

How might the above interaction be viewed differently than the following student/school counselor interaction below?

Student:	*Hi Mr. M. Have a great summer. Since this is the last day of school, I wanted to give you this basket and tell you thank you for all your help this year. You really helped me a lot.*
School Counselor:	*Wow, this is very kind of you, but I don't want you or your parents to think you have to bring gifts for me. This looks like quite a large basket. Tell me a little about it.*
Student:	*I know I don't have to bring gifts, but it's something I really wanted to do. You were an incredible help to me this year, and it's my small way of letting you know how much I appreciate all you do. Plus, it's not much—just a mug, some coffee and a gift card. I bought it for you because every time I see you, you're drinking coffee.*
School Counselor:	*Again, this is very kind of you, and I wouldn't feel comfortable keeping this all to myself, but I also know you put some serious thought into this gift and want to express my appreciation. I would like to keep the coffee mug and I can put the coffee in our counselor's lounge for everyone to share. However, I don't feel as though it would be ethical of me to accept this gift card. How about if I keep these two (coffee and mug) and give this card back to you?*
Student:	*Well I guess, but I bought it all for you. I won't tell anyone if you want to keep it all.*
School Counselor:	*I sincerely appreciate your thoughtfulness, but it really wouldn't be right for me to accept all of this. I will definitely use this coffee mug, and I know all of our counselors will enjoy the coffee, but you keep the gift card.*

Finally, in Scenario 5 a client presents her counselor with an inscribed bookmark. At first glance, this would most likely be appropriate or ethical for the counselor to accept the gift. However, the counselor would still want to be sure to engage in conversation with the client to determine the client's motivation in giving the gift.

In addition to this information, Welfel (2010) provides additional criteria to consider when determining the ethicality of accepting a gift: (1) Does the gift promote rather than endanger the client's welfare? (2) Does accepting the gift compromise the counselor's ability to be objective? (3) Is the gift consistent with the client's cultural norms? (4) Is the gift a one-time event, or does the client continually bring gifts? (p. 233).

Bartering

According to Merriam-Webster's online dictionary, bartering is trading or exchanging one commodity for another. For professional counselors, bartering is trading counseling services for something other than money (i.e., trading counseling for electrical work, dental work, lawn care, printing services, babysitting, etc.). The ACA Code of Ethics (2014) addresses bartering in Standard A.10.e. (see Text Box 8-5 for APA standards related to this issue).

ACA Standard A.10.e. (2014) Bartering: Counselors may barter only if the bartering does not result in exploitation or harm, if the client requests it, and if such arrangements are an accepted practice among professionals in the community. Counselors consider the cultural implications of bartering and discuss relevant concerns with clients and document such agreements in a clear, written contract.

TEXT BOX 8-5

American Psychological Association

APA Standard 6.05 (2010) Barter With Clients or Patients: Barter is the acceptance of goods, services, or other nonmonetary remuneration from clients or patients in return for psychological services. Psychologists may barter only if (1) it is not clinically contraindicated, and (2) the resulting arrangement is not exploitative.

American Association for Marriage and Family Therapists

The AAMFT does not address giving or receiving gifts in their code of ethics.

Consider Annie's dilemma in Case Illustration 8-9 as she determines whether to barter with her client, trading counseling services for baked goods.

CASE ILLUSTRATION 8-9

Annie is a professional counselor working in private practice. Her practice is located in a small, traditional community. Annie's first appointment today is Jessica. Jessica owns a local bake shop and self-referred due to symptoms of depression. At the end of their session, Jessica looks through her purse and is very embarrassed realizing she forgot her wallet back at her bakery. She is very apologetic and offers to leave her license with Annie, while she goes back to her shop to retrieve her wallet. Annie responds with a smile and seems satisfied with Jessica's solution to the problem. As Jessica is leaving, Annie mentions she is very fond of the pastries Jessica makes at her bakery. Annie asks Jessica if she would be willing to deliver two dozen of her pastries to Annie's office every Monday in exchange for her counseling. Jessica happily agrees, and the two shake hands on the agreement.

> *Do you believe Annie acted in an ethical manner? Why, or why not?*
>
> *If unethical, what could Annie have done to align her actions more closely with ethical expectations?*

The first question in Case Illustration 8-9 inquires about the ethicality of Annie's actions. Even though Jessica agreed to the arrangement, Annie's actions would most likely be considered unethical for the following reasons: (1) The code of ethics is very clear that the client (not the counselor) should be the one requesting to barter. In Case Illustration 8-9, Annie is the one requesting to barter with Jessica; (2) Annie did not discuss possible concerns with Jessica (i.e., How long must Jessica provide pastries for Annie? What happens if either of the two [Jessica or Annie] is not satisfied with the services the other is providing? What, if any, possible conflicts might arise?); (3) and there is no indication Annie and Jessica have a written agreement concerning the services each will provide. It is Annie's responsibility to document the bartering agreement.

The second question asks about the steps Annie would need to take to act more ethically. One of the primary concerns with Annie's actions in Case Illustration 8-9 is in how the bartering agreement first came about. Annie made the first suggestion of bartering rather than the request coming from Jessica. For this to be considered ethical, the initial request would have needed to come from the client, Jessica. Once Jessica made the inquiry, Annie would need to engage in conversation with Jessica to determine any possible conflicts caused by the bartering for services. Annie would also need to discuss the possible pros and cons of the relationship, and finally, Annie must document the agreement and the decision-making process used in making the final decision.

Conclusion

Appropriate boundaries are a difficult tightrope walk for counselors to navigate. Counselors who are too rigid in the boundaries they keep with clients may come across as cold and lack the ability to build solid working alliances. Conversely, counselors who are too flexible in the boundaries they keep may be guilty of inappropriate or unprofessional relationships with clients. In navigating these relationships, the ACA Code of Ethics offers broad guidelines requiring counselors to use critical-thinking skills in determining whether to extend counseling boundaries.

Throughout Chapter 8 the authors described various examples of possible boundary extensions, including social relationships with clients, sexual and romantic relationships, relationships with former romantic partners, giving and receiving gifts, and bartering with clients. Regardless of the type of extension, counselors must use an ethical decision-making process to determine an appropriate action, include clients in the decision-making process, and fully document their decision. Use the information learned in Chapter 8 to address the ethical dilemma and discussion questions presented in Exercise 8-1.

EXERCISE 8-1

Rebecca is a licensed professional counselor who owns her own private practice. Although her practice is still quite small, she has seen some growth and added many new referral sources. Rebecca has come to realize that renting office space from a larger practice in town will no longer fit her needs. Knowing this, she has begun to look for a small house or other type of office space to purchase and turn into her permanent location. Because she feels strongly about being very transparent with clients, Rebecca has begun letting her clients know about her potential move and the possible change in her office location. She wants to let her clients know far enough in advance, so she can provide appropriate referrals to any clients not wanting to or not having the ability to travel to her new office.

Today Rebecca is meeting with Krystal, who has been Rebecca's client for approximately six months; the two have a strong rapport. When Rebecca mentions her intentions of buying a new place, Krystal seems very intrigued and excited for her. Krystal asks many questions, including whether Rebecca has a real estate agent helping her with the process. When Rebecca says that she doesn't, Krystal mentions that her sister works in real estate and would probably be happy to help her. Krystal even mentions her sister would probably work for her at a reduced price. Rebecca graciously thanks Krystal and offers to think about it.

At her next scheduled session, Krystal brings her sister along to the visit and introduces her to Rebecca. Krystal's sister, Melissa, tells Rebecca about how Krystal had told her all about Rebecca's plans to move and how she would be willing work with her at a reduced cost. Melissa is very appreciative of the help Rebecca has provided to Krystal and wants to be helpful in any way she can. She tells Rebecca, "I don't want to be too pushy and put pressure on you, but I do want you to know I will help you find a new place for your business in any way I can. I know this area very well, and because you have been so helpful to my sister, I will work for you at a reduced fee." While talking, Melissa hands Rebecca a folder full of information about homes and offices for sale in the area. She says, "I did some research this past week and looked up as many listings as I could find. Even if you don't decide to use me, this may be helpful to you."

Rebecca again graciously thanks Melissa and Krystal for their concern and mentions to Melissa she will think about it and get back to her. Over the next few days Rebecca thinks about the offer from Melissa. She knows she needs to be careful about exploiting her clients and doesn't want to overextend the boundaries of her professional relationship with Krystal. On the other hand, she knows Krystal and Melissa approached her, and it wasn't something she propositioned them about. She is also very aware every penny is valuable, and she is always trying to cut costs to better help her business. Finally, after looking through the information Melissa provided, it is very evident Melissa is a very skilled real estate broker and could no doubt help her find the right place at the right cost.

Do you believe it would be ethical for Rebecca to accept Melissa's offer to act as her real estate agent? Why, or why not? (Be sure to use an ethical decision-making process to aid you in your decision.)

If Rebecca declines Melissa's offer, how might if affect the counseling relationship between Krystal and Rebecca?

If Rebecca accepts Melissa's offer, how might if affect the counseling relationship between Krystal and Rebecca?

If Rebecca decides to hire Melissa, what (if any) type of discussion should she have with Krystal about her decision?

If Rebecca declines Melissa's offer, what (if any) type of discussion should she have with Krystal about her decision?

Keystones

- Boundary crossings and violations are one of the most common ethical concerns for professional counselors.
- Professional counselors are prohibited from having sexual or intimate relationships with clients.
- When determining whether or not a boundary extension is ethical, counselors must consider the possible benefits and consequences of the extension.
- Counselors must document their decision to extend counseling boundaries prior to the extension taking place.
- Counselors will have clients with whom they feel sexually attracted and must be able to appropriately address their feelings before they become an ethical concern.
- When deciding whether or not to counsel a friend or family member, counselors must consider possible risks and benefits to the client and whether or not the counselor is able to remain objective throughout the counseling process.
- The general rule in accepting gifts from clients is the gift should not be more than $50 in value.
- Counselors understand that in some cultures, gift giving is a sign of respect.
- Counselors may barter with clients if the client requests it and the bartering does not exploit the client in any way.

Additional Resources

Barnett, J. E. (2014). Sexual feelings and behaviors in the psychotherapy relationship: An ethics perspective. *Journal of Clinical Psychology, 70*(2), 170–181.

Everett, B., MacFarlane, D. A., Reynolds, V. A., & Anderson, H. D. (2013). Not on our backs: Supporting counsellors in navigating the ethics of multiple relationships within queer, two spirit, and/or trans communities. *Canadian Journal of Counselling and Psychotherapy, 47*(1), 14–28. Retrieved from http://search.proquest.com/docview/1420143870?accountid=7122

Gonyea, J. L. J., Wright, D. W., & Earl-Kulkosky, T. (2014). Navigating dual relationships in rural communities. *Journal of Marital and Family Therapy, 40*(1), 125–136. doi:http://dx.doi.org/10.1111/j.1752-0606.2012.00335.x

References

American Association for Marriage and Family Therapy. (2015). *Code of ethics.* Retrieved from https://www.aamft.org/iMIS15/AAMFT/Content/legal_ethics/code_of_ethics.aspx

American Counseling Association. (1995). *Code of ethics.* Alexandria, VA: Author.

American Counseling Association. (2005). *Code of ethics.* Alexandria, VA: Author.

American Counseling Association. (2014). *Code of ethics.* Alexandria, VA: Author.

American Psychological Association. (2010). *American Psychological Association ethical principles of psychologists and code of conduct.* Retrieved from http://www.apa.org/ethics/code/principles .pdf

Anderson, J. (2011, June). Is it better to give, receive, or decline? The ethics of accepting gifts from patients. *JAAPA-Journal of the American Academy of Physicians Assistants, 24*(6), 59+. Retrieved from https://login.libweb.lib.utsa.edu/login?url=http://go.galegroup.com/ps/i.do?id=GALE%7CA 263440650&v=2.1&u=txshracd2604&it=r&p=HRCA&asid=59f7f433125796272a943eba9f986f38

Bartering. (n.d.). In *Merriam-Webster* online. Retrieved from http://www.merriam-webster.com/ dictionary/bartering

Brendel, D. H., Chu, J., Radden, J., Leeper, H., Pope, H. G., Samson, J., . . . Bodkin, J. A. (2007). The price of a gift: An approach to receiving gifts from patients in psychiatric practice. *Harvard Review of Psychiatry, 15*(2), 43–51. doi:10.1080/10673220701298399

Meyers, L. (2014). A living document of ethical guidance. *Counseling Today, 56*(12), 32–42.

Pope, K. S., Keith-Spiegel, P., & Tabachnick, B. G. (1986). Sexual attraction to clients: The human therapist and the (sometimes) inhuman training system. *American Psychologist, 41*, 147–158.

Remley, T. P., & Herlihy, B. (2014). *Ethical, legal, and professional issues in counseling* (4th ed.). Upper Saddle River, NJ: Pearson.

Welfel, E. R. (2010). *Ethics in counseling & psychotherapy: Standards, research, and emerging issues.* Belmont, CA: Brooks/Cole.

9

Ethics and Technology

*I've missed more than 9,000 shots in my career. I've lost almost 300 games. 26 times,
I've been trusted to take the game winning shot and missed. I've failed over and over
and over again in my life. And that is why I succeed.*

—Michael Jordan

hapter 9 examines the evolution of the practice of counseling through the lens of
technology infusion. "Technology infusion" is a phrase used to gauge the extent
to which someone uses technology in his/her counseling practice. For this chapter,
think of technology as any tool, digital or otherwise, a counselor will or could use with
a client. Technology is not just computers, tablets, or smartphones; technology is a way
of thinking about solutions to problems. As technology continues to evolve exponentially,
counselors must also evolve to address the issues clients face with the tools currently and
potentially available. In the introduction to Section H of the 2014 ACA Code of Ethics
(Distance Counseling, Technology, and Social Media), counselors are directed to "actively
attempt to understand the evolving nature of the profession with regard to distance counseling, technology, and social media" (ACA, 2014, p. 17). Therefore, even those counselors
who have no interest in integrating distance counseling into their own practice must
attempt to understand ethical implications of using technology in general (e.g., e-mail,
text, cloud storage, cell phones, and laptops or tablets).

Technological issues arise when technologies are used incorrectly or used without
proper training or experience. In Chapter 9, the reader is asked to think about technology as a solution to problems of the past while preparing for potential problems of the
future. The terminology included in this discussion may be confusing. Distance counseling, online counseling, and Internet counseling all imply the use of technology, whereas
face-to-face and live counseling imply in-person counseling. The distinction between

distance and live is where the ethical threats may exist. At the forefront of these ethical threats is client confidentiality, which tends to drive ethical textbooks and articles concerning technology. Because data is a hot commodity in a digital world, there are some security concerns in using untested technologies. Chapter 9 addresses not only confidentiality concerns but also the use of distance counseling, supervision, consultation, and the entire technological evolution available to professional counselors.

Technological evolutions concern social media, distance counseling relationships, and taking the counseling session outside the therapy room. Taking the session out of the therapy office has been done for decades through various isolated means such as written correspondence, the telephone, and e-mail. However, only recently has communication technology been reliable enough for mainstream use of distance technologies. As this chapter progresses it will encourage the reader to process the technological tools currently available to counselors and will encourage the counseling profession to continue to evolve in the use of technology. Specifically, at the conclusion of chapter nine, readers will be able to do the following:

1. Define ethical obligations related to technology as a whole.

2. Understand laws vary by state and counselors must consider the related laws in their state concerning distance counseling as well as ethical guidelines.

3. Explain ethical obligations in providing informed consent when practicing distance counseling.

4. Discuss how to develop their own informed consent document to use when providing distance counseling services.

5. State the limits of confidentiality as related to the use of technology.

6. Explain the benefits and limitations of using technology-assisted counseling.

7. Explain the importance of meeting encryption standards related to technology.

8. Explain technological concerns related to record storage when using technology.

9. Define ethical obligations related to the use of mobile devices.

10. Define ethical obligations related to web maintenance.

11. Define multicultural concerns related to access and usability for all clients.

The ACA Code of Ethics includes a new section for 2014. Titled Section H (Distance Counseling, Technology, and Social Media) it broadly covers concerns with the central theme of using technology ethically. Technological aptitude varies with each counselor. Some may be more hesitant to use it, and others may feel more comfortable and feel as though technology makes their practice run more smoothly. Regardless, all counselors use technology to some degree. Consider Case Illustration 9-1 and how Danny responds to a request from his client about the use of distance counseling.

CASE ILLUSTRATION 9-1

Danny is a licensed professional counselor and a national certified counselor who works at a mental health facility in a city with 45,000 residents. Jeremy is a 23-year-old male who is dealing with an undefined, undiagnosed anxiety problem. His parents, with whom he lives, have referred Jeremy to counseling. Jeremy's parents have become frustrated with his lack of motivation and given him an ultimatum. For him to remain living in their home, Jeremy's parents have made a stipulation; he must participate in counseling sessions on a regular basis. His parents are worried about Jeremy because he never leaves the house and he seems to have no friends.

Jeremy has entered into a counseling relationship with Danny at Danny's office. The two have met weekly for almost two months, and Jeremy still appears to lack focus and seems disinterested in counseling. At one session Jeremy inquires about the option of distance counseling using his computer at home. Jeremy claims meeting face-to-face is intimidating to him, and he might be able to relax more if he were able to sit in his own house.

Danny is familiar with videoconference applications, and considers himself to be a person with higher-than-average technology aptitude, knowledge, and skills, but has never formally provided distance counseling. As he discusses different distance counseling options, he notices Jeremy becoming interested in counseling for the first time since the beginning of counseling a month ago. After again talking about his anxiety, Jeremy shares that he would like to participate in distance counseling because he believes it would help him better engage in counseling by not having to leave his house.

Ethically speaking, if a client asks for a change of counseling treatment modality, in this case distance counseling, is the counselor (Danny) obligated to provide the requested treatment if it will help the client?

How might Danny proceed in this situation with Jeremy?

Related to the first question in Case Illustration 9-1, no, Danny is not obligated to change his counseling treatment unless he believes the new technique will help Jeremy. Even then Danny must also follow Standard C.2.a. (Boundaries of Competence), directing him to practice only within the boundaries of his competence based on his education, training, supervised experience, state and national professional credentials, and appropriate professional experience. Because Danny has higher-than-average technology aptitude, knowledge, and skill, he might feel comfortable moving to distance counseling. Still, Danny would also want to seek training to assist him in the transition from face-to-face to technology-assisted counseling.

If Danny did not have the confidence in his technological skills, nor did he wish to provide distance counseling, the most ethical thing for him to do would be to discuss the situation further with his client. Depending on Jeremy's wishes, Danny could either continue to meet with him in face-to-face sessions or provide appropriate referrals to counselors who would provide distance counseling services.

The second question inquires as to what Danny's next steps might be in providing distance counseling. Danny would first want to review ACA Ethical Standard H.1.a. (Knowledge and Competency). Standard H.1.a. requires that "counselors who engage in the use of distance counseling, technology, and/or social media develop knowledge and skills regarding related technical, ethical, and legal considerations (e.g., special certifications, additional course work)" (ACA, 2014, p. 17). Related to Case Illustration 9-1, Danny would first want to make sure he is competent to provide the distance counseling services he has mentioned to his client. Additionally, he would want to be sure all his credentials were current and he had the technology needed to provide the services.

Next, Danny would want to review Standard H.1.b. (Laws and Statutes), which states:

> Counselors who engage in the use of distance counseling, technology, and social media within their counseling practice understand that they may be subject to laws and regulations of both the counselor's practicing location and the client's place of residence. Counselors ensure their clients are aware of pertinent legal rights and limitations governing the practice of counseling across state lines or international boundaries. (ACA, 2014, p. 17)

Depending on the state in which Danny practices, and the state where Jeremy resides, the rules may coincide or conflict. Although not specifically addressed in the ACA Code of Ethics, it is critical counselors understand states are beginning to draft governing laws and statutes to address the physical location of the counselor. Professional counseling organizations have addressed this debate by calling for a national certifying credential for counselors who wish to provide distance counseling. Still, as of this book's publication, states have focused on the need to first meet the mental health concerns of their own citizens. By creating a rule regulating how and when a counselor will counsel, state legislators may interfere with mental health services being readily available to the residents of the state.

Related to Case Illustration 9-1, Danny must have awareness of laws and regulations of where the counselor is located and where the client resides. Both Danny and Jeremy reside in the same state, and counseling services will be provided in the state where Danny is licensed. Therefore, Danny must worry only about the one state.

Informed Consent

Even though the authors reviewed the informed consent process thoroughly in Chapter 5, it is necessary to revisit informed consent again as it relates to the use of distance counseling. When counselors provide technology-assisted services, they must include additional information in the informed consent process as required by ACA Ethical Standard H.2.a.

ACA Standard H.2.a. (2014) Informed Consent and Disclosure: Clients have the freedom to choose whether to use distance counseling, social media, and/or technology within the counseling process. In addition to the usual and customary protocol of informed consent between counselor and client for face-to-face counseling, the following issues, unique to the use of distance counseling, technology, and/or social media, are addressed in the informed consent process:

- *Distance counseling credentials, physical location of practice, and contact information;*
- *Risks and benefits of engaging in the use of distance counseling, technology, and/ or social media;*
- *Possibility of technology failure and alternate methods of service delivery;*
- *Anticipated response time;*
- *Emergency procedures to follow when the counselor is not available;*
- *Time zone differences;*
- *Cultural and/or language differences that may affect delivery of services;*
- *Possible denial of insurance benefits; and*
- *Social media policy.*

Review the sample consent form provided in Case Illustration 9-2, and pay close attention to the information included. In addition to covering the information specifically named in Standard H.2.a., the sample that follows also includes requirements of standards H.2.b. and H.2.c.

ACA Standard H.2.b. (2014) Confidentiality Maintained by the Counselor: Counselors acknowledge the limitations of maintaining the confidentiality of electronic records and transmissions. They inform clients that individuals might have authorized or unauthorized access to such records or transmissions (e.g., colleagues, supervisors, employees, information technologists).

ACA Standard H.2.c. (2014) Acknowledgement of Limitations: Counselors inform clients about the inherent limits of confidentiality when using technology. Counselors urge clients to be aware of authorized and/or unauthorized access to information disclosed using this medium in the counseling process.

CASE ILLUSTRATION 9-2

Informed Consent

Counseling is no longer bound by physical proximity. As a therapist I strive to serve my clients and stay current on counseling issues as well as with how technology can play an important role in the accomplishment of counseling goals. I use technology to communicate with clients such as e-mail, text messaging, phone calls, and voice calls and mail. As such, I participate in professional organizations, accreditation bodies, and professional development opportunities providing the knowledge and skills required for delivering distance counseling services and staying current in technology trends. The organizations to which I belong include the American Counseling Association, the American School Counselor Association, the Association for Counselor Education and Supervision, and the National Board for Certified Counselors.

As a distance counselor I must ensure you are intellectually, emotionally, physically, linguistically, and functionally capable of using the technologies and applications required for

(Continued)

(Continued)

participation in distance counseling. Please complete the technology competencies questionnaire listed in Appendix 1.

I utilize social media to connect with potential clients. However, I do not use social media with clients. I do understand the role social media plays in the lives of clients, and I will respect your privacy by not "friending" or connecting with you through any form of social media. One piece of counseling essential to success is congruence. With this in mind, what is stated using social media (e.g., Facebook, Twitter, Instagram, LinkedIn, Pinterest, and Tumblr) is in the public domain, in other words, available to the whole of the Internet community. I will not search for you on social media without your consent. If you would like to consent to this practice please initial here _____. I will treat any and all information gathered online as confidential just as if you are sharing the information with me in a counseling session.

Because our counseling relationship will require a high use of technology, the following issues must be addressed:

This relationship is subject to laws between my practicing state of _____ and your place of residence, which is: _____. I will need to read the legal requirements and ethical standards of your place of residence before we enter into this counseling relationship.

My distance counseling credentials consist of the following:

1. *Distance Credentialed Counselor*

2. *Systems Security Certified Practitioner (SSCP)*

3. *Certified Information Systems Security Professional (CISSP)*

The physical location of my practice is: _____

You can contact me using the following methods: _____

The risks and benefits of engaging in the use of distance counseling, technology, and/or social media include: _____

Anything mechanical fails eventually. The technology I use in counseling is mechanical; therefore, it may fail during our counseling sessions. In the event that technology does fail, please use the following protocol:

Our main method of service delivery is videoconference using _____. If this method does not work, we will use an alternate method of service delivery such as phone calls, voice-over Internet protocol (VOIP) calls, or FaceTime audio and video. Face-to-face meetings and referrals can be arranged if needed.

You can anticipate a response from a phone call, e-mail, and/or text message within 24 hours during the weekdays and 48 hours over the weekend. If you have a scheduled weekend appointment, you can expect a 24-hour response to your communication. Please understand that none of the interactions we use are 100 percent safe from deliberate, malicious individuals. Therefore, when leaving a message, e-mail, or text, I will never disclose personal information. I ask that you limit your personal disclosure of information in e-mails, phone calls, and text messages.

If you have an immediate emergency concerning your safety, please contact your local law enforcement at this number: _____ or your local 911. Here are emergency procedures to follow when the counselor is not available:

My office is located in the central time zone. You are a resident of the _____ time zone. This means that you are _____ hour/s _____ from central time.

Technology sometimes creates new opportunities for communication. However, sometimes differences in culture and/or language may affect the delivery of my counseling services, especially if our communication is not clear. Please ask me questions at any time if something I say or write does not make sense to you.

Currently, in my state (Texas), insurance will not reimburse for distance-delivered counseling services. After we discuss financial arrangements, you agree to pay _____ per session.

You will be given a client number once we begin our counseling. Your client number is: _____. I create and save your case notes using the _____ software program. The files are saved on my computer using encryption software that requires a password to access. Your file is saved on a drive that is in a ventilated, locked cabinet that is secured to the floor in my office building. Every effort has been made to protect your records. It would be very difficult for someone to steal your case file from my office as it is difficult for someone to identify the location, but it is not impossible. The computer I use to create, save, and review your file is not connected to the Internet or networked in any way, which includes Wi-Fi, Bluetooth, or cabled connections. I use a stand-alone computer that is purely used for case notes. Even though I use encryption software to secure your files, there may be ways to exploit the encryption using noncommercially available methods. This means that a person would be acting in a deliberate, malicious manner to be able to access your file. It would be tremendously difficult for anyone other than me to access your files but not impossible.

One method that may be of consequence to your confidentiality is the device or devices you use to communicate with me. That is, every person who has access to this device or devices has access to your communications. My website is non-encrypted because it contains only information and no way for you to add information to the site. However, your browser history may store my website, which may be available to other people who use your computer or device. Please read and follow the attached checklist for ensuring your personal files are safe when using a computer that is not secure.

Attachment 1

I must ensure you are who you say you are. Therefore, I contract with a service called _____. Once you are a client, you will be given an access code. Your access code is: _____. Instructions will be sent to your e-mail.

My e-mail communications with you are always encrypted using ciphertext. You will need a password to confirm you are the intended recipient. Your password for accessing my e-mails is: _____.

Client Name and Signature: _____

Counselor Name and Signature: _____

In addition to the standards discussed prior to Case Illustration 9-2, the consent also includes other valuable information required by the 2014 ACA Code of Ethics. Examine the example consent provided in Case Illustration 9-2 again, and see if you are able to determine how the authors included additional information about the distance counseling relationship. Specifically, the authors included information required by the following seven standards.

ACA Standard H.3. (2014) Client Verification: Counselors who engage in the use of distance counseling, technology, and/or social media to interact with clients take steps to verify the client's identity at the beginning and throughout the therapeutic process. Verification can include, but is not limited to, using code words, numbers, graphics or other nondescript identifiers.

ACA Standard H.4.a. (2014) Benefits and Limitations: Counselors inform clients of the benefits and limitations of using technology applications in the provision of counseling services. Such technologies include, but are not limited to, computer hardware and/or software, telephones and applications, social media and Internet-based applications, and other audio and/or video communication or data storage devices or media.

ACA Standard H.4.b. (2014) Professional Boundaries in Distance Counseling: Counselors understand the necessity of maintaining a professional relationship with their clients. Counselors discuss and establish professional boundaries with clients regarding the appropriate use and/or application of technology and the limitations of its use within the counseling relationship (e.g., lack of confidentiality or times when not appropriate to use).

ACA Standard H.4.c. (2014) Technology-Assisted Services: When providing technology-assisted services, counselors make reasonable efforts to determine that clients are intellectually, emotionally, physically, linguistically, and functionally capable of using the application and that the application is appropriate for the needs of the client. Counselors verify that clients understand the purpose and operation of technology applications and follow up with clients to correct possible misconceptions, discover appropriate use, and assess subsequent steps.

Standard H.4.d. (2014) Effectiveness of Services: When distance counseling services are deemed ineffective by the counselor or client, counselors consider delivering services face-to-face. If the counselor is not able to provide face-to-face services (e.g., lives in another state), the counselor assists the client in identifying appropriate services.

ACA Standard H.4.e. (2014) Access: Counselors provide information to clients regarding reasonable access to pertinent applications when providing technology-assisted services.

ACA Standard H.4.f. (2014) Communication Differences in Electronic Media: Counselors consider the differences between face-to-face and electronic communication (nonverbal and verbal cues) and how these may affect the counseling process. Counselors educate clients on how to prevent and address potential misunderstandings arising from the lack of visual cues and voice intonations when communicating electronically.

Security Standards

As stated previously, security is a primary concern when incorporating technology into counseling. Any device with the ability to connect to the Internet is vulnerable to being hacked. While it is impossible for counselors to completely protect documents and information from all threat, it is important for counselors to take necessary steps in protecting technology-based communications and documents. Review Ethical Standard H.2.d. (see Text Box 9-1 for more information about AAMFT and standard related to technology), and consider Case Illustration 9-3 in which June is setting up her new office space.

ACA Standard H.2.d. (2014) Security: Counselors use current encryption standards within their websites and/or technology-based communications that meet applicable legal requirements. Counselors take reasonable precautions to ensure the confidentiality of information transmitted through any electronic means.

CASE ILLUSTRATION 9-3

June has been in private practice and has kept her office in the same place for almost 10 years. Over the past 10 years, the town where she lives and has her practice has grown dramatically. In an effort to revitalize her practice and update her working space, June is planning to move into a different office complex across town. The new office complex houses many different professional offices, a few restaurants, and a coffee shop. The coffee shop provides free Wi-Fi to customers. Because June is setting up her office with utilities, she decides against having Internet access in her office because she can get a Wi-Fi signal for free from the coffee shop in the office complex. Prior to making her decision, June speaks to the coffee shop owner about using the free Wi-Fi. The coffee shop owner has no problem with her using the connection from the shop and welcomes her to the complex.

What information does June need to have concerning the Wi-Fi provided by the coffee shop?

What steps can June take to ensure the data and client information kept on her computer is safe while using the community Wi-Fi?

In Case Illustration 9-3, June is in the process of setting up her new office. She is able to save on expenses by connecting to the wireless network of a coffee shop in the same office complex. June is careful to ask the coffee shop owner for permission, and he happily agrees. In addition to acquiring the permission from the coffee shop owner, June should also be aware of a few other concerns related to connecting to the coffee shop Wi-Fi. Wireless networking, or Wi-Fi, is typically the fastest wireless network June could use but is drastically different from the traditional wired network June had at her previous office. When June was using a wired network, it was extremely difficult for someone to steal her bandwidth, but wireless signals are significantly easier to access. Other individuals may be able to access the Internet using June's broadband connection while they are sitting in a booth across the room from her at the coffee shop. It may also be possible for others to connect to her broadband when they are as far away as a neighboring building. Simply stated, it is much easier for someone to "hack" into June's computer files when she uses a wireless network. The practice described in the case study is also known as "piggybacking" and is bad for two reasons:

1. *It will decrease June's Internet access speed because she is now sharing the same Internet connection with other users.*

2. *It can create a security hazard because others may hack her computer and access her personal files through her unsecured wireless network.*

In Case Illustration 9-3, June would want to take a few simple steps to ensure her wireless network was secure. Doing so will both prevent others from stealing her Internet and will also prevent hackers from taking control of her computer through her own wireless network. To secure her Wi-Fi, June should take the following steps:

Step 1. June would want to open her router settings page and access her wireless router's settings by typing in "192.168.1.1" into her web browser. The number, 192.168.1.1 is a universal IP address and is a common gateway address for most routers. She could then enter her correct user name and password for the router. This is different for each router, so June would first want to check the user manual for her router to determine the correct username and password for her router.

Step 2. Once June has logged into her router, the first thing she would want to do is secure her network by changing the default password of the router to something more secure. Doing so will prevent others from accessing the router, and she can easily maintain the security settings she wants.

Step 3. Next, June would want to change her network's SSID name. The SSID (or Wireless Network Name) of a wireless router is usually predefined as "default" or is set as the brand name of the router (e.g., Inksys). Although this will not make the network fundamentally more secure, changing the SSID name of the network would be a good idea as it would make it more obvious for others to know the network to which they are connecting.

Resetting the network's SSID name is usually done by accessing the information under the basic wireless settings in your router's settings page. Once June sets hers, she will always be sure she is connecting to the correct wireless network, even if there are multiple wireless networks in her area. To protect her privacy, June would not want to use her name, home address, or other personal information in the SSID name. In addition, June should consult with computer experts to ensure she utilizes proper and appropriate available security procedures and techniques. In Chapter 3 the authors discussed the importance of consulting a legal expert when needing to make a legal decision. Similarly, when making decisions related to technology, it is always best to consult with an expert in technology.

Case illustration 9-3 examined June's efforts to properly secure the network at her new office space and prevent others from accessing sensitive information. Security threats may occur in situations such as June's but may also be present with other devices and in other everyday activities. Consider Case Illustration 9-4 and Camille's efforts to secure her cell phone.

CASE ILLUSTRATION 9-4

To save money, Camille, a private practitioner, uses her smartphone (mobile) as her primary number for her practice. She also uses the same phone for personal calls, text messaging, e-mail, applications, and video watching. Camille also has a young child who occasionally uses the phone to play games and watch streaming videos. The phone keeps track of all calls, and the counselor has saved all client contact information in the phone's contact list for her company.

What are the potential problems with others in her family using Camille's phone?

What could Camille do to mitigate someone accessing her phone if lost?

In Case Illustration 9-4, Camille uses her cell phone for both business and personal calls. By using her personal phone for business, Camille could possibly be acting in an unethical manner, violating Standard H.2.d. requiring her to "take reasonable precautions to ensure the confidentiality of information transmitted" (ACA, 2014). Camille has all of her contact information (including client names and phone numbers) open to anyone using her phone. Specifically with her family, Camille needs to discuss the importance of privacy and how all the information on her phone is private. Camille must stress to her daughter to never answer the phone if it should happen to ring while she is watching videos and playing games. Similarly, if a text message comes in, Camille's daughter should immediately hand the phone to Camille. Ideally, Camille would not let anyone in her family use the phone she uses to communicate with clients. If Camille does let her daughter use her phone for other activities, it is critical she set firm boundaries with her daughter regarding usage and how to respond if a call or text should come in.

The second question asks how Camille might protect the information on her phone if it were to be lost. The ACA Code of Ethics (2014) states counselors must take reasonable steps to protect client information. The easiest way Camille could protect her information would be to add an automatic lock and password to her phone. Camille could adjust the settings on her phone, so it would automatically lock after sitting idle for a few seconds. Therefore it would take a password to enter the phone's interface, thus minimally protecting Camille's information.

TEXT BOX 9-1

American Psychological Association

The APA does not include standards specific to technology-assisted services in their ethical guidelines.

(Continued)

(Continued)

American Association for Marriage and Family Therapists

The AAMFT includes six standards concerning technology-assisted services. The standards provide guidance related to informed consent, competence, confidentiality, documentation, and location of practice. See the following for specific standards.

AAMFT Standard 6.1 (2015) Technology-Assisted Services: Prior to commencing therapy or supervision services through electronic means, marriage and family therapists ensure that they are compliant with all relevant laws for the delivery of such services. Additionally, marriage and family therapists must: (a) determine that technologically-assisted services or supervision are appropriate for clients or supervisees, considering professional, intellectual, emotional, and physical needs; (b) inform clients or supervisees of the potential risks and benefits associated with technologically-assisted services; (c) ensure the security of their communication medium; and (d) only commence therapy or supervision after appropriate education, training, or supervised experience using the relevant technology.

AAMFT Standard 6.2 (2015) Consent to Treat or Supervise: Clients and supervisees, whether contracting for services as individuals, dyads, families, or groups, must be made aware of the risks and responsibilities associated with technology-assisted services. Therapists are to advise clients and supervisees in writing of these risks and of both the therapists' and clients' or supervisees' responsibilities for minimizing such risks.

AAMFT Standard 6.3 (2015) Confidentiality and Professional Responsibilities: It is the therapist's or supervisor's responsibility to choose technological platforms that adhere to standards of best practices related to confidentiality and quality of services and that meet applicable laws. Clients and supervisees are to be made aware in writing of the limitations and protections offered by the therapist's or supervisor's technology.

AAMFT Standard 6.4 (2015) Technology and Documentation: Therapists and supervisors are to ensure that all documentation containing identifying or otherwise sensitive information that is electronically stored and/or transferred is done using technology that adheres to standards of best practices related to confidentiality and quality of services and that meets applicable laws. Clients and supervisees are to be made aware in writing of the limitations and protections offered by the therapist's or supervisor's technology.

AAMFT Standard 6.5 (2015) Location of Services and Practice: Therapists and supervisors follow all applicable laws regarding location of practice and services and do not use technologically assisted means for practicing outside of their allowed jurisdictions.

AAMFT Standard 6.6 (2015) Training and Use of Current Technology: Marriage and family therapists ensure that they are well trained and competent in the use of all chosen technology-assisted professional services. Careful choices of audio, video, and other options are made to optimize quality and security of services and to adhere to standards of best practices for technology-assisted services. Furthermore, such choices of technology are to be suitably advanced and current so as to best serve the professional needs of clients and supervisees.

Social Media

With the emergence of Internet user-created content (Web 2.0), social media has become a fundamental part of life for many. Prior to Internet user-created content, users were required to have knowledge of programming languages like HTML, and the ability to create content was limited to people who had the technological expertise to create websites and maintain online servers. This is no longer the case with the growing Internet. Novice users of Internet technologies can post their own pictures, thoughts, and comments on everything from news articles to the clothes a celebrity wears or a public event. The person's ability to share his/her ideas and thoughts is what makes social media the leading type of social networking activity.

Social media companies continually emerge in the United States. There are so many social media applications and companies that it may be difficult for many counselors to understand how to choose the most appropriate ones to use. Subsequently, a counselor might find it challenging to protect him/herself when he/she does not know where the threat lies or if it even exists.

In the following illustrations, social media refers to applications accessed through various mediums allowing users to generate and distribute content to a social network. Consider Case Illustration 9-5 in which Lori must determine how to react to being "tagged" in a picture on Facebook.

CASE ILLUSTRATION 9-5

Lori is a professional counselor who considers social media to be a great way to stay in touch with friends and family. She uses her Facebook page to stay in touch with many people with whom she grew up as well as her friends from college. Lori also uses her Facebook page to advertise and promote her counseling practice. She knows it would be unethical to post any information about specific clients but routinely posts pictures of the outside of her office. She also posts information about new counseling groups she is starting and has a habit of changing her "status" each morning to a new inspirational message.

Lori has even started receiving "friend" requests from a few of her clients, and she accepts the requests as long as her clients do not have a history of criminal or aggressive behaviors. Lori knows she never posts any inappropriate messages or pictures and believes Facebook is a good way to give her clients access to her when they are not in session. Lori feels as though she has nothing to hide and hopes the inspirational quotes and information about her practice will be helpful to her clients.

Is Lori acting in an ethical manner by accepting her clients' "friend" requests?

Should Lori discontinue her use of social media?

The first question in Case Illustration 9-5 asks if Lori is behaving ethically by communicating with her clients on her Facebook page. The simple answer is no; she is not acting in an ethical manner. By communicating with clients, friends, and family all through the use of one Facebook account, Lori is not in compliance with Ethical Standard H.6.a.

ACA Standard H.6.a. (2014) Virtual Professional Presence: In cases where counselors wish to maintain a professional and personal presence for social media use, separate professional and personal webpages and profiles are created to clearly distinguish between the two kinds of virtual presence.

If Lori would like to continue to use social media to connect with her clients, she must have separate accounts: one for her friends and family members and the other for her professional practice. By communicating with all parties via one account, Lori is exposing herself and her clients to various security threats (e.g., breach of confidentiality).

In response to the second question and whether Lori should discontinue all social media usage, no. Lori is able to continue her usage of social media sites and may continue to connect with her clients. If she chooses to do so, she will want to review Ethical Standard H.6.b. and integrate her social media policy into her regular informed consent document.

ACA Standard H.6.b. (2014) Social Media as Part of Informed Consent: Counselors clearly explain to their clients, as part of the informed consent procedure, the benefits, limitations, and boundaries of the use of social media.

The term "professionalism" should come to mind for counselors considering using social media (i.e., counselors must use it in a professional manner). In Case Illustration 9-5, Lori must be cognizant of the conceivable harm of informal uses of social media and other related technology with clients, former clients and their families, and personal friends. Before deciding to continue her use of social media, Lori must consider all ethical implications, including confidentiality, privacy, and multiple relationships. She would want to develop written practice procedures related to social media and digital technology and incorporate them into the informed consent form provided to clients before or during the initial session.

Although the use of social media is new to most people, it has been around for more than a decade. Counselors are implored to be congruent between public and private self on social media. Social media is not private and should be discussed with clients during the informed consent part of the counseling process. The ethical concerns raised in Case Illustration 9-5 are based on Lori's lack of preparation and implementing preventive measures prior to using social media.

Social media gives individuals a chance to share parts of their lives with friends and family members. Social media also gives individuals the opportunity to glance inside the lives of others. Given the opportunity, it may be tempting for professional counselors to look up current or past clients. Concomitant to the social media ethical concerns presented previously, counselors have a duty to respect client's rights to privacy on social media. Simply stated, counselors should not view their clients' information or make any attempt to contact clients via social media unless given written consent.

ACA Standard H.6.c. (2014) Client Virtual Presence: Counselors respect the privacy of their clients' presence on social media unless given consent to view such information.

To exemplify Ethical Standard H.6.c. please consider Case Illustration 9-6, and determine the appropriateness of Clyde's behaviors.

CASE ILLUSTRATION 9-6

Clyde is the director of a clinic with five full-time licensed professional counselors and two office staff. He is a licensed professional counselor and a national certified counselor. Over the last five years he and the counselors he supervises have provided counseling services on a sliding fee scale to clients ranging from a minimum of $25 to a maximum of $135 a session. Clyde's clinic also provides counseling services to three large companies in the area through an employee assistance program. A year ago the clinic began taking insurance from clients because the cash flow was not sufficient to stay in business. The office staff at Clyde's clinic is also very active on social media. After receiving approval from Clyde, the office staff developed an office Facebook page and regularly updates the page with relevant office information. The staff also reaches out to new clients by looking them up on Facebook and asking them to "like" the office Facebook page. Unbeknownst to Clyde, the office staff also routinely searches the backgrounds of each client at the clinic. They use court records, tax records, online public files, and social media to research potential clients and existing clients to get demographic information they may be able to use to track down clients if they do not pay for services.

Is it ethical for the clinic office staff to reach out to clients via Facebook or other social media sites?

Is it ethical for the clinic office staff to research the backgrounds of clients on the Internet?

In other professions such as construction, real estate, and finance, background information of clients is essential. There is a potential for loss if a construction company builds an office building and the company hiring the company cannot pay; a real estate company sells a house to someone who can't afford the house; or a loan officer provides a personal loan to someone who cannot afford to pay the money back. Why should counseling be any different? According to Standard H.6.c. (Client Virtual Presence), the actions taken by Clyde's office staff would most likely be considered unethical. In this case, the people seeking counseling services are not technically clients yet; therefore, it would not be unethical according to the written word of the code of ethics. However, it could be argued that someone seeking counseling services should be considered a client at first contact. In such cases, the office staff should not examine social media and should not reach out to clients without first having the client's written permission. Although nothing in the code addresses gathering online information outside of social media (e.g., tax records and court records), it is all in the public domain. The ethical counselor would discuss social media and public profiles with clients if needed. In addition, Clyde is responsible for the actions of his office staff. Therefore he must inform his subordinates who do have physical and electronic access to information of the importance of maintaining privacy and confidentiality. Clyde would want to direct his staff to avoid contacting clients or potential clients via digital technology and social media sources (e.g., Facebook, LinkedIn, Twitter, etc.) in accordance with established practice procedures provided to clients at the beginning of starting counseling services.

Records Storage

Records and storage of records was discussed in detail in Chapter 5 along with other counselor responsibilities. In this section the authors address record storage specifically related to storing electronic documents. The ACA Code of Ethics provides guidance in Ethical Standard H.5.a. (Records).

ACA Standard H.5.a. (2014) Records: Counselors maintain electronic records in accordance with relevant laws and statutes. Counselors inform clients on how records are maintained electronically. This includes, but is not limited to, the type of encryption and security assigned to the records, and if/for how long archival storage of transaction records is maintained.

Review Case Illustration 9-7 as an example of how Standard H.5.a. might help Tony determine how to best store e-mails and other client documents.

CASE ILLUSTRATION 9-7

Tony, a counselor at a rural nonprofit agency, has clients who are located over a large geographical area. He has discovered the best way to effectively communicate with his clients is to utilize e-mails, phone calls, videoconferencing, and text messaging. Most of Tony's clients use the various communication avenues sparingly and mainly as a means to confirm or reschedule appointments. Although, Tony has one client who regularly sends rather detailed and elaborate e-mails. Recently, Tony's client sent an e-mail concerning her reaction to side effects of a new drug she was prescribed to treat her seasonal depression. The e-mail is longer than any he has ever received. It contains insight into her thought processes under this new drug as well as details of her intimacy issues, parenting problems, substance use, compulsive video gaming, and her desire to get better from the injuries she sustained as a result of a recent car accident. Tony typically responds to all e-mails and then deletes them, but he is concerned about the detail of his client's correspondence and believes he should begin keeping them. Tony wonders how he might store his e-mails and for how long he should keep them.

How might Tony determine the best way to store his communication with clients?

In Case Illustration 9-7, Tony is concerned about how to store e-mails he receives from clients. According to Ethical Standard H.5.a., Tony is held to local, state, and federal laws regarding how long he maintains records. Therefore Tony would need to search for online record storage laws for the state in which he lives or seek the assistance of a legal expert to aid him in the search. In addition to adhering to those laws, Tony is responsible for notifying his clients about such standards and how he is making sure his records conform to the level of security required. Notifying clients of how records are stored is often done through the informed consent process.

Web Maintenance

Professional websites are a common tool for professional counselors to advertise services and connect with clients. Websites vary in structure and depth; however, there are some specific requirements identified by the ACA Code of Ethics and all counselors and agencies must conform.

ACA Standard H.5.b. (2014) Client Rights: Counselors who offer distance counseling services and/or maintain a professional website provide electronic links to relevant licensure and professional certification boards to protect consumer and client rights and address ethical concerns.

Counselors who maintain a professional website or provide distance counseling must provide the links to all relevant licensure and certification boards. In striving toward aspirational ethics, professional counselors should have links in an area easily accessible to clients.

ACA Standard H.5.c. (2014) Electronic Links: Counselors regularly ensure that electronic links are working and are professionally appropriate.

Similar to Standard H.5.b., H.5.c. requires clients to regularly check links on their professional websites to ensure all are functioning and up-to-date. This requirement is of all links and not just those to licensure boards. Simply stated, in acting professionally, counselors monitor their webpages to make sure they are properly maintained. See Case Illustration 9-8 as an example of how Sabra maintains her website.

CASE ILLUSTRATION 9-8

Sabra is a licensed professional counselor in Texas and considers herself to have average technological skills and expertise. She does not provide distance counseling to clients but does maintain a webpage to advertise and communicate with clients and the general public. On her site, Sabra lists information about her practice, has copies of her consent forms, and also describes her general beliefs about counseling. Sabra also has a section of her webpage dedicated to providing referrals and resources for clients. In this section she typically includes links to various community websites (e.g., United Way, Boys and Girls Club, Department of Health and Family Services, Domestic Violence websites, etc.).

Sabra also prides herself on being conscientious and ethical in her practice. Knowing the requirements of the ACA Code of Ethics, she includes links to the Texas State Board of Examiners

(Continued)

(Continued)

for Professional Counselors, Texas Counseling Association, and the ACA at the bottom of her main webpage. Finally, Sabra is careful to make sure her office manager checks and updates every link listed on her webpage on the first day of every month.

Would Sabra's actions be considered sufficient according to ACA Ethical Standards H.5.b. and H.5.c.?

In response to the question in Case Illustration 9-8, yes, Sabra's actions would most likely be sufficient in covering Ethical Standards H.5.b. and H.5c. Sabra provides links to all relevant licensure boards for the state in which she lives (i.e., Sabra lives in Texas and provides a link to the Texas licensure board). Sabra also provides links to her state and national professional counseling associations. In accordance with Ethical Standard H.5.c., Sabra also has a process for checking and updating all links on her webpage (i.e., she directs her office assistant to verify and update all links on the first day of every month).

Multicultural and Disability Considerations

ACA Standard H.5.d. (2014) Multicultural and Disability Considerations: Counselors who maintain websites provide accessibility to persons with disabilities. They provide translation capabilities for clients who have a different primary language when feasible. Counselors acknowledge the imperfect nature of such translations and accessibilities.

When counselors work in areas where multiple languages are spoken (e.g., the primary language spoken is English but approximately 40 percent of the population is English/Spanish bilingual), they provide translations on their websites. Additionally, professional counselors are cognizant to use software that is compatible to any devices that may be used by clients or consumers that may have a visual or other impairment. Consider Case Illustration 9-9 and how Mark sets up a webpage to advertise the opening of his new private practice.

CASE ILLUSTRATION 9-9

Mark is a licensed professional counselor and licensed marriage and family therapist. He has recently moved into his own private practice and is struggling to make ends meet. Mark has marketed his services to several surrounding school districts and doctor's offices but is still struggling to fill his caseload. As a result he has decided to develop a webpage to attract more clients. Mark has limited knowledge related to technology and therefore goes online to search for the best bargain in creating a professional webpage. Mark is able to find an inexpensive package in which he will be able to develop his own webpage and link to a maximum of three other webpages.

Is Mark acting in an ethical manner by creating his webpage?

In Case Illustration 9-9, it is difficult to say for sure if Mark is acting ethically or not. Mark wanted to save money and therefore sought out the least expensive way to create a professional webpage. He is able to link his page to three other sites, giving him the ability to list credentialing bodies and professional associations. The main ethical concern is related to Mark's ability to develop his webpage and make it accessible to various populations. For example, is someone who is visually impaired able to access his page? Is the information on Mark's webpage written in a way accessible to those speaking various languages?

Conclusion

The development of distance technology continues to evolve. From letters being sent back and forth between client and counselor in the early 1900s to live distance professional services, threats and opportunities exist. In regard to technology, the ethical counselor will actively attempt to understand the changes to counseling with the infusion of technology into the counseling relationship. Counselors, like most other individuals, likely use technology throughout most of their everyday activities (i.e., cell phones, computers, social media, video games, and automobiles). As technology continues to expand and new opportunities become available to the general public, it will also continue to grow in the counseling profession. The future growth of technology will bring more changes and understanding. Concepts of confidentiality, data security, and distance professional services will continue to be at the forefront of ethical concerns. It is up to each and every counselor to understand the threats and opportunities technology presents to clients, students, and supervisees.

Use the information learned in Chapter 9 to address the ethical dilemma and discussion questions presented in Exercise 9-1.

CASE EXERCISE 9-1

Ronald is a newly licensed professional counselor and has been working as an independent contractor with several agencies for almost six months. Ronald is an avid user of technology and believes in using technology to aid in the growth of his counseling practice. Therefore he

(Continued)

(Continued)

has developed a webpage marketing his counseling practice. Ronald is careful to follow all ACA ethical guidelines by monitoring his webpage closely, including links to licensure boards, and regularly checking to make sure all links work appropriately. As with many new counselors, Ronald contracts with various agencies as a way to build up his own reputation and clientele. He would eventually like to open his own private practice and views his contract work with agencies as a stepping stone.

Because Ronald travels between home visits and various offices, he tries to keep the amount of "stuff" he needs to a minimum. He uses his personal laptop to store all client records and uses his personal cell phone as his business phone to contact clients. Upon getting his license Ronald splurged and bought a new car because he knew he would need reliable transportation. While traveling from one office to another, Ronald finds the "hands-free" Bluetooth phone function very helpful. All of his phone contacts are stored in his car, and he can easily call to confirm or reschedule appointments while on the road.

At a recent home visit, one of Ronald's clients mentioned she has been receiving random e-mails from Ronald's e-mail address. She claims to have received five or six e-mails in the past week and worries Ronald's computer or e-mail may be infected with a virus. After checking with several other clients, Ronald determines that most of his clients have been receiving the same e-mails, and he needs to get his laptop scanned to make sure all viruses are removed. Consequently, Ronald must find a place to take his computer to be fixed.

Where should Ronald take his computer to be fixed if he can't remove the viruses on his own?

If Ronald does take his computer to a shop, how can he be sure his clients' confidentiality will be maintained by the individual(s) working on his laptop?

What, if any, are other potential ethical concerns regarding his usage of his laptop to store client records?

Ronald drives a newer model car and is able to download his phone contacts to his car via the car's Bluetooth technology. What, if any, potential ethical concerns exist by him doing this?

If Ronald ever decides to sell his car, do his phone contacts (i.e., client names and numbers) stay on the car's hard drive? If so, does that pose a threat to client confidentiality?

Discussion Questions

What is your general comfort level when using technology as a whole?

Do you believe distance counseling is something you plan on providing in your own practice?

What do you believe are the main benefits of providing distance counseling?

What do you view as the primary drawbacks of distance counseling?

Using the example given in this chapter and any other examples or references you may have, take time to construct your own informed consent form for use with distance counseling clients.

Keystones

- Section H, newly added to the 2014 ACA Code of Ethics, relates to distance counseling, technology, and social media.
- Technology can be a valuable tool for counselors but also poses many threats to confidentiality.
- Counselors using distance counseling or technology to assist in their counseling practice must be competent to use the technology.
- Counselors using distance counseling or technology to assist in their counseling practice must be aware of related ethical and legal considerations.
- Clients have the freedom to choose whether or not they wish to participate in distance counseling.
- Counselors providing distance counseling must provide clients with informed consent including: the counselor's credentials, physical location of the counselor's practice, benefits and drawbacks related to distance counseling, possibility of technology failure, time zone differences, cultural or language differences, possible denial of insurance benefits, social media policy, and anticipated response time.
- Counselors providing distance counseling must take steps to verify the client's indemnity throughout the therapeutic process.
- Counselors must take reasonable measures to assure client information is kept confidential when using technology-based communication.
- Counselors should take preventative measures to assure client confidentiality is respected.
- If counselors choose to participate in social media websites, they must keep firm boundaries between personal and professional accounts.
- Clients are prohibited from spying on clients via social media without having written consent from clients to do so.
- Counselors who maintain a professional webpage must continually monitor their webpage, making sure all links are properly working.
- Counselors who maintain a professional webpage must include links to all applicable licensure boards and professional associations.
- Counselors who maintain a professional webpage must be sure to use appropriate software when designing the webpage, making sure all information is accessible to various populations.

Additional Resources

American Psychological Association. (2010). *American Psychological Association ethical principles of psychologists and code of conduct.* Retrieved from http://www.apa.org/ethics/code/principles.pdf

Center for Credentialing and Education. (2014, November 1). Retrieved from http://www.cce-global.org

Gonyea, J. L. J., Wright, D. W., & Earl-Kulkosky, T. (2014). Navigating dual relationships in rural communities. *Journal of Marital and Family Therapy, 40*(1), 125–136. doi:http://dx.doi.org/10.1111/j.1752-0606.2012.00335.x

National Board for Certified Counselors. (2012). *Code of ethics*. Retrieved from http://www.nbcc .org/assets/ethics/nbcc-codeofethics.pdf

National Board for Certified Counselors. (2012). *Policy regarding the provision of distance professional services*. Retrieved from http://www.nbcc.org/Assets/Ethics/NBCC Policy Regarding the Practice of Distance Counseling –Board – Adopted Version – July 2012-PDF.pdf

Rousmaniere, T., & Frederickson, J. (2013). Internet-based one-way-mirror supervision for advanced psychotherapy training. *The Clinical Supervisor, 32*(1), 40–55. doi:http://dx.doi.org/10.1080/07 325223.2013.778683

References

American Association for Marriage and Family Therapy. (2015). *Code of ethics*. Retrieved from https://www.aamft.org/iMIS15/AAMFT/Content/legal_ethics/code_of_ethics.aspx

American Counseling Association. (2014). *Code of ethics*. Alexandria, VA: Author.

10

Ethics in Group Work, Couples, and Families

You cannot plough a field by turning it over in your mind.

—Author Unknown

This chapter will discuss ethical issues related to counseling and working with couples, families, and groups in a therapeutic setting. Each of the populations mentioned has special considerations when addressing confidentiality, consent, and the relationships among all parties involved. The authors will also discuss pertinent ethical codes and general laws related to domestic violence and intimate partner violence. As with the previous chapters in this text, ethical dilemmas and application of knowledge will encourage readers to examine how they would react in real-life clinical situations rather than in the academic classroom. Discussion questions will be tailored to challenge students to evaluate how they decide on their ways to act rather than their actual actions.

Specifically, after reading this chapter the reader will be able to do the following:

1. Explain ethical concerns when counseling couples, families, and groups.

2. Describe situations when a counselor may need to make an informed ethical decision to ensure a family or group member's safety and/or well-being.

3. Define characteristics of confidentiality and consent specific to working with groups, couples, and/or families.

4. Discuss the importance of screening group members prior to the start of group counseling.

Ethics in Group Work

The ACA Code of Ethics (2014) has sections that directly address working with groups (Section A.9. [Group Work]) and couples and families (Section B.4. [Groups and Families]); however, most issues that arise in group counseling and/or family and couple counseling situations are covered by other sections of the code. Throughout this chapter, the authors will discuss issues related to working with groups, families, and couples while also addressing how other, more general, sections of the ACA Code of Ethics may apply to working with these populations. Though families and couples are contained in the same phrase in the ACA Code of Ethics, readers should be aware that there are differences in treating couples compared to families.

As mentioned previously, there are few standards included in the 2014 ACA Code of Ethics specific to group work (Welfel, 2010). Standards A.9.a., A.9.b., and B.4.a. are the only three standards that speak specifically to working in group settings. What follows are descriptions of each and examples related to how the standards may be applied in real-world situations.

ACA Standard A.9.a. (2014) Screening: Counselors screen prospective group counseling and therapy participants. To the extent possible, counselors select members whose needs and goals are compatible with the goals of the group, who will not impede the group process, and whose well-being will not be jeopardized by the group experience.

Similar to the idea that all professional counselors prescreen clients to assure the client's area of counseling need falls within the counselor's area of competence, counselors working in group settings must follow the same or similar procedures. Additionally, counselors who conduct group counseling must also ensure all active group members are compatible with each other and the overall goals for the group. Review Case Illustration 10-1 as an example of the importance of prescreening group members.

CASE ILLUSTRATION 10-1

A professional school counselor is forming a psychoeducational group for students who have recently had a parent or guardian die and fails to screen potential group members. At the first group meeting, school students are individually invited to share about themselves and their interest in group participation. During a discussion one student says her mother has not died yet but has just been diagnosed with a terminal illness; she thought this group might help her prepare for her mother's eventual death. Another student says he has just had his dog die and wanted to be able to talk to other people that were grieving the loss of someone or something they loved.

How might these differences in group members possibly have a negative impact on the overall success of the group?

While there is no way to immediately determine if this group will be successful or not, it is feasible to say some of these students are dealing with completely different types of grief. If the group were to proceed with the member issues outlined in Case Illustration 10-1, the group members dealing with recent deaths of parents or guardians may likely have different concerns than the group members dealing with the recent loss of a pet or the recent diagnosis of a terminal illness. Those differences in goals would likely have a detrimental impact on the overall group. By prescreening group members, the school counselor would have been able to identify the two students grieving the loss of a pet and the foreseeable death of a parent and possibly either develop another group to address their needs or fit them into a different school counseling group. In summary, goals need to be made apparent for all group participants prior to the beginning of the group. Prescreening group members will enable the group facilitator to assure all group members' needs fit the goals of the group.

Case Illustration 10-2 serves as another example of the importance of screening group members prior to the first session. In this case illustration, the facilitator rushes to get a counseling group started and fails to screen to ensure balance among group members.

CASE ILLUSTRATION 10-2

A clinical mental health counselor publicizes a "developing healthy relationships" group at the request of his counseling supervisor. Because he is in a hurry to get the group started, he neglects to fully screen potential group counseling members. On the first night of the counseling group, seven males (ages 19–21) attend the group and one female (age 18) attends. During the group session it is obvious that the female participant is uncomfortable being the only female, and she is very quiet and hesitant to share with the counseling group. After the first meeting, she fails to show up for any more group sessions without calling or notifying the group counseling facilitator.

How might it have benefited the group if the counselor would have taken time to screen potential group members?

In Case Illustration 10-2, screening might have helped identify an adequate balance of male and female participants and even participants of similar ages. By not screening for these variables, the counselor failed to include members who were potentially more compatible for the group that would have increased group counseling efficacy. There is not a specific number of males or females needed to appropriately balance a group, but screening would have alerted the facilitator to the clear imbalance and allowed him/her to make appropriate changes to increase the comfort level of all participants.

ACA Standard A.9.b. (2014) Protecting Clients: In a group setting, counselors take reasonable precautions to protect clients from physical, emotional, or psychological trauma. Simply stated, counselors are responsible for their clients. Counselors should not allow group members to harass or physically or emotionally abuse one another. It is the counselor's role to be the facilitator and moderate the interactions between members. This includes setting up rules and standards for communication outside of the counseling setting. Namely, with the continual and increasing use of technology, an informed counselor may need to set social media and technology-aided communication guidelines for group participants. Review Case Illustration 10-3, and see how understanding ACA Ethical Standard A.9.a. might have been beneficial to Heath in dealing with an altercation during group.

CASE ILLUSTRATION 10-3

Heath is a counselor at a long-term care facility in which boys between the ages of 10 and 17 are placed (typically by child protective services or juvenile probation). The general length of stay for clients is between 6 and 12 months, and during that time, group counseling is a staple in the therapeutic process. Heath has been working at the facility for approximately three years and is one of the more senior counselors at the facility.

During a weekly staff meeting, Heath brings up an incident that occurred during one of his groups earlier in the week. Heath explained that the incident started when one of the older boys (Ray) was called out by a few of the younger boys as being a bully. Ray denied the allegations and simply laughed them off. As a result, all of the other seven members of the group seemed to gang up on Ray, calling him out on his actions. The group continued to escalate and eventually got to the point where group members were insulting Ray, and the group turned into a personal attack of Ray.

When questioned about the eventual outcome and his role as the facilitator, Heath said that Ray was fine. Heath explained the attack only lasted about five minutes, and he thought Ray "had it coming to him. After all, Ray is a bully, and he does the same thing to the younger kids all the time. It's about time he got a taste of his own medicine." Heath further explained Ray was alright; he cried a little at the end but he needs to get "punked" every once in a while, so he doesn't get too cocky.

Do you believe Heath acted ethically in letting the "attack" occur?

What could Heath have done differently to still address Ray's bullying behavior but prevent Ray from being verbally attacked as he was?

Related to the first question associated with Case Illustration 10-3, Heath would be considered as acting in an unethical manner. As previously stated in ACA Standard A.9.b., the counselor, Heath in this case, must take precautions to protect every client from being harmed. Whether the attack was physical, emotion, or verbal, it was Heath's responsibility to put a stop to it at first notice.

The second question inquires as to how Heath might have addressed Ray's bullying behavior differently in group while still being sure to protect him from any type of trauma. There are many ways Heath might have addressed the behaviors differently. The simplest of these may have been to slow the group members down and review group rules and expectations at the first notice of escalating behaviors:

I hear you all becoming very angry with Ray. You feel as though he bullies you all the time and even now, when it is brought up with the whole group, you feel as though he's not even paying attention. I can tell the way all of you are sitting and chomping at the bit that you want to get back at Heath and put him in his place. I can certainly understand your feelings, and I want you all to be able to speak your mind. At the same time I want to make sure we still abide by our group rules and norms. As the leader, I won't just sit back and let you tear into another member. How about we give each person a chance to talk? Ray, I think this may be important for you to pay attention to. I can't force you to listen, but it will certainly give you a sense of what everyone else thinks about you.

This is only one example of many. The goal for Heath would be to provide a safe group atmosphere for all group members (including Ray) to speak and be listened to. In Case Illustration 10-4, the authors explore the case of Heath in more depth and discuss additional areas of the ACA Code of Ethics that may be appropriate in considering the entire situation.

CASE ILLUSTRATION 10-4

Following the staff meeting in which Heath shared the incident occurring during his group, he is called in for a meeting with his clinical supervisor. During the meeting the supervisor questions Heath further about his actions or lack thereof during the group altercation. Heath again explained that he felt as though Ray had it coming, and it wasn't like he let the other kids beat him up. No one ever physically touched Ray; they were only words. As Heath continues to talk with his supervisor, Heath reveals he was bullied on many occasions growing up, so he knows what the other kids feel like when Ray picks on them. Heath says it gives the victims a feeling of power if they are allowed to stand up for themselves. Heath continues to stand by his decision to allow the verbal abuse to continue for a short amount of time.

What part(s) of the ACA Code of Ethics may be appropriate to reference in this situation?

Responding to the discussion question associated with Case Illustration 10-4, ACA Standard A.4.b. (Personal Values) would be important to reference in this situation. Standard C.2.g. might also be appropriate to consider. Case illustration 10-4 gives the reader more insight into Heath's background, and it is determined that he was bullied at a young age, similar to the bullying he sees Ray do to the other clients. Counselors must be aware of their own "stuff" and understand how past issues can affect the counselor's ability to work with clients.

Self-awareness is a concept talked about multiple times throughout this text. The case of Heath provides another example of the need for self-awareness and counselors' understanding their own morals, values, beliefs, and experiences. In this case, if Heath were to have been self-aware and in touch with his strong beliefs about bullies, he would have been extra sensitive to his tendencies. Instead of allowing the verbal abuse to occur,

Heath might have been expecting his strong feelings to come up and might have been extra careful to protect "the bully" (Ray). Without self-awareness and understanding, Heath rationalizes his actions as Ray "getting what he deserves" and has jeopardized his ability to be an objective and ethical group facilitator.

As mentioned in previous chapters, professional counselors must be able to be vulnerable, understanding both their strengths and areas for improvement. Standard C.2.g. is appropriate to keep in mind if Heath feels as though his countertransference toward those who bully others is a constant concern. According to ACA Standard C.2.g., Heath should monitor himself and seek assistance if his issues with bullies become a more prominent concern.

ACA Standard B.4.a. (2014) Group Work: In group work, counselors clearly explain the importance and parameters of confidentiality for the specific group.

See Text Box 10-1 for the APA standard related to group therapy.

TEXT BOX 10-1

American Psychological Association

APA Standard 10.03 (2010) Group Therapy: When psychologists provide services to several persons in a group setting, they describe at the outset the roles and responsibilities of all parties and the limits of confidentiality.

American Association for Marriage and Family Therapists

The AAMFT 2015 Code of Ethics does not specifically address group work.

At the onset and throughout the life of the group, counselors continually explain the importance of confidentiality and limits of confidentiality. When conducting individual counseling, counselors can provide assurances to the client that confidentiality will be kept (except in cases of harm to self or others or other state-required exceptions). However, in group counseling settings, where there are multiple members, the counselor cannot provide such assurances because the counselor cannot completely assure how each group member will act outside of the group—online or in person. As such, it is important that the counselor continues to remind members of the importance of confidentiality and how sharing another member's confidential information may have considerable consequences for the group. These rules should be arranged prior to the start of the group counseling sessions.

Case Illustration 10-5 shows how group counseling involves various sections of the 2014 ACA Code of Ethics other than those specific areas already discussed.

CASE ILLUSTRATION 10-5

Georgia, a licensed professional counselor, is currently forming a psychotherapeutic group for children focusing on families of divorce. She is advertising using a radio spot, an online advertisement, and flyers passed out to local clinics, churches, and schools. The advertisements make known that the cost per family is $100 for a four-week, 20-hour treatment process consisting of four week nights and one Saturday. The payment must be made prior to the first evening.

Are Georgia's recruiting methods ethical?

Advertising on the radio, on the Internet, and through other media such as passing out flyers in the community are all ethical ways of advertising as long as Georgia follows Standard C.3.a. (Accurate Advertising). This section requires Georgia to accurately represent her credentials as a licensed professional counselor in a manner that "is not false, misleading, deceptive, or fraudulent" (ACA, 2014, p. 9). For this group specifically, the wider a counselor can cast a marketing net, the better the response rate of potential participants and group members. Advertising will change as marketing professionals create new media, and advances in technology are diffused across communities.

Georgia consulted Standard A.10.c. (Establishing Fees) and took into account the low- to middle-class income status of the population where the agency is located. She consulted with other counselors and determined $100 was an acceptable fee. Still, Georgia must also be prepared with external referrals should potential clients call and ask for comparable services that might be more affordable for clients unable to afford her fees. A major benefit of group counseling is that it is considered to be one of the most financially sound clinical efforts a counselor can make as well as a better value for clients. The cost is lower than individual sessions for the client, and the financial return for the counselor is better than individual sessions for time spent in session. However, in the case of Georgia, her fees could keep some people from getting the counseling services they may need. Typically, the price point is solely left up to the counselor, and at the time of this text, there is no limit on the price for counseling from a private payer. However, insurance companies may have planned and contracted prices available for counselors and clients to assess for affordability.

Georgia chooses to require prepaid services to help avoid the occurrence of client attrition in the group before the conclusion of the final session. She believes premature termination by one (or more) of the members could potentially be disruptive to other counseling group members. The question of cost is worth discussing related to what happens if a client needs to drop out. Georgia's refund policy must be stated up front before any sort of payment is made (Section A.2 [Informed Consent]). This information must be reviewed in the informed consent, which must occur prior to any services and must be signed. Additional changes in fees must be given in writing to clients prior to any change in fee structure for services rendered.

The case of Georgia brings to light the need for informed consent to occur for all counseling services prior to beginning services. The case also brings up the concern of financial arrangements having the ability to screen out potential group membership because some individuals may not be able to afford services at a certain price point. If Georgia does not have enough respondents to her initial marketing of the group, she may want to drop her price point to increase the potential group participation.

In group work, the code of ethics must be followed at all times prior to creating a counseling group and once the group is created. Screening is paramount to group work to help avoid problems, specifically harm, prior to the occurrence of such issues. Case Illustration 10-6 demonstrates how counselors may choose to screen participants prior to entering into a group counseling treatment relationship.

CASE ILLUSTRATION 10-6

Mark, a licensed professional counselor, created a therapeutic group to address the grief experienced upon the death of a loved one (e.g., a grandparent, parent, sibling, child, aunt, uncle, or cousin). He advertised the group as a grief support group and stated it was open to anyone who is dealing with the death of a loved one. Mark mailed flyers and posters to funeral homes, churches, hospices, hospitals, and area school counselors. He received about 30 inquiries for the group, and he spoke with each person on the phone quickly about their needs. He referred a few potential participants to other clinics because the group was not right for them. Specifically, he did not want people needing hospice care, dealing with the loss of a family pet, or people suffering from severe depression. The first time the group met, 18 people showed up. His group therapy room seats about 20 people, so space was limited in his little clinic. The first few group counseling sessions focused on the establishment of trust, allowing members to talk personally and honestly. During those sessions, each individual was asked to make a personal commitment to the group and its goals to foster a sense of belonging and promote group trust.

At that point, Mark realized the grief experiences of the participants ranged widely. Some members were dealing with the death of a spouse after a long-term illness; others dealing with the sudden loss of a child, the loss of a parent or grandparent, the loss as a result of violent crimes, or loss by suicide. He realized the group members did not exactly complement each other through the therapeutic process. Mark had originally set up the group as a general loss group rather than a loss-specific group.

What could Mark have done ethically to have created a loss-specific group rather than a general loss group?

In this situation what is the best thing Mark might do to mitigate the problem?

Mark initially believed he had followed Standard A.9.a. (Screening) and had screened the participants by accepting only the clients who had suffered the loss of a loved one. Therefore he accepted everyone who was grieving in some way. In doing so, the needs and goals of some of the group members were incompatible with the goals of the whole group. For example, the extreme anger and a need to take revenge felt by some members who might have lost a loved one due to a violent crime would be significantly different than the sorrow and loss felt by a family who had lost a loved one to a long-term illness. Those differences impeded the overall therapeutic group process. Mark may have been able to avoid this by requiring all potential participants to attend a pre-group screening. A pre-group screening and orientation session would have allowed Mark to meet with all group participants and screen them for appropriateness before the group began. As a group counseling facilitator, it is difficult to rescreen clients once the group has started. Preliminary screening would have provided information to prospective participants about the group and helped determine if group therapy fit each person's current needs. Mark was not thorough enough on the telephone. Setting up a prescreening is paramount to the ethical delivery of group counseling and would have followed in line with the expectations set forth by Standard B.4.a.

The second question in Case Illustration 10-6 inquires as to what Mark might have done to mitigate the problem. Standard A.9.b. (Protecting Clients) reminds Mark about his ethical responsibility to take reasonable precautions to protect participants from emotional and psychological trauma. Mark believes the participants are vulnerable at this point in their grief work and are not yet ready to process the anger issues shared by those who suffered loss due to homicide. Rather than referring and eliminating troublesome group members, he decides to first conduct skills groups rather than a therapy group. The skills group will most likely be more structured than a therapy group and have more of a workshop format than a counseling format. In the skills group, Mark may provide psychoeducational information and opportunities for participants to apply the concepts they are learning in group counseling to their real, everyday lives. Following the six-week skill group on grief, Mark may invite the participants to regroup into more specific grief or loss groups, which may allow the participants to work with others who share a more common grief concern. In these groups members may talk about their specific losses and give feedback and support in a safe, supportive, copacetic environment. These interactions might offer group members an opportunity to learn more about the way they interact with others and try out new ways of dealing with their specific grief.

In addition to screening potential group members, confidentiality and beneficence are two important issues that should also be addressed prior to beginning any counseling group. They are specifically demonstrated in Case Illustration 10-7.

CASE ILLUSTRATION 10-7

Amy, an experienced professional counselor, has established a group for unemployed individuals who are faced with the prospect of losing a job and losing a way of life. Along with the job loss and unemployment, the group deals with the confusion of setting a new career direction and

(Continued)

(Continued)

the stress associated with searching for a new job. Most of her clients find the process to be extremely difficult and feel as if they are on an emotional roller coaster. This often proves true for the clients' families and also for the counselor who is trying to offer assistance. Amy meets once a week for two hours with the group and has been successful in assisting her group members in developing or changing career directions. The goals of her group are to help members do the following:

- Develop communication and other skills needed to gain pertinent information related to their fields of interest.
- Acquire information about the current economic climate and labor market opportunities in the city.
- Develop self-confidence adequate to be more self-sustaining in moving toward their goals of finding employment.

The group is open to everyone, but the majority of the group members are referrals from the local workforce commission, which is funded by the state and provides unemployment benefits.

One day, Amy receives a call from one of the job coaches at the workforce commission asking for information about a group member. The job coach asks about a client's attendance record because the client, as part of her continued unemployment benefits, must attend weekly jobless support groups. Amy is asked to confirm the client has consistently been attending sessions each week. According to the job coach, if Amy can't confirm the client has been attending weekly sessions, the client will lose unemployment benefits.

Can Amy break confidentiality and give the information to the job coach?

How does beneficence play in this ethical dilemma?

The answer to the first question in Case Illustration 10-7 is yes *but only* because Amy had the group members sign an informed consent form and a release of information form during the first meeting. The counselor consulted A.2.a. (Informed Consent) and "has reviewed in writing and verbally with clients the rights and responsibilities of both counselors and clients. Informed consent is an ongoing part of the counseling process, and counselors appropriately document discussions of informed consent throughout the counseling relationship" (ACA, 2014, p. 4). Amy's signed informed consent form indicates that the client understands Amy maintains confidentiality in accordance with the ethical guidelines and legal requirements of her counseling profession and in the state where she practices. It also states providing effective counseling services sometimes requires counselors to share confidential information with other professional counseling and service staff members to coordinate continuation of care. In the case of this particular client, Amy reviews his consent form and release of information and sees this client has specifically given permission for Amy to release information to the identified job coach. If the client had not signed a release specifically to the previously mentioned job coach, she would have needed to get a signed release prior to sharing any information with the coach.

For the second question Amy refers to the ACA Code of Ethics (2014) preamble, which identifies five ethical principles related to counseling: respect for autonomy, nonmaleficence, beneficence, justice, and fidelity. The ACA Code of Ethics defines beneficence as "working for the good of the individual and society by promoting mental health and well-being."

Amy meets individually with her client to share the request that has been made by the workforce commission job coach. In addition to sharing the information about the request, Amy also wants to solicit her client for ideas as to how she might be helpful in the future. The client has missed two sessions, which will influence the continual payment of unemployment compensation once the job coach is informed. The absences were due to the client's inability to secure care for his two young children, who were home sick with chicken pox. The client's wife is deceased, and he is the sole support for his two children. If his unemployment compensation is reduced, his family's welfare will be adversely affected. Amy explains to her client that she, as an ethical counselor, is expected to do what is best for him, but if unable to assist, she will offer appropriate alternatives.

The counselor will respond to the job coach but, with the client's permission, will follow A.7.a. (Advocacy), which directs Amy to "address potential barriers and obstacles that inhibit access and/or the growth and development of clients." The client and the counselor meet with the job coach to follow A.7.b. (Confidentiality and Advocacy) and to attempt to find alternatives to discontinuing the client's unemployment compensation as his absences were due to extenuating circumstances.

Amy practices career counseling, which may be an individually based therapeutic intervention. Her use of group career counseling in this case could have been a reaction to the closing of a large manufacturing plant in her city. She adjusted her services to meet the needs of the community in a way that helps both her and her clients. The ethical counselor will modify costs in writing with clients.

Counseling Couples and Families

Similar to what was discussed at the beginning of this chapter concerning group counseling and the minimal number of standards directly addressing group settings specifically, the same is true for couples and family counseling. There is only one standard in the ACA Code of Ethics (2014) specifically mentioning couples and family counseling (see Text Box 10-2 for the APA's guidelines).

ACA Standard B.4.b. (2014) Couples and Family Counseling: In couples and family counseling, counselors clearly define who is considered "the client" and discuss expectations and limitations of confidentiality. Counselors seek agreement and document in writing such agreement among all involved parties regarding the confidentiality of information. In the absence of an agreement to the contrary, the couple or family is considered to be the client.

TEXT BOX 10-2

American Psychological Association

APA Standard 10.02 (2010) Therapy Involving Couples or Families: (a) When psychologists agree to provide services to several persons who have a relationship (such as spouses, significant others, or parents and children), they take reasonable steps to clarify at the outset (1) which of the individuals are clients or patients and (2) the relationship the psychologist will have with each person. This clarification includes the psychologist's role and the probable uses of the services provided or information obtained. (b) If it becomes apparent that psychologists may be called on to perform potentially conflicting roles (such as family therapist and then witness for one party in divorce proceedings), psychologists take reasonable steps to clarify and modify, or withdraw from, roles appropriately)

Case Illustration 10-8 is an example of how Standard B.4.b. might be applied to an actual situation.

CASE ILLUSTRATION 10-8

Michael, a licensed professional counselor who works in an agency setting, faces a complicated family counseling ethical dilemma. He is working with the Sanchez family (husband, José; wife, Claudia; children, Joey (12) and Roberto (10). They originally came to counseling to work on the constant conflicts existing in the family relationship.

José and Claudia have been married for 16 years and were high school sweethearts. José is an executive in a local manufacturing company, and Claudia is a full-time homemaker who spends much of her time as a community volunteer. Her volunteering is mostly at Roberto's school and her church. During the telephone intake interview, Claudia shares with Michael that she feels the discord in her relationship comes from the fact that José is absent quite often from the family because he is constantly working long hours. He travels 60 percent of the time, and she believes that when he isn't in his office, he brings work home with him. Claudia also believes José's absence from the family has caused problems with Joey and Roberto who show disrespect for her, constantly argue with each other, and are not doing well academically in school.

Joey's middle school counselor, who is a friend of Michael's from graduate school, referred the family for family counseling. The school counselor was concerned about Joey because of his drop in grades and numerous referrals to the office for acting out in the classroom and fighting with his peers. Claudia shared that it took some coercing, but she had finally talked Josè into attending family counseling sessions.

During the initial session, Josè shares that he believes the children's misbehavior is a result of Claudia's spoiling them and giving them whatever they want. Conversely, Claudia feels the children's misbehavior is due to Josè's constant absence from the family. During this session and in front of the children, Josè yells at Claudia, saying that if she wasn't so cold and distant to him, he might want to be home more often. Claudia begins to cry, and the children glare at their father. The children remain silent during most of the session, and when Michael attempts to bring them into the discussion, Roberto finally interjects, "See, this is the way it always is at home. My parents are always disagreeing and yelling at each other." Roberto shakes his head and shares that he usually goes to his room and plays video games when his parents argue. At this point Michael realizes the arguing and yelling in the session has lasted so long that he was not able to complete the client informed consent for treatment forms or the assessment of family-of-origin history gathering. Prior to the end of the session, he has the family complete the informed consent forms, and both counselor and family decide they will complete family history assessment at the next scheduled meeting.

Before the scheduled second session, Josè calls the counselor and explains that he is on the verge of having an affair with a female colleague with whom he travels regularly. They have not yet had any sexual contact, but he has very strong emotions for her and reports, "She is so easy to be around. My relationship with Claudia is like being in a war zone." Josè asks Michael not to say anything to Claudia and asks to schedule an individual counseling session to clarify his feelings and options.

Josè's call is followed by a telephone call from Claudia. She tells Michael she is two months pregnant, and Josè is not aware of the unplanned pregnancy. She is considering a termination of the pregnancy as a way to get even with Josè for being so accusing and unavailable to her. In addition, she shares that the abortion will really hurt Josè because he has always wanted a daughter, and Claudia is sure that this baby is a girl.

Michael does not know where to begin with the family or what to do with all of the secrets.

Who is the client? Why?

Do Michael's clients have an expectation of privacy in family counseling sessions about things discussed in individual counseling sessions?

The answer to the first question of Case Illustration 10-8 is that the family is the client during family therapy. Because Michael does not have signed documentation and no specific individual within the family was previously identified as "the client," the family is considered the client according to Standard B.4.b. (Couples and Family Counseling).

In addition to following Standard B.4.b., Michael could also refer to Standard A.8 (Multiple Clients) and realize that he could also simply ask and clarify the expectations of the family who they might identify as the "client." During the course of treatment, if it ever were to become apparent that Michael may be called upon to perform potentially conflicting roles, he should also clarify, adjust, or withdraw from roles appropriately (ACA, 2014, p. 6).

Michael has a "no secrets" policy in his informed consent form, which he was able to complete with all family members at the end of the first session. As such, Michael is now in a situation where he knows José is secretly contemplating an affair and Claudia is secretly considering terminating her unplanned pregnancy. It could be unethical or at least problematic for Michael to have such information and continue to work with the couple, knowing each member is not being an honest and active participant in the family counseling, with each client having contradictory agendas. Michael's signed policy addresses the situations in which information is shared with the counselor by one member of the couple or family unit outside the presence of the other member of the couple or family unit. This "no secrets" policy states that information shared with the counselor *could* be shared with the other member(s) of the couple or family unit, as the counselor thinks is appropriate. This assures Michael that he will not allow himself to be put in the position of holding the secrets of one party participating in family therapy.

This case typifies the triangulation that may occur between the counselor and a couple or family. Triangulation occurs when someone being treated in the family or group singles out the counselor and shares information that might be either damaging or therapeutic for the family system or group. The ethical counselor must make every effort to explain triangulation prior to entering into the therapeutic relationship. Even though the ethical counselor will try and prevent this from happening, it may still occur. If it does occur, the ethical counselor will have prepared the family through informed consent to choose the best way to use the triangulated information. The code of ethics does not address triangulation directly, but in Section B, the code discusses confidentiality. In the family setting, the family is the client; therefore, nothing is confidential among family members. Unless the information is deemed nontherapeutic, or damaging to another family member, the information will, and should, be shared therapeutically with the family.

Case Illustration 10-9 is an extension of Case Illustration 10-8 and further explores Michael's ongoing counseling relationship with the Sanchez family.

CASE ILLUSTRATION 10-9

The Sanchez family continues to work with Michael in counseling. However, the mode of therapy has evolved into couple's therapy, and the children, Joey and Roberto, are now being seen together with Amanda, a licensed professional counselor who specializes in play therapy and to whom Michael referred them. José and Claudia have committed to work together to save their marriage. Claudia is now eight months pregnant, and José has changed offices at his company and is no longer in contact with the female counterpart he found so alluring. During today's couples sessions, Claudia shares that José has been unusually tense, angry, and depressed since the last counseling session. He has lost his temper several times this week and one night struck her in the face and pushed her off of the bed. Michael noted that her cheek was swollen and she had applied extra makeup to cover a black eye. As she speaks, José holds his head in his hands and stares at his feet. Michael shares with the couple that abuse may begin or may increase during pregnancy. However, pregnancy is a particularly perilous time for an abused woman because not only is Claudia's health at risk but also the health of their unborn child. José entered into the discussion and described what appeared to be normal irritations, frustration, changes, and adjustments that were part of living with a pregnant partner and two active sons. He shares that lately his way of dealing with these events, however, is to not deal with them. He states that recently he seems to be unaware of his feelings and has made no attempt to discuss with Claudia what he was going through emotionally. He started smoking again and spends significant amounts of time browsing the Internet in isolation.

Because José doesn't want to bother his wife during her pregnancy, he keeps everything inside himself. During the night in question, José stated that the children were spending the night with their grandparents across town, and he and his wife were spending a night in their home and had ordered out for dinner. He was unaware of any anger or conflict that was occurring in the relationship at that time. When asked what led him to hit his wife and push her off of the bed, he again lowered his head. He quietly replied that Claudia had eaten the last piece of pizza, and that had set him off. He said his reaction happened so quickly that he did not have time to think about his behavior before it occurred. When asked, Claudia and José say that after the event, they were both OK with not reporting it to the police, as it was an isolated incident, and they want to work on it in counseling.

Even though Claudia did not report the abuse to the city police, is Michael mandated to call the police and make a report of domestic violence?

What other steps should Michael take in resolving this ethical and legal dilemma?

What information would be helpful in this situation?

To answer the first question in Case Illustration 10-9, the counselor reviews B.1.c. (Respect for Confidentiality), which reinforces his decision to protect his clients' confidentiality. Clearly the answer to this question is negative. At the beginning of every couples counseling session, Michael reviews B.1.d. (Explanation of Limitations) and reminds the couple that he will respect confidentiality as long as they do not make a threat to harm themselves or others. Even though Michael understands that B.2.a. (Serious and Foreseeable Harm and Legal Requirements) allows him to "break confidentiality to protect clients or identified others from serious and foreseeable harm or when legal requirements demand that confidential information must be revealed," he knows that in his state, professional counselors are mandated reporters for incidents of child abuse, but they are not mandated to report issues between two adults.

To find the answer to the second question, Michael again follows the suggestions in B.2.a. (Serious and Foreseeable Harm and Legal Requirements) directing him to "consult with other professionals when in doubt as to the validity of an exception." He consults with several other counseling professionals at his agency and comes to the conclusion to maintain the confidentiality and continue working with José and Claudia in couples counseling.

For the third question Michael believes this violent incident was isolated and will not be repeated as the couple continues in therapy. But as a precautionary measure, he shares with Claudia a list of resources:

1. With an immediate threat or emergency, 911 or local emergency lines

2. With no immediate danger:

   a. National Domestic Violence Hotline

   b. Local hospital or crisis center

   c. Local court to help with a court order of protection

3. Books and online resources

Learning more about how to cope with your situation and communicating with others who understand what you're going through can help you make strong choices. Some online forums may help Claudia and José see that other people have worked through this difficult taboo predicament. If an online resource or book is given, the ethical counselor must make sure to thoroughly review the materials prior to passing the resource along to the client.

José and Claudia responded well to couples therapy, which included domestic violence treatment. Over time, José developed the ability to identify and express an array of emotions, not just anger and rage. He learned more about how to speak the language of feelings and became comfortable identifying stressors, irritations, and his resulting thoughts and feelings on an ongoing and daily basis. His communication skills and ability to be respectfully direct and assertive in his relationship with Claudia were instrumental in saving their marriage.

When it comes to breaking confidentiality in the couples setting, the ACA Code of Ethics (2014) Section B.1.c. states that "counselors protect the confidential information of prospective and current clients. Counselors disclose information only with appropriate consent or with sound legal or ethical justification" (p. 7). Though this is in the code of ethics, this is not a duty, legally, in every state (see Texas Supreme Court case *Thapar v. Zezulka*, 1999). The ethical counselor will know and understand the difference between ethical and legal issues in his/her respective state and consult a legal expert when necessary.

As mentioned in Case Illustrations 10-1 and 10-2, screening is vital to good group counseling outcomes. In Case Illustration 10-10, screening takes on a different form to include inclusionary and exclusionary screening. The counselor must identify who fits and who does not fit.

CASE ILLUSTRATION 10-10

Roger is a licensed professional counselor who has a contract with the clinic to provide premarital counseling groups. Roger facilitates this group after the winter holidays for six weeks and charges $150 per couple. This group is intended and designed to examine issues for people prior to getting married. To qualify for the group, the participants must have a date set for their wedding. The curriculum includes a personality assessment, a relationship assessment, lessons on empathy, physical and emotional intimacy, communication, and conflict resolution. It also includes financial planning, family of origin conversations, and future planning.

Is the screening process comprehensive enough?

Which couples would not qualify to be in the group?

Would a mixture of same-sex and heterosexual couples be a good fit for this group?

Every potential group member must be screened for an appropriate fit into the main group. According to A.9.a. (Screening) each participant must meet the needs and goals of the group. If the screening is inclusionary, then there may be an issue letting in all couples. Imagine the lack of focus if there was a mixture of premarital couples and couples who wanted to save their marriage.

The answer to the third question in Case Illustration 10-10 depends on the makeup of the group. Specifically, when screening for the group, Roger may want to ask this question. If the people who are screened for the group have the goal of building a strong relationship with their partner, there should be no issue with a mixture of people. Actually, the diversity of the group makeup could create a more meaningful relationship counseling experience for all participants.

Conclusion

The ethical considerations in group work, families, and couples therapy, as shown in this chapter, may be diverse. Taking into account the cost for services, who owns confidentiality, and when to break confidentiality lead the ethical issues in this area. Practicing ethically within these specialized fields of counseling requires professional counselors to use thorough and rigorous decision-making processes. As with all other areas, counselors are also encouraged to reflect on their actions and maintain self-awareness. Finally, counselors must continue to seek out professional development opportunities as a way to stay current on rapidly changing expectations.

To end this chapter and reinforce what you have read, the authors would like to invite you to complete Exercise 10-1, which includes an ethical dilemma, specific discussion questions related to the dilemma, and some overarching discussion questions.

EXERCISE 10-1

In your own practice, how do you feel about secrets, and how might you address secrets that are shared with you during or between sessions by one or more members of a family?

In group counseling, there is often talk about expressing the importance of confidentiality to members of the group. However, there is no way a counselor can guarantee confidentiality. If you were in charge of a group, how might you deal with a situation in which one group member was sharing the confidential information of other group members? If you were to remove that person from the group, is it possible it could be seen as client abandonment?

In couples and family counseling, it is important that all members of the couple or family feel as though the counselor understands and respects their point of view. Considering all people have varied morals, values, and beliefs, can you think of any situations or presenting concerns for which it may be difficult for you to remain neutral?

Use an ethical decision-making process to determine how you might act if you were the counselor in the following scenario.

You are a counselor working with a couple for issues related to communication. After several sessions working with both husband and wife, it becomes apparent to both you and the couple that the main issues are related to the husband's violent temper and his inability to control his anger (the husband admits to pushing, shoving, and hitting his wife on multiple occasions). As a result, the husband continues to meet with you for individual counseling, but his wife only attends sessions once a month (every fourth visit). During your first few individual meetings with the husband, you notice that he seems more relaxed, and he reports fewer times losing his temper at home. When you ask him about how he is making such progress, he claims that he was feeling caged up at home, as if he had lost all his freedom. He hesitantly reveals that several evenings each week when he claims to be working late, he has started going out to bars to meet other women. He claims that there is an incredible sense of excitement and risk in these encounters and only on a few occasions have they involved anything sexual. He says that the extramarital excitement has really helped him control his anger at home. He reports that there is no emotional attachment to the individuals and that he simply needs a sexual outlet sometimes because his wife has no sex drive lately. As you talk about his newfound "anger management" strategy more, he says he loves his wife and knows that if she found out about these extramarital affairs, she would leave him for sure (and take his two kids away from him too). He says he wasn't going to tell you but then remembered that you can't say anything to his wife because you have to keep things confidential.

At your next meeting, both husband and wife arrive and seem to be in good spirits. As you sit down to start the session, the wife begins by telling you how great things are at home and thanks you for all that you have done. She claims that you have "transformed him back into the loveable man that she married." She openly admits to both you and her husband that she thought he might never change. She then asks you how you were able to help him so quickly.

How might you respond to her questions?

How might your response(s) be affected by your own morals, values, and beliefs related to marriage, relationships, and or fidelity?

Discussion Questions

Some counselors choose to work primarily in group settings, and others choose to focus more on individual work. What do you see as the biggest benefits and drawbacks of group counseling?

Couples and family counseling often involve value-laden topics (e.g., premarital or extramarital sexual activity, abortion, religion, spirituality, drugs or alcohol, and/or extreme sexual practices). Which, if any of these may be the most difficult for you to work with? Why?

Keystones

- Counselors who provide group counseling services must prescreen clients prior to the beginning of the group. Screening is not only an ethical responsibility but also promotes a healthy and effective group.
- In couples and family counseling, if there is not an identified individual(s) as the client, then the entire family or couple is considered the client.
- There are only a few standards in the ACA Code of Ethics (2014) specifically addressing counseling couples, families, and groups.
- When facilitating a counseling group, it is the counselor's responsibility to protect all members from physical, emotional, and psychological harm.
- Confidentiality cannot be guaranteed in group settings.
- Like every other aspect of counseling, working with groups, families, and couples requires professional counselors to have self-awareness and avoid imposing values onto clients.

Additional Resources

Association for Specialists in Group Work. (2007). *Best practice guidelines.* Retrieved from http://www.asgw.org/PDF/Best _Practices.pdf

Burlingame, G. M., Fuhriman, A., Johnson, J. (2004). Process and outcome in group counseling and group psychotherapy. In J. L. DeLucia-Waack, D. A. Gerrity, C. R. Kalodner, & M. T. Riva (Eds.), *Handbook of group counseling and psychotherapy* (pp. 49–61). Thousand Oaks, CA: Sage.

Wilcoxon, S. A., Gladding, S. T., Remley, T. P., Jr., & Huber, C. H. (2007). *Ethical, legal, and professional issues in the practice of marriage and family therapy* (4th ed.). Englewood Cliffs, NJ: Prentice Hall.

References

American Association for Marriage and Family Therapy. (2015). *Code of ethics.* Retrieved from https://www.aamft.org/iMIS15/AAMFT/Content/legal_ethics/code_of_ethics.aspx

American Counseling Association. (2014). *Code of ethics.* Alexandria, VA: Author.

American Psychological Association. (2010). *American Psychological Association ethical principles of psychologists and code of conduct.* Retrieved from http://www.apa.org/ethics/code/principles .pdf

Thapar v. Zezulka, 994 S.W. 2d 635 (Tex. 1999).

Welfel, E. R. (2010). *Ethics in counseling & psychotherapy: Standards, research, and emerging issues.* Belmont, CA: Brooks/Cole.

11

Ethics in School Counseling

It is in fact a part of the function of education to help us escape, not from our own time—for we are bound by that—but from the intellectual and emotional limitations of our time.

—T. S. Eliot

The ASCA Ethical Standards, like the ACA Code of Ethics, is broken up into various sections (e.g., confidentiality, responsibilities to the profession, technology, responsibilities to clients/students, etc.). However, the ASCA Code of Ethics specifically addresses requirements for professional school counselors. The ACA Code of Ethics has merely two standards (i.e., B.5.a. [Responsibilities to Clients] and B.5.b. [Responsibilities to Parents and Legal Guardians]) addressing ethical issues with minors and students, whereas the ASCA Code of Ethics is an entire document. The remainder of Chapter 11 will not explore every standard of the ASCA Code of Ethics due to the many similarities between the ASCA Ethical Code (2010) and the ACA Code of Ethics (2014). Often the only difference between the two being the term "student" used in place of "client." Review Case Illustration 11-1 to see examples of similarities between the ACA and ASCA Codes of Ethics.

CASE ILLUSTRATION 11-1

Referrals

Both the ACA and ASCA Codes of Ethics encourage professional counselors to make referrals when working with the client or student would be outside his/her competence. Additionally, both codes of ethics discuss the importance of terminating services when the counselor determines the client or student is no longer in need of services.

Dual Relationships

Both the ACA and ASCA Codes of Ethics discuss the importance of firm boundaries and avoiding relationships that may harm the client or student or interfere with the counselor's ability to work objectively with the client or student.

Diversity

Both the ACA and ASCA Codes of Ethics discuss diversity and the importance of being sensitive to diversity.

Counselor Competence

Both the ACA and ASCA Codes of Ethics discuss professional competence, expressing the need for counselors to monitor their own effectiveness and their own mental and physical wellness. Additionally, both codes stress the importance of membership in professional organizations and the need for professional counselors to pursue continuing education.

Ethical Decision Making

Both the ACA and ASCA Codes of Ethics require professional counselors to use an ethical decision-making model when faced with ethical dilemmas.

The complete Ethical Standards for School Counselors can be found in Appendix B. While the authors encourage readers to examine and become familiar with the entire document of the ASCA Code of Ethics, only specific areas will be addressed in this chapter. Specifically, after reading chapter eleven, readers will be able to accomplish the following:

1. Define the basic tenets on which the ASCA Code of Ethics is built.

2. Explain the informed consent process in a school setting and how to provide informed consent to students, teachers, parents, and other stakeholders.

3. Explain the importance of developing positive working relationships with school faculty and staff.

4. List ethical requirements related to confidentiality in schools.

5. Define ethical obligations for sharing information with parents, faculty, and school administration.

6. Explain the difference between student educational records and sole possession records.

To begin, professional school counselors are defined in the Ethical Standards for School Counselors as "advocates, leaders, collaborators and consultants who create opportunities for equity in access and success in educational opportunities by connecting their programs to the mission of schools" (ASCA, 2010, p. 1). A professional school counselor is the primary mental health supporter of all students on his/her campus. Additionally, professional school counselors have an ethical responsibility to abide by the following five tenets as listed in the preamble of the ASCA Code of Ethics (2010):

Each person has the right to be respected, be treated with dignity and have access to a comprehensive school counselor program that advocates for and affirms all students from diverse populations including: ethnic and racial identity, age, economic status, abilities or disabilities, language, immigration status, sexual orientation, gender, gender identity or expression, family type, religious or spiritual identity and appearance.

School counselors are ethically obligated to facilitate a comprehensive school counseling program. Additionally, professional school counselors are responsible for providing services to all students regardless of differences in race, gender, socioeconomic status, family structure, and so on:

Each person has the right to receive the information and support needed to move toward self-direction and self-development and affirmation within one's group identities, with special care being given to students who have historically not received adequate educational services. (ASCA, 2010)

Similar to the first tenet, professional school counselors help all students move toward achieving each students' own educational, career, and life goals. There is also specific wording in this tenet that school counselors are careful to be sensitive to the needs of students and families who may have previously not received adequate educational services:

Each person has the right to understand the full magnitude and meaning of his/her educational choices and how those choices will affect future opportunities. (ASCA, 2010)

Professional school counselors help students and families understand the choices they make related to the students' education and educate students and families on how those choices may benefit or impede them in the future:

Each person has the right to privacy and thereby the right to expect the school-counselor/student relationship to comply with all laws, policies, and ethical standards pertaining to confidentiality in the school setting. (ASCA, 2010)

As with professional counselors working in a clinical mental health setting, school counselors are expected to respect the privacy and confidentiality of students and families (with certain exceptions):

Each person has the right to feel safe in school environments that school counselors help create, free from abuse, bullying, neglect, harassment, or other forms of violence. (ASCA, 2010)

School counselors are responsible for collaborating with other school officials to create a safe learning environment for all students.

Informed Consent

Informed consent is a primary concern and emphasis for all professional counselors, not only those working in a school setting. However, professional school counselors work in a unique environment and have many different considerations than those working in more clinical settings. Perkins, Oescher, and Ballard (2010), describe school counselors as professionals who must assume many different roles and attend to the needs of various stakeholders (i.e., parents, school administrators, students, community members, and other professional counselors).

ASCA Standard A.2.a. (2010): Professional school counselors inform individual students of the purposes, goals, techniques, and rules of procedure under which they may receive counseling. Disclosure includes the limits of confidentiality in a developmentally appropriate manner. Informed consent requires competence on the part of students to understand the limits of confidentiality and, therefore, can be difficult to obtain from students of a certain developmental level. Professionals are aware that even though every attempt is made to obtain informed consent, it is not always possible and when needed will make counseling decisions on students, behalf.

ASCA Standard A.2.b. (2010): Professional school counselors explain the limits of confidentiality in appropriate ways such as classroom guidance lessons, the student handbook, school counseling brochures, school website, verbal notice, or other methods of student, school, and community communication in addition to oral notification to individual students.

Similar to informed consent for professional counselors working outside of a school, professional school counselors must also provide clients or students with informed consent regarding the school counselor's role, what counseling entails, and how one can make arrangements to meet with the school counselor. For clinical mental health counselors, this process typically occurs at the first meeting or "intake session." For a school counselor, meeting with each student individually may likely be impossible considering the number of students at the school (400–500 students). Therefore, school counselors may choose alternate options for providing informed consent. Review the ways in which the school counselors in Case Illustration 11-2 provide informed consent to students.

CASE ILLUSTRATION 11-2

Example 1

Over the course of the first two weeks of every school year, an elementary school counselor schedules times to meet with every classroom throughout the school (i.e., Monday she meets with all five first-grade classrooms for 15 minutes each, Tuesday all four second-grade classrooms, etc.). During her time with each class, she introduces herself and describes where her office is, how students may schedule a time to meet with her, confidentiality, limits to confidentiality, and overall what the school counselor is all about. With the younger students, the counselor typically uses puppets to help her explain everything as a way to make it more fun and understandable to the younger kids. Additionally, throughout the year, when students visit her office, the counselor always quickly reviews confidentiality, purpose of counseling, and her role in the school just to make sure students are fully aware.

Example 2

At the beginning of every school year a high school counselor schedules a time to visit all of the health classes at her high school. She visits the health classes because she knows it is a requirement for all ninth-grade students. During her 15- to 20-minute visit, she talks about counseling and some of the topics for small groups that she is thinking about for the upcoming year. The counselor also discusses confidentiality, that is, how and why information discussed in counseling might be shared with others. The counselor notifies all students where her office is and invites everyone to stop by if they have any questions or concerns. Additionally, the counselor sets up an information table during all lunch periods. In addition to the handouts she has related to the school counseling office, the counselor also has pens, pencils, and other giveaway items to attract students to come and visit her table to ask questions. Finally, the school counselor maintains a website that is linked to the school's main webpage, which includes full information about the school counseling program.

In Case Illustration 11-2, the school counselors use a variety of methods of informing students about the counseling process, confidentiality, and limits of confidentiality. In addition to the large-scale efforts described, school counselors would also want to be sure to review informed consent orally to individual students (i.e., each time a student visits the school counselor's office, a quick review of the counselor's role within the school, confidentiality, and limits of confidentiality).

Similar to the informed consent provided to students, school counselors must also discuss the same information with parents or guardians as stated in ASCA Standards B.1.a., B.1.d., and B.2.a.

ASCA Standard B.1.a. (2010): Professional school counselors respect the rights and responsibilities of parents/guardians for their children and endeavor to establish, as appropriate, a collaborative relationship with parents or guardians to facilitate students' maximum development.

ASCA Standard B.1.d. (2010): Professional school counselors inform parents of the nature of counseling services provided in the school.

ASCA Standard B.2.a. (2010): Professional school counselors inform parents or guardians of the school counselor's role to include the confidential nature of the counseling relationship between the counselor and student.

Parents and guardians are vital members of the school community. As such, school counselors must reach out to parents and guardians and inform them of the counselor's role and the counseling process. Schools and school districts may vary in the ways in which they reach out to parents, and policies may likely be influenced by various state laws. For instance, some districts may simply include the counselor's role and counseling process in the school handbook (assuming parents will read the school handbook), while others may require each student to have a parent or guardian sign an informed consent prior to that student being able to have ongoing visits with the counselor. Whatever the process, the code of ethics clearly states school counselors should work to establish relationships with parents and guardians, inform them of the counseling process, and speak to the confidential nature of counseling. Consider the interaction in Case Illustration 11-3 between a school counselor and parent.

CASE ILLUSTRATION 11-3

At the conclusion of talking with Drake, a sixth-grade boy, about his anger outburst during class, the school counselor, Mr. Arnold, notifies Drake he will be giving Drake's parents a call just to let them know the two met today. Mr. Arnold says he will not tell Drake's parents anything in great detail but feels it is important to let them know and include them in the conversation. After their discussion, Drake goes back to class and Mr. Arnold calls the parents on the phone. Mr. Arnold introduces himself as the counselor of the school and mentions that he had the opportunity to meet with Drake today. Mr. Arnold also shares a little bit about the counseling office, counseling in general, and confidentiality. Specifically Mr. Arnold says, "I always do my best to have open communication with all parents. I believe parents play a vital role in students' lives."

Case illustration 11-3 is a brief example of how a counselor might begin to establish a relationship and communicate with parents. Some parents or guardians may be more or less interested in their child's interactions with school counselors; however, it is the counselor's responsibility to reach out to all guardians and make sure all know the role of the school counselor.

In addition to students and parents or guardians, the ASCA Code of Ethics (2010) also discusses the importance of establishing relationships with other school personnel and connecting the school counseling program with the overall school community. Consider the following standards.

ASCA Standard C.1.a. (2010): Professional school counselors establish and maintain professional relationships with faculty, staff, and administration to facilitate an optimum counseling program.

ASCA Standard C.1.c. (2010): Professional school counselors recognize that teachers, staff, and administrators who are high functioning in personal and social development skills can be powerful allies in supporting student success. School counselors work to develop relationships with all faculty and staff to advantage students.

ASCA Standard C.2.a. (2010): Professional school counselors promote awareness and adherence to appropriate guidelines regarding confidentiality, the distinction between public and private information, and staff consultation.

In these standards, school counselors are given general guidelines for building relationships with other members of the school community, promoting the school counseling program and beginning the conversation regarding confidentiality and the types of information that the school counselor may share with teachers, administrators, and/or other school personnel. As with most codes of ethics, general guidelines and vague statements are given to help school counselors understand what is "appropriate" or "correct" behavior. Review Case Illustration 11-4 for one example as to how a school counselor might adhere to the requirements of Standards C.1.a., C.1.c., and C.2.a.

CASE ILLUSTRATION 11-4

Jolie is one of three school counselors at her middle school. During the days prior to the first day of school (teacher workdays) and several other days throughout the school year, Jolie and her co-counselors provide a small continental breakfast for all the teachers and staff at the school. The cost of providing the breakfast is quite small compared to the enormous benefit they feel it provides. The school counselors advertise the breakfast to other school personnel, and when teachers and administrators stop by for breakfast, the counselors are able to meet everyone and share a little about the school counseling program. Additionally, the counselors developed a short video and PowerPoint presentation describing the counseling office, the services they provide for students, and ways in which the counselors are able to contribute to everyday classroom activities. Jolie and her co-counselors play the video while everyone is coming and going. Finally, as everyone leaves, Jolie hands each person a "goodie bag" containing the counselors' names, contact information, and a description of the services they provide.

Has Jolie fulfilled the ethical requirements set by Standards C.1.a., C.1.c., and C.2.a.?

In response to the question posed in Case Illustration 11-4, yes, Jolie has fulfilled the requirements. Jolie and her co-counselors provided an event for their colleagues to establish relationships with other faculty and staff. During the breakfast, Jolie was able to advocate for her program by notifying faculty about the services the counselor office provides. Similar to the informed consent school counselors provide to students and parents, Jolie and her co-counselors were providing informed consent about their counseling program to faculty and staff.

Confidentiality

Confidentiality is a tremendous issue with many areas left up to interpretation. The issue is intensified when working with minors because there is not merely one stakeholder (the client) but instead the client and the client's parent or guardian. Some minors may not mind information being shared with parents, and others may wish to have complete confidentiality when talking to a counselor. Collins and Knowles (1995) found that many minors may be hesitant to visit a counselor at all due to fears of inappropriate breach of confidentiality. Counselors working in schools must consider another stakeholder. School counselors must be cognizant of obligations to the student, parent, and the school community (i.e., teachers and administrators). Moyer and Sullivan (2008) described confidentiality as a "tightrope act between being an effective helper and acting as an informant to parents and administrators." As such, the ASCA Code of Ethics (2010) provides some guidance to school counselors in navigating confidentiality in schools.

ASCA Standard A.7.b. (2010): Professional school counselors report risk assessments to parents when they underscore the need to act on behalf of a child at risk: Never negate a risk of harm as students sometimes deceive to avoid further scrutiny and/or parental notification.

If for any reason a professional counselor feels the need to do a risk assessment, no matter how minor it may seem, the counselor must pass that information along to parents. Consider Case Illustration 11-5 and how Theo handles student concerns.

CASE ILLUSTRATION 11-5

Theo is a school counselor at a relatively large high school, and although he interacts with all students, he is primarily assigned to working with 10th graders. Today during a lunch period, two 11th graders stop by the counseling office. Because Theo is the only counselor available, they step into his office and mention that they are worried about their friend Remi, who has been acting very strange lately. The two students also mention Remi has talked in passing about hurting himself and seems very withdrawn. Finally, the two ask Theo to talk to their friend to make sure he is alright. Theo, having never met the two students in his office or their friend Remi, agrees to talk to him.

Later in the day, Remi arrives at Theo's office with a pass from his teacher. Remi seems a bit confused and wonders why he was called out of class. Theo informs Remi that a couple of his friends came down and expressed concern he was not doing well. Remi smiles in disbelief and downplays his friends' concern. Remi further explains his friends were just messing with him and trying to get him in trouble. Remi denies ever wanting to hurt himself and laughs at the idea.

What should Theo do in this situation?

In Case Illustration 11-5, Theo is put in an awkward situation. He has two students with whom he is not familiar report that their friend Remi, with whom Theo is also not familiar, is acting strange and possibly going to hurt himself. Although Remi completely denied ever wanting to hurt himself, Theo still must contact Remi's parents and notify them of the interaction and concern from Remi's friends. If Theo fails to contact Remi's parents, he is in clear violation of Standard A.7.b., and if anything were to happen to Remi, would most likely be held liable. Theo's notification to Remi's parents may look something like the following:

"Hi, my name is Theo and I'm the counselor at Remi's school. I'm calling because I had the opportunity to talk with Remi today. I just wanted to fill you in on a few things we talked about. It was brought to my attention earlier today that Remi has been talking to some of his friends about hurting himself. However, when I talked to Remi, he seemed to not think anything of it. I don't want to scare you about anything, but I did want to let you know. Please let me know if you have any questions or if there is anything I can do to be helpful."

ASCA Standard A.7.c. (2010): Professional school counselors understand the legal and ethical liability for releasing a student who is a danger to self or others without proper and necessary support for that student.

Using the same scenario depicted in Case Illustration 11-5 (Remi and Theo) and assuming Remi admitted to wanting to hurt himself rather than denying it, Theo would have needed to adjust his actions. Theo would have been ethically required to notify Remi's parents; however, according to Standard A.7.c., Theo would have needed to provide "proper and necessary support" for Remi as well. Therefore, instead of sending Remi back to class while he notified his parents, Theo might have kept Remi in his office, had him sit in another counselor's office, and so on. The key component to Standard A.7.c. is to ensure students are not left unattended when they pose a danger to themselves or others.

Clear and Foreseeable Harm

Similar to the ACA Code of Ethics and the information provided in Chapter 6 (Confidentiality and Privileged Communication), the ASCA Code of Ethics requires school counselors to breach confidentiality when doing so would prevent serious and foreseeable harm to students. Still, the question remains, what constitutes clear and foreseeable harm? Whereas the ASCA 2004 version of the Ethical Standards for School Counselors included a fairly broad statement (i.e., A counselor keeps information confidential unless disclosure is required to prevent clear and imminent danger to the student or others or when legal requirements demand that confidential information must be revealed. Counselors will consult with appropriate professionals when in doubt.), the 2010 standards include more specifics in determining the appropriateness of a breach. Counselors must consider context, age, setting, and nature of the harm. While helpful, there is still much room for interpretation, thus highlighting the need for counselors to use an ethical decision-making process.

ASCA Standard A.2.c. (2010): Professional school counselors recognize the complicated nature of confidentiality in schools and consider each case in context. Keep information confidential unless legal requirements demand that confidential information be revealed or a breach is required to prevent serious and foreseeable harm to the student. Serious and foreseeable harm is different for each minor in schools and is defined by students' developmental and chronological age, the setting, parental rights, and the nature of the harm. School counselors consult with appropriate professionals when in doubt as to the validity of an exception.

Consider whether or not you believe the student behaviors described in Case Exercise 11-1 constitute clear and imminent danger and would require a breach of confidentiality.

CASE EXERCISE 11-1

A 14-year-old student admits to sneaking into his/her parents' liquor cabinet and taking shots of alcohol when friends come over on weekends.

A 15-year-old admits to stealing gum and Gatorade from a local grocery store on his/her way home from school from time to time.

An 11-year-old admits to going home each day, sitting on his/her couch and eating multiple bags of potato chips while watching television all afternoon and night until his/her parents get home.

A 17-year-old admits to racing his/her car on Saturday nights on remote city streets in an effort to make extra cash to pay for clothes, food, and so on.

A 7-year-old student admits to stealing his/her parents' cigarettes and smoking five to six cigarettes a week.

A 16-year-old student admits to making multiple cuts on his/her arm several times a month as a way to cope with stress and anxiety.

For each of the scenarios in Case Exercise 11-1, arguments can be made for both maintaining and breaching confidentiality. All three key terms ("clear," "foreseeable," and "harm") in this standard may be interpreted in various ways. A student who steals merchandise from a store may be harming the store and placing herself in harm's way by committing a crime. A student who cuts his arm to cope may be harming his skin and body. A student who sits in front of a television all day and eats fatty foods may be harming his brain and long-term health. There is oftentimes not a "right" or "wrong" action but rather more appropriate and less appropriate actions. To determine the most appropriate action, school counselors must have self-awareness, determine their motivation in choosing one action over another, avoid imposing their own morals and values onto students, and always use an ethical decision-making model.

ASCA Standard A.7.a. (2010): Professional school counselors inform parents or guardians and/or appropriate authorities when a student poses a danger to self or others. This is to be done after careful deliberation and consultation with other counseling professionals.

When it is determined "clear and foreseeable danger" does exist, parents are notified of the risk. Due to their work in a school setting, most all of the students with whom school counselors work will be minors. Because parents or/guardians are the legal representative for said minors, they must be notified.

ASCA Standard D.1.b. (2010): Professional school counselors inform appropriate officials, in accordance with school policy, of conditions that may be potentially disruptive or damaging to the school's mission, personnel, and property while honoring the confidentiality between the student and the school counselor.

As mentioned previously, school counselors have many stakeholders to whom they are accountable. Occasionally, a student's behavior may be considered clear and foreseeable harm and be against school policy (e.g., a high school student reveals to her school counselor that she frequently brings alcohol to school and will drink with friends in between classes). In other cases, students may participate in behaviors that may not be deemed as "clear and foreseeable harm" but still may be against school policy or may be considered disruptive to the school's mission (e.g., a student claims to cheat on tests and reveals to his counselor that many students cheat on tests in some specific classes). Consider Case Illustration 11-6 and Case Illustration 11-7 as two examples related to Ethical Standard D.1.b.

CASE ILLUSTRATION 11-6

Sarah, a high school junior, meets with her counselor Mrs. M. and reveals that she believes she has a drinking problem. Sarah also reveals that she frequently brings vodka to school in her water bottle and drinks throughout the day. Sarah even admits to once getting so drunk at school that she had trouble walking home.

After consulting and using an ethical decision-making model, Mrs. M. determines Sarah is in clear and foreseeable harm and she must notify Sarah's parents. Mrs. M. first discusses her concerns with Sarah and asks her which way she thinks may be best to share the information with her parents. Although Sarah does not agree with Mrs. M's decision to contact her parents, Sarah decides she would like to sit in the office with her, while Mrs. M. makes the call.

Additionally, Mrs. M. realizes this is a behavior that is against school rules and is damaging to the school's mission. After much thought and going through yet another ethical decision-making model, Mrs. M. decides to talk to the principal and campus security. During the meeting she shares, "I've heard some information leading me to believe we may have some issues with students drinking during the school day. Students may be camouflaging vodka and other alcoholic drinks in their water bottles and other drink containers. Because it would impossible to monitor unless we test everyone's drinks, I'm wondering if anyone has any ideas about ways to keep our students safe. I wanted to bring it your attention because I would hate for any students to get hurt. What can we do?"

Did Mrs. M. do the right thing in telling Sarah's parents, the school principal, and security?

Should Mrs. M. have shared Sarah's name with the school principal and security guard?

It is difficult to say definitively if Mrs. M's actions were right or wrong in Case Illustration 11-6, but her actions would most likely be considered ethical. Mrs. M. used an ethical decision-making model and determined Sarah's actions constituted clear and imminent danger. Once that determination was made, Mrs. M. knew she must ethically notify Sarah's parents. In adhering to Standard A.2.e., Mrs. M. promoted Sarah's autonomy by having a "discussion about the method and timing of the breach" (ASCA, 2010). Finally, Mrs. M. also notified her school administration because she determined Sarah's actions were potentially damaging to the school's mission.

The second question asks if Mrs. M. should have revealed Sarah's name to school administration. In reviewing Standard D.1.b., it clearly says school counselors should "honor the confidentiality between the student and the school counselor." Therefore, no, Mrs. M. should not have shared Sarah's specific name. Mrs. M. notified appropriate officials of the behaviors and potential harm and maintained confidentiality with her student.

CASE ILLUSTRATION 11-7

Thomas is meeting with his middle school counselor, Mr. A. Mr. A. questions Thomas about his dramatic improvement in math from last semester to the current one. Thomas sheepishly replies that he has had help. Mr. A. seems a bit confused by Thomas's hesitant answer and reviews confidentiality again and how information shared with the school counselor is confidential except for certain limitations. Thomas further explains, "Well, if you want the whole story, my math teacher had me stay after school some last semester, and I was supposed to work on my homework in his classroom. Most of the time my teacher wasn't even in there; he would go and do other things. So, I got bored one time and started looking at his computer. I saw a file on his desktop that said 'tests' and opened it. Inside were all his tests for the year and the answers, so I took out my phone and took pictures of all of them. Now, I don't even have to study much. I just memorize all the tests before I take them."

Does Mr. A. have an obligation to breach confidentiality and let someone else know about this new information about cheating?

If Mr. A. decides to break confidentiality, how might he do it while also honoring the confidentiality he has with Thomas (as required by Standard D.1.b.)?

The answer is maybe. If Mr. A. believes cheating on the tests is a "condition that may be potentially disruptive or damaging to the school's mission, personnel, and property," then yes, he needs to take action. If he does not believe it is such a condition, then Mr. A. is not required to act in any way and is ethically obligated to keep the information confidential.

Oftentimes knowing how to act and actually acting are very different. Therefore, the second question inquires as to how Mr. A. might share information with other school officials while also respecting Thomas's confidentiality. There are a number of ways Mr. A. may notify school officials. He may send a general reminder out to all teachers mentioning rumors of cheating going on in many subjects and encouraging all teachers to revise any future tests they give. However, Mr. A. chooses to share information, it is important he maintain Thomas's confidentiality and not identify him individually.

Confidentiality and Sharing Information With Parents and School Personnel

In addition to clear and foreseeable harm, there are other times in which school counselors must determine when, how much, and to whom information should be shared. In such cases Ethical Standard A.2.d. offers some guidance.

ASCA Standard A.2.d. (2010): Professional school counselors recognize their primary obligation for confidentiality is to the students but balance that obligation with an understanding of parents' or guardians' legal and inherent rights to be the guiding voice in their children's lives, especially in value-laden issues. Understand the need to balance students' ethical rights to make choices, their capacity to give consent or assent, and parental or familial legal rights and responsibilities to protect these students and make decisions on their behalf.

This standard addresses issues that may not appropriately fit under Standard A.2.c. (Clear and Foreseeable Harm). Consider the scenario in Case Illustration 11-8 and the school counselor's rationale and actions.

CASE ILLUSTRATION 11-8

Ms. Darla, a high school counselor, conducts groups with both girls and boys throughout the school year. She enjoys conducting groups because she feels as though she is able to reach more students than when she tries to meet with everyone face-to-face. Ms. Darla is currently running a group with 16- and 17-year-old girls focusing on healthy relationships. At today's group, several girls begin talking about current relationships and how they know their partner truly cares for them. Jenna, a 17-year-old junior, begins to share that she knows her boyfriend loves her because he always wants to be around her and is always touching and hugging her. Jenna continues that her parents are going to be out of town this weekend, and her boyfriend is planning on coming over to stay the night. She is hoping they will have sex for the first time; she is convinced it will make their relationship stronger than it already is.

As the group ends, everyone heads back to their classes, except for Jenna. Ms. Darla asks her to stay for a few minutes after the group. Ms. Darla expresses her concern about Jenna's plans to be sexually active with her boyfriend. Ms. Darla shares her belief sex will probably not make Jenna and her boyfriend's relationship better and may even hurt it. Ms. Darla also shares that she would feel most comfortable if she were to notify Jenna's parents because she feels

(Continued)

(Continued)

Jenna is participating in risky behaviors. Jenna seems a bit upset and wonders why Ms. Darla feels she has to call. Jenna says her parents know she is sexually active already, and they are "cool" with it. Jenna wonders why Ms. Darla doesn't believe her and needs to bother them at work. Jenna also argues that she thought everything was confidential in group. Ms. Darla agrees with her but counterargues that Jenna is participating in a risky behavior, and her parents deserve to know because they are the "guiding voice" in her life.

Jenna leaves the office feeling betrayed and goes back to class. Ms. Darla picks up the phone, calls Jenna's mom, and shares Jenna's plans for the weekend with her mom. Ms. Darla finishes by mentioning that although Jenna may have felt a bit betrayed, she felt the need to call because she would want to know as a parent. Jenna's mom thanks Ms. Darla for calling but explains that she and Jenna's dad already knew Jenna was sexually active and had a good idea of what was going to happen over the weekend. Jenna's mom further shares that they know Jenna is going to be sexually active, and they make sure she is safe by providing her with contraceptives.

Was it ethical for Ms. Darla to breach confidentiality and notify Jenna's parents?

What could Ms. Darla have done differently to increase the ethicality of her actions?

In Case Illustration 11-8, the ethicality of Ms. Darla's behavior is difficult to determine, and arguments for both sides could be made regarding whether she had an obligation to share Jenna's plans for the weekend with her parents. Depending on the reader's own morals, values, and beliefs, he/she may feel more or less obligated to notify the parents. For example, a school counselor who was him/herself sexually active as a teenager may feel as though "all" teenagers are sexually active and sex is just a part of growing up. On the reverse side, a school counselor with more conservative views related to teenage sexual behaviors or someone who had a negative experience as a teenager related to sexual activity may feel quite different. It seems clear in this example that Ms. Darla's values are quite different than the values of Jenna and her parents. It is critical for all professional counselors to avoid imposing values onto students or their families.

The second question inquires as to how Ms. Darla could have acted differently to be more ethical. There no doubt are numerous things Ms. Darla could have done differently. A few suggestions include the following: (1) Ms. Darla could have been much more detailed in her informed consent with the girls in her group, explaining more thoroughly under which circumstances she would need to breach confidentiality and share information with parents or others. (2) Ms. Darla could have followed Standard A.2.e. and included Jenna in the decision-making process:

> *"Jenna, I know this is difficult to hear, and you're wondering why I need to call your parents when you believe they already know. I feel very strongly that they need to know, but if they already know, I don't see any reason to call them. How about if I give*

you the next two days to talk to them and get them to give me a call so that I know you talked to them. I will wait until then. If they call and let me know you talked to them, then we will leave it there. If they don't call me, then I will give them a call and follow up with them. Does that sound fair to you?"

(3) Ms. Darla would want to use an ethical decision-making model and look at all possibilities prior to breaching confidentiality.

ASCA Standard B.2.d. (2010): Professional school counselors provide parents or guardians with accurate, comprehensive, and relevant information in an objective and caring manner, as is appropriate and consistent with ethical responsibilities to the student.

Standard B.2.d. simultaneously includes both very direct and vague guidance at the same time. In Standard B.2.d., counselors are encouraged to provide parents with "accurate and comprehensive information." However, one sentence later counselors are reminded to adhere to ethical responsibilities to students. Consider Case Illustration 11-9 related to providing information to parents.

CASE ILLUSTRATION 11-9

Mr. Ceyas, a high school counselor, meets with William, a sophomore, today for the first time. During the conversation the two talk about many different topics. William shares that he is making new friends easily and is even thinking about asking a girl in his class to go to the homecoming dance. He also shares that he has experimented with drugs in the past but doesn't use them anymore. Finally, William shares information about his family and how he likes playing hockey with his older brother. At the end of the conversation, Mr. Ceyas thanks William for coming in and writes him a pass back to class.

The next day Mr. Ceyas receives a call from William's father. William's father thanks Mr. Ceyas for talking with William and asks what they talked about and if William shared anything important. Mr. Ceyas describes his conversation with William in detail, saying, "William said he is making friends and even likes a girl in one of his classes enough to ask her out to homecoming. William also shared that he likes playing hockey with his brother. Finally, William said that he used to experiment with marijuana, but he doesn't do it anymore. I don't think you should worry too much."

Was Mr. Ceyas's response ethical according to Standard B.2.d.?

In Case Illustration 11-9, it is difficult to say for sure if Mr. Ceyas acted in an unethical manner. However, he may have been too careful to share "accurate, comprehensive information" with William's father and neglected to remember his "ethical responsibilities to the student" (i.e., William) (ASCA, 2010). Instead, Mr. Ceyas may have chosen to respond in a way to better balance the two parts of this standard. For example, Mr. Ceyas could have responded with the following:

Hi. Yes, William and I spoke yesterday, and he seems like a wonderful student. We talked a little about how school is going and his new friends. He also shared some about his family and various activities and hobbies that he likes. If there is anything I can do in the future to be helpful, please let me know.

In this example, Mr. Ceyas shares information with William's father but also remembers that his primary obligation is to William.

ASCA Standard B.2.e. (2010): Professional school counselors make reasonable efforts to honor the wishes of parents and guardians concerning information regarding the student unless a court order expressly forbids the involvement of a parent. In cases of divorce or separation, school counselors exercise a good-faith effort to keep both parents informed, maintaining focus on the student and avoiding supporting one parent over another in divorce proceedings.

Considering this example related to Mr. Ceyas and William, if Mr. Ceyas were aware William's parents were separated or divorced, he would want to make sure he made attempts to contact William's mother as well and share the same information with her as he did with William's father. Mr. Ceyas would want to share information with both parties unless there was a specific court order forbidding disclosure of information to one parent or the other.

ASCA Standard C.2.e. (2010): Professional school counselors recognize the powerful role of ally that faculty and administration who function highly in personal and social development skills can play in supporting students in stress and carefully filter confidential information to give these allies what they "need to know" to advantage the student. Consultation with other members of the school counseling profession is helpful in determining need-to-know information. The primary focus and obligation is always on the student when it comes to sharing confidential information.

School teachers, administrators, and other personnel are vital to the success of any comprehensive school counseling program. Therefore, open communication is a necessity (Freeman, 2000). However, providing too much information, or information that is not considered "need to know" as stated in Standard C.2.e., may be detrimental to school counselors' abilities to build trusting relationships with students. As mentioned earlier in this chapter, school counselors must balance obligations to parents and school personnel with losing trust with students and being seen as an informant to parents and teachers. Consider the example given in Case Illustration 11-10 and whether you believe the information in the illustration would be considered "need-to-know" information for teachers or other school personnel. Also, if you consider the information "need to know," how might you share the information to protect the confidentiality of the student to the greatest extent possible?

CASE ILLUSTRATION 11-10

Johnny, a middle school student, shares with his school counselor that his father moved out of the house, and now it is just him and his mother living together. Since his father moved out, it has been difficult for Johnny to get to school on time because his mom leaves for work well before he gets up in the morning. Johnny informs his school counselor that his dad used to take him to school, but now he has to walk. Johnny says he is worried about getting too many tardy slips and getting sent to after-school detention, which would make things even harder on his mom.

The information shared by Johnny in Case Illustration 11-10 would most likely be helpful for the teacher to know about as the teacher is the one giving out tardy slips. The counselor would first want to be sure to check with Johnny and verify whether or not he would be "OK" with the school counselor sharing the information with his teacher. If Johnny agrees, the counselor might share something such as the following:

Hi, I was wondering if I may talk to you for a moment about Johnny. He talked to me this morning and let me know that there are a lot of things going on at home right now affecting his ability to get to school on time. He is really worried about getting detention due to his tardy slips. I'm wondering if it might be possible to give him some leniency for a week or two until we can figure out some strategies for him and his family. Thanks, and I will definitely keep you informed if anything new comes up.

Responsibilities to the School

ASCA Standard D.1.c. (2010): Professional school counselors are knowledgeable and supportive of their school's mission and connect their program to the school's mission.

Professional school counselors and school counseling programs are an active and vital component of each school's community. As such, school counselors should be knowledgeable of their school's mission and work to interweave the school's mission throughout the school counseling program.

ASCA Standard D.1.d. (2010): Professional school counselors delineate and promote the school counselor's role and function as a student advocate in meeting the needs of those served. School counselors will notify appropriate officials of systemic conditions that may limit or curtail their effectiveness in providing programs and services.

Just as professional school counselors are to know the missions of their schools, they are also required to notify officials when school conditions affect the counselors' abilities to implement or maintain effective programs. A frequent occurrence in schools is for the school counselor to be assigned duties commonly referred to as "non-guidance activities" (i.e. coordinator of standardized testing or assigned to "cover" a classroom when a teacher or substitute does not show up, etc.). In such situations, it is the school counselor's responsibility to advocate for his/her position. Whether it occurs at the campus or district level, it is the school counselor's responsibility to make sure everyone knows the school counselor's role and function.

Advocating for one's position may be awkward and difficult if the school counselor does not do so in an organized and planned manner. Consider Case Illustration 11-11, where Mary tries to advocate for her position as a professional school counselor. ·

CASE ILLUSTRATION 11-11

Mary, an elementary school counselor at a large, urban school, has been at her current school for almost three years. Over the first couple years, she has been hesitant to embrace her role as a school counselor because her principal often viewed her as another administrator, frequently assigned Mary to lunch or bus duty, and turned to Mary when a teacher or substitute was running late or absent during the day. Mary has never wanted to "rock the boat."

This past summer, Mary went to several school counselor conferences and spent many hours listening to other counselors talk about "advocating for her position as a school counselor." At the beginning of this school year, Mary felt motivated to make changes and was confident in advocating for her position. During the second week of school, the principal approached Mary and asked her to cover a classroom until a long-term substitute could be hired. Mary, feeling inspired, said to her principal, "I need to advocate for my position, and I don't feel as though being a substitute is part of my job description. Please find someone else to cover the class. I would like to try to organize a small-group activity instead."

Was Mary ethical in her actions according to Ethical Standard D.1.d.?

In Case Illustration 11-11, Mary may have been acting ethically according to Standard D.1.d., but she would likely not be very effective in her method. Mary must remember school administration and faculty are allies, and she must work with school personnel. Mary must also be organized and strategic in the way she informs faculty, administration, and other stakeholders about the school counseling programs. Consider Case Illustration 11-12 as Mary again tries to advocate for her school counseling program.

CASE ILLUSTRATION 11-12

Mary, an elementary school counselor at a large, urban school, has been at her current school for almost three years. Over the first couple years, she has been hesitant to embrace her role as a school counselor because her principal often viewed her as another administrator, frequently assigned Mary to lunch or bus duty, and turned to Mary when a teacher or substitute was running late or absent during the day. Mary has never wanted to "rock the boat."

This past summer, Mary went to several school counselor conferences and spent many hours listening to other counselors talk about "advocating for her position as a school counselor." At the beginning of this school year, Mary felt motivated to make changes and was confident in advocating for her position. Prior to the beginning of school, Mary reflected on some of the major concerns affecting students at her school. She researched small-group activities on topics such as military deployments, bullying, and self-injurious behaviors. Mary then organized her school counseling calendar and planned for when she might be able to implement her groups. During teacher in-service days, Mary invited all the teachers to enjoy small breakfast treats, coffee, and handouts. Her handouts included the mission of the school and how her proposed small groups fit in. Mary asked teachers to keep her groups in mind and asked teachers if they could think of any students who might be appropriate for the groups. Mary then scheduled a meeting with her principal and shared information about how the groups might help with student academics and attendance and promote an overall healthier school environment.

During the fourth week of school, the principal approached Mary and asked her to cover a classroom until a long-term substitute could be hired. Mary responded, "I would really like to help out. Unfortunately I have two of my groups scheduled for this afternoon. I believe the students in the groups would be very disappointed if I had to cancel. If you really need me in the classroom, I'm willing to do so. However, I will need a few minutes to notify the students and their parents I will no longer be able facilitate the counseling groups as I will need to go into a classroom."

How did Mary act differently in Case Illustration 11-12 as opposed to Case Illustration 11-11?

In Case Illustration 11-12, Mary still confronted her principal when asked to fill in for an absent teacher. However she was more strategic and organized about her method. In Case Illustration 11-11, Mary simply said, "That's not in my job description." She didn't have other options planned. In Case Illustration 11-11, Mary also didn't explain her counseling program to other stakeholders as encouraged by ASCA Ethical Standard C.1.a. In Case Illustration 11-12, Mary was organized and notified her school faculty and staff of the programs she would like to implement. Mary explained her programs to her administrators and described how the school counseling program aligned with the overall mission of the school. Regardless of whether Mary was able to continue the groups or was forced to cancel them and go into the classroom, she was still advocating for her students and notifying school administration of barriers to the program's success.

ASCA Standard D.1.g. (2010): Professional school counselors assist in developing: (1) curricular and environmental conditions appropriate for the school and community; (2) educational procedures and programs to meet students' developmental needs; (3) a systematic evaluation process for comprehensive, developmental, standards-based school counseling programs, services, and personnel; and (4) a data-driven evaluation process guiding the comprehensive, developmental school counseling program and service delivery.

Simply stated, professional school counselors are active participants in developing and implementing a comprehensive school counseling program.

Student Records

Similar to the ACA Code of Ethics (2014), the ASCA Code of Ethics (2010) requires professional school counselors to "maintain and secure records necessary for rendering professional services to the student as required by laws, regulations, institutional procedures and confidentiality guidelines." However, professional school counselors have a responsibility to take care of two types of records "student records" and "sole-possession records." Sole possession records are those kept in the sole possession of the school counselor and typically used only as a personal memory aid. To be considered a sole-possession record, it must not be accessible or reviewed by anyone else. Ethically speaking, Standard A.8.b. requires professional school counselors to "keep sole-possession records or individual student case notes separate from students' educational records in keeping with state laws" (ASCA, 2010). Concomitantly, Standards A.8.c. and A.8.d. obligate school counselors to recognize the limits of personal memory aids and determine a reasonable time frame for destroying such records. Suggested time frames include destroying the memory aids when the student transitions to another school or upon the student's graduation.

Conclusion

Similar to all other professional counselors, school counselors must have knowledge of and abide by ethical requirements. While some areas of the ASCA Ethical Standards for School Counselors are very similar to the ACA Code of Ethics, other areas are quite different. School counselors must fulfill obligations to many stakeholders (parents, teachers, and administrators) all while acting in the best interests of their students. Counselors may often find themselves in a balancing act, navigating the thin line between keeping student information confidential and acting as an informant to parents and teachers. Use the information you have learned in Chapter 11 to respond to the ethical dilemma and the corresponding discussion questions presented in Case Exercise 11-2.

CASE EXERCISE 11-2

Keenan is a 10th-grade student at a relatively large high school. He comes from an upper middle-class family, typically makes As and Bs on his report cards, and seems to be well liked by his peers and school staff. One day, Keenan stops by the school counselor's office and "wants to talk." Keenan explains that he is having a great deal of anxiety and feels "overstressed" by his classes. Further discussion reveals Keenan is really worried he won't be able to keep up his typical good grades and his parents will make him quit the school baseball team. Keenan also reveals that he hasn't been honest with his teachers or parents about his grades, and he worries everything will come crashing down on him. He says that for the past year, he has been cheating on tests and having other students complete his homework to maintain his high grades.

Keenan explains his parents used to buy him whatever he wanted as long as he kept his grades up. As a result, he typically traded or sold extra pairs of shoes, shirts, and pants in exchange for homework and test answers. Keenan says his parents have started asking questions, and now he isn't able to keep up his normal routine. He is stressed about having to start taking tests on his own without help from others. He begs you not to tell anyone and asks you to help him figure out ways to deal with his current stress.

Do you see any ethical dilemmas in this scenario?

If you were Keenan's counselor, how might you respond to his request that you not tell anyone?

How might you balance confidentiality with Keenan while also reporting behaviors jeopardizing the school's mission?

Keystones

- The ACA and ASCA Codes of Ethics contain many similar ethical requirements.
- School counselors provide informed consent to various stakeholders including parents, administrators, faculty, and students.
- School counselors respect the rights of parents to be the guiding force in their child's life.
- School counselors balance student confidentiality and providing parents with relevant and accurate information.
- Counselors maintain positive working relationships with students and administration.
- Counselors do not leave students alone when they pose a risk to themselves or anyone else.
- When determining "clear and foreseeable harm," school counselors are sure to understand their own values and avoid imposing them onto students.
- School counselors provide equal information to both parents unless a court order specifically prohibits one or both parents from receiving student information.
- School counselors share confidential information with faculty and administration when necessary to benefit students. When doing so, school counselors always understand their primary obligation is to the student.
- School counselors must keep records necessary to provide services to students.

Additional Resources

Family Educational Rights and Privacy Act (FERPA) of 1974, 20 U.S.C. § 1232g (1974).

Froeschle, J., & Crews, C. (2010). An ethics challenge for school counselors. *Journal of School Counseling, 8*(14). Retrieved from http://www.jsc.montana.edu/articles/v8n14.pdf

Mitchell, R. W. (2007). *Documentation in counseling records: An overview of ethical, legal, and clinical Issues* (3rd ed.). Alexandria, VA: American School Counselor Association.

Moyer, M. S., Sullivan, J. R., & Growcock, D. (2012). When is it ethical to inform administrators about student risk-taking behaviors? Perceptions of school counselors. *Professional School Counseling, 15*(3), 98–109.

References

American Counseling Association. (2014). *Code of ethics*. Alexandria, VA: Author.

American School Counselor Association. (2004). *Ethical standards for school counselors*. Alexandria, VA: Author.

American School Counselor Association. (2010). *Ethical standards for school counselors*. Alexandria, VA: Author.

Collins, N., & Knowles, A. D. (1995). Adolescents' attitudes toward confidentiality between the school counselor and the adolescent client. *Australian Psychologist, 30*, 179–182.

Freeman, S. J. (2000). *Ethics: An introduction to philosophy & practice*. Belmont, CA: Wadsworth.

Moyer, M., & Sullivan, J. (2008). Student risk-taking behaviors: When do school counselors break confidentiality? *Professional School Counseling, 11*(4), 236–245.

Perkins, G., Oescher, J., & Ballard, M. (2010). The evolving identity of school counselors as defined by the stakeholders. *Journal of School Counseling, 8*(31). Retrieved from http://www.jsc.montana.edu/articles/v8n31.pdf

12

Ethics in Counselor Education

Education is the ability to listen to almost anything without losing your temper or your self-confidence.

—Robert Frost

C hapter 12 is designed to educate students on the ethics behind teaching in a counselor education program and the guidelines counselor education programs must follow. The authors will address ethics related to admissions, student evaluation, and curriculum. Additionally, standards and expectations set forth by the CACREP will be discussed. Finally, the authors will cover ethical guidelines related to faculty competence and relationships with students. Chapter 12 will give students an understanding of the ethics expected of the faculty teaching in counselor education programs and counselor education programs as a whole. Specifically, after reading this chapter, students will be able to do the following:

1. List the overall ethical responsibilities of counselor education programs.

2. Explain ways in which counselor education programs provide informed consent to students.

3. Explain ethical responsibilities of counselor education programs related to student evaluation.

4. Discuss ethical standards related to assisting students with remediation.

5. Explain ethical requirements related to diversity in counselor education programs.

6. Define competency requirements for counselor educators.

7. Explain ethical guidelines related to the use of case examples.

8. Define ethical standards related to relationships between counselor educators and students.

Responsibilities of Counselor Education Programs

Counselor education programs have the distinct role of preparing and training future professional counselors. Although the literature directly related to the ethics of counselor education is quite sparse, there is some direct attention given to this topic in the ACA Code of Ethics (2014). Standards F.7, F.8, and F.9 discuss responsibilities of counselor education programs (see Text Box 12-1 for APA guidelines).

ACA Standard F.8.a. (2014) Program Information and Orientation: Counselor educators recognize that program orientation is a developmental process that begins upon students' initial contact with the counselor education program and continues throughout the educational and clinical training of students.

TEXT BOX 12-1

American Psychological Association (APA)

APA Standard 7.02 (2010) Descriptions of Education and Training Programs: Psychologists responsible for education and training programs take reasonable steps to ensure that there is a current and accurate description of the program content (including participation in required course- or program-related counseling, psychotherapy, experiential groups, consulting projects, or community service), training goals and objectives, stipends and benefits, and requirements that must be met for satisfactory completion of the program. This information must be made readily available to all interested parties.

Program orientation is a critical aspect of counselor education programs. It is the informed consent (Welfel, 2010), providing students with information needed to be successful in the program. Similar to the informed consent professional counselors discuss with their clients (see Chapter 5), counselor education programs are ethically required to provide information to students. This "informed consent" is initiated at the student's first contact with the program and revisited throughout the training program. Review Case Illustration 12-1, and see an example of how a counselor education program might provide informed consent throughout a student's course of study.

CASE ILLUSTRATION 12-1

Dan is a high school teacher interested in furthering his education; specifically he wants to pursue a degree in school counseling. Searching online for school counseling degree programs in his area, Dan is able to find a program at the local college. On the college's website he is able to find information about the admissions process, the number of hours needed to complete the program, and the specific classes he must take.

After being accepted to the program, Dan is invited to a "new student orientation." At the orientation Dan is able to meet some of the faculty who teach in the program. During the presentation, the coordinator of the school's school counseling program covers material related to: program goals and objectives, ethical responsibilities of school counselors, technology needed to complete the classes, the ways in which students are typically evaluated, ways in which students are supervised throughout the program, and employment opportunities for graduates who receive their degree in school counseling.

At the beginning of each class, throughout his graduate training, Dan is given a course syllabus. The syllabus covers a detailed description of the expectations and evaluation procedures for each specific course in addition to some general expectations of the department and college.

In Case Illustration 12-1, the school counselor education program in which Dan is enrolled uses the college website, new student orientation, and course syllabi to fulfill the requirements of ACA Standard F.8.a. Dan's first contact with the program (the college website) provides him with "informed consent" related to the training program. After he is admitted to the program, Dan is again provided with "informed consent" during the new student orientation. Finally, at the beginning of each of his classes, Dan is provided with "informed consent" material, so he is able to understand what to expect in the upcoming semesters.

F.9.a. (2014) Evaluation of Students: Counselor educators (counselor education programs) clearly state to students, prior to and throughout the training program, the levels of competency expected, appraisal methods, and timing of evaluations for both didactic and clinical competencies. Counselor educators provide students with ongoing feedback regarding their performance throughout the training program.

See Text Box 12-2 for APA's standards regarding this topic.

TEXT BOX 12-2

American Psychological Association (APA)

APA Standard 7.06 (2010) Assessing Student and Supervisee Performance: (a) In academic and supervisory relationships, psychologists establish a timely and specific process for providing

(Continued)

(Continued)

feedback to students and supervisees. Information regarding the process is provided to the student at the beginning of supervision. (b) Psychologists evaluate students and supervisees on the basis of their actual performance on relevant and established program requirements.

Ethical counselor educators and counselor education programs provide ongoing feedback to students. Additionally, faculty and programs seek to be transparent in their evaluation of students. While no direct formula is given, goals, objectives, expectations, and timelines related to student evaluation should be clearly stated and made available. Consider whether you believe the activities of the counselor education program depicted in Case Illustration 12-2 are ethical or not.

CASE ILLUSTRATION 12-2

Dr. Pop is a faculty member who typically teaches a counseling theories course each semester as one of his course assignments. On the course syllabus, Dr. Pop clearly states students are expected to complete three theory papers during the semester, but he does not include any other explanation or guidelines. His rationale for not including more information is that he believes "students should be able to think on their own and not be spoon-fed information all the time." When students turn in their papers, Dr. Pop typically has them graded and returned to students within one or two weeks, but when students receive their papers back, there is typically no feedback given other than a letter grade. Dr. Pop rationalizes his decision because he feels students only care about grades anyway. He believes that if students want feedback on their papers, they will come and ask him. In those cases, Dr. Pop is happy to share feedback with students but does not want to waste his time or energy if students do not initiate the contact.

Do you believe Dr. Pop is acting ethically in providing feedback?

In Case Illustration 12-2, the authors would argue that Dr. Pop would most likely be guilty of unethical practices. While some may argue he provides feedback to students by way of providing them with a grade and will gladly talk to students if they initiate the discussion, the feedback given is minimal at best. Dr. Pop may be able to argue he follows the letter of the standard, but he certainly does not fulfill the spirit of Standard F.9.a. Moreover the directions given for the assignments do not adequately fulfill the ethical requirement that counselor educators inform students of "the level of competency expected or appraisal methods" as described in Standard F.9.a. (ACA, 2014, p. 15). A more appropriate way for Dr. Pop to act might be to (1) list the due dates of the theory papers clearly in the syllabus, (2) include a brief description of the paper expectations along with the assignments, and (3) provide feedback on all papers along with the stated grade.

ACA Standard F.9.b. (2014) Limitations: Counselor educators, through ongoing evaluation, are aware of and address the inability of some students to achieve counseling competencies. Counselor educators do the following: (1) assist students in securing remedial assistance when needed, (2) seek professional consultation and document their decision to dismiss or refer students for assistance, and (3) ensure that students have recourse in a timely manner to address decisions requiring them to seek assistance or to dismiss them and provide students with due process according to institutional policies and procedures.

There are several components to the standard listed here (F.9.b.). The initial section requires counselor education programs to conduct "ongoing" evaluations. This means students should be evaluated throughout their program of study rather than once at either the beginning or end of their program. Second, counselor educators (counselor education programs) provide students with remedial assistance. Ethical counselor education programs work in tandem with students who may be struggling in achieving counseling competencies. Next, counselor educators and counselor education programs are careful to consult with others when determining whether to dismiss a student or refer them for remedial assistance. Finally, counselor education programs ensure students receive feedback in a timely manner to adequately address the remediation expectations. Consider Case Illustration 12-3 in which a student, Christian, is asked to meet with a committee to discuss some faculty concerns.

CASE ILLUSTRATION 12-3

Scenario 1

Christian, a student pursuing his degree in counselor education, receives feedback (like all students in his program) throughout the program. His program has a policy of providing students with a "fitness review" at various times (i.e., after students' second course and fifth course and during each practicum or internship course). Christian has received positive feedback on his first three fitness reviews; however, at his fourth review his instructor indicated he was lacking in skills needed to allow him to better connect with clients. Additionally, his instructor expressed concern Christian had become sloppy in his note taking and treatment plans.

As a result, Christian was invited to a formal meeting in which Christian, his instructor, and two other faculty members discussed the identified concerns. Christian was notified he will be required to receive additional supervision in which his rapport-building skills and documentation will be the primary focus. Christian was then notified which faculty member would provide him with the additional supervision and given a written copy of the committee's expectations. He was also given a chance to respond to the committee and made aware of the appeal process. Finally, the committee informed Christian that they will reconvene in six weeks to review his progress and determine whether additional remediation will be required. Christian was encouraged to contact any of the fitness committee members if he had any questions or concerns regarding his remediation plan and ways he can be successful in completing the plan.

(Continued)

(Continued)

Scenario 2

Christian, a student pursuing his degree in counselor education, received an e-mail from the department chair of his program at the end of his second year. The e-mail informed Christian that several faculty in the department (over the course of the last year) had expressed concern about Christian becoming sloppy in his note taking and treatment plans. The faculty also noted that Christian seemed to lack the skills necessary to build rapport with clients. Christian was invited to a formal meeting in which Christian, the department chair, and two other faculty members were in attendance. During the meeting each committee member read aloud the concerns he/she had noticed over the past year, but Christian was not given a chance to speak, nor was he provided with any written documentation of the concerns. At the end of the meeting Christian was simply told he must "fix his mistakes and work harder to improve his skills with clients." Christian was told he had one week to fix any errors or sloppiness in his client files, and he must locate someone to provide assistance in strengthening his counseling skills.

In Case Illustration 12-3, two scenarios are provided. In both scenarios Christian has the same deficiencies and must meet with a "fitness review" committee. However, in Scenario 1 the counselor education program has a policy of reviewing students throughout the program (i.e., ongoing evaluation) and provides Christian with feedback during the semester it was noticed. Additionally, during the "fitness review" meeting, Christian was provided with documentation of the faculty's concerns and was given assistance in remediation. Finally, Christian was given adequate time to address the concerns identified by the fitness review committee before being reevaluated. Even though the committee members are direct and specific about the changes Christian must make, the faculty in Scenario 1 provide students with support and the necessary resources to be successful as described by Remley and Herlihy (2014).

Conversely, in Scenario 2, the program did not have an ongoing evaluation policy, and Christian was not made aware of the concerns until several semesters later. Christian was not given any assistance in remediation, nor was he given any documentation to help him understand faculty concerns. Christian was simply told to "fix any errors or sloppiness." The program in Scenario 2 may likely be seen as unethical according to Standard F.9.b. (ACA, 2014).

ACA Standard F.8.d. (2014) Addressing Personal Concerns: Counselor educators may require students to address any personal concerns that have the potential to affect professional competency.

If counselor educators determine students have personal issues inhibiting their counseling effectiveness, educators may choose to require students to address such concerns in remediation plans. Addressing concerns may be done in many different ways including requiring personal counseling as a part of the remediation process. Personal counseling is not a requirement in regard to addressing personal concerns but a viable option for counselor educators to consider.

ACA Standard F.9.c. (2014) Counseling for Students: If students request counseling, or if counseling services are suggested as part of a remediation process, counselor educators (education programs) assist students in identifying appropriate services.

Related to the previous standards (F.9.b. and F.8.d.), when students are encouraged to seek out counseling services as a part of remediation, it is the responsibility of the counselor education program and faculty to assist students in locating services. Additionally, if students request counseling on their own, counselor educators and counselor education programs ethically should assist them in finding a counselor. This standard does not imply that counselor education programs pay for the services or provide the services themselves, rather programs simply provide assistance. In many cases this may mean notifying students of counseling services available to all students through the university's student support services or other offices. Review Case Illustration 12-4 and how Dr. J helps a student locate counseling.

CASE ILLUSTRATION 12-4

Dr. J is a full-time faculty member teaching in a small, rural counselor education program. As part of her usual course load, Dr. J typically teaches an Introduction to Counseling Skills course. During the course, students practice basic attending skills with each other and take turns acting as the client and counselor. This semester Dr. J has some concerns about one of the students in the class, Tiago. Tiago has had trouble most of the semester discussing feelings during the mock sessions, and Dr. J has expressed her concerns to Tiago on several occasions. Worrying Tiago will not have the skills to move forward and be successful in his upcoming clinical classes and frustrated due to what she feels is his lack of accepting and implementing feedback, Dr. J refers Tiago to a faculty review committee. During the faculty review meeting, Tiago reveals he has been dealing with the recent death of his mother. He does not feel safe addressing feelings with clients because he worries it may trigger uncontrollable feelings of his own.

Is the faculty review committee able to require Tiago to seek out counseling as a part of his remediation plan?

If the faculty review committee does require Tiago to seek out mental health counseling, what obligations do they have in helping find a counselor?

The simple answer to the first question in Case Illustration 12-4 is yes; the review committee is ethically able to require Tiago to attend counseling. Tiago's lack of ability to address emotions with clients is clearly something affecting his professional competency. Therefore, according to Ethical Standard F.9.b., the review committee may make such a requirement. If the committee does decide to require Tiago to visit a counselor, the committee has an obligation to assist him in locating a counselor. Many counselor education programs may have a list of potential resources for such occasions.

Review Case Illustration 12-5 as yet another example of how counselor education programs act as gatekeepers to the counseling profession.

CASE ILLUSTRATION 12-5

Dr. Gonzalez teaches in a counseling department containing three different CACREP accredited programs, a school counseling program, a clinical mental health counseling program, and an addictions counseling program. Dr. Gonzalez's expertise is in addiction-related disorders. In addition to his teaching responsibilities, he also practices clinically in an intensive outpatient program (IOP), where he conducts individual and group counseling sessions. This semester Dr. Gonzalez is teaching an advanced addictions course that is a required class for all students in the addiction counseling program. One of the class assignments requires students to attend four addiction-related self-help groups in the community. Because Dr. Gonzalez is himself a recovering alcoholic, he shares his group experiences with his students as a teaching moment and further encourages his students to fully participate in the groups they attend. Dr. Gonzalez also attends a weekly meeting of alcoholics anonymous. One week as he is attending his regular weekly group, Dr. Gonzalez notices one of his students come in and sit in the back of the room. Although Dr. Gonzalez typically shares his past experiences with alcohol and drugs, he decides not to speak at this particular meeting so as not to divulge too much personal information in front of his student. On the other hand, Dr. Gonzalez's student decides to share her addiction to alcohol. During her testimonial the student talks about her past struggles with alcoholism and further reveals she has relapsed in the past week and feels as though she is out of control again with her drinking. Hearing his student's testimonial and knowing this particular student is also currently enrolled in practicum and working with clients dealing with their own addictions, Dr. Gonzalez wonders if he has a responsibility to share this new information with other faculty in the department.

Should Dr. Gonzalez address the concept of an impaired counselor with the student?

What responsibility does Dr. Gonzalez have to protect the clients this student is seeing in her practicum course?

In Case Illustration 12-5, Dr. Gonzalez hears one of his current students discuss her own battle with addictions and her current relapse. Additionally, Dr. Gonzalez knows the student is completing her practicum and working with clients who are dealing with addictions. Question 1 in Case Illustration 12-5 inquires whether Dr. Gonzalez should address the issue of impairment with his student. The answer is yes; Dr. Gonzalez should definitely discuss counselor impairment with his student. Counselor educators are responsible for educating students about ethical standards and making sure students do not harm their clients. In Chapter 13, related to ethics in counselor supervision, the authors discuss supervisors' responsibilities in ensuring supervisees are knowledgeable of and follow ethical guidelines. In Case Illustration 12-5, Dr. Gonzalez is acting in a supervisory role and therefore should address the issue with his student.

In the second question the authors pose a question about Dr. Gonzalez's responsibility to protect the clients the student is counseling in her practicum course. Again, as will be discussed in Chapter 13, counselor supervisors have a responsibility not only to their supervisees but also to their supervisee's clients. In this case, the counselor education program has a duty to protect, as best they can, the clients seen by students.

Related to Ethical Standard F.8.d., F.9.c., and F.9.d., Dr. Gonzalez may see his student's addiction and recent relapse as a situation limiting her ability to competently work with clients. In such a case, Dr. Gonzalez (along with other faculty members) may require her to attend counseling to address her addiction issues prior to continuing her work with her own clients. If Dr. Gonzalez or other faculty members were to require such counseling, they must assist the student in locating appropriate resources to provide the necessary counseling.

ACA Standard F.8.b. (2014) Student Career Advising: Counselor educators provide career advisement for their students and make them aware of the opportunities in the field.

Simply stated, counselor educators and counselor education programs are responsible for talking with students about career opportunities. This may occur in various formats (e.g., classroom discussions, individual meetings, etc.), but as mentors and teachers, counselor educators ethically should work with students in some way to prepare them for a career in professional counseling.

Curriculum

Curriculum is an integral part of any counselor education program. While some programs may look to state licensure boards to inform their course work, others may use current CACREP standards to guide curriculum (Schweiger, Henderson, & Clawson, 2007; Bobby, 2013). In addition to the aforementioned entities, the ACA Code of Ethics (2014) also provides course work requirements. The following four standards address ethics related to the course work provided by counselor education programs.

ACA Standard F.7.c. (2014) Infusing Multicultural Issues and Diversity: Counselor educators infuse material related to multiculturalism and diversity into all courses and workshops for the development of professional counselors.

Understanding and learning to work with diverse populations is a must for all professional counselors. Cottone and Tarvydas (2007) describe multiculturalism as "critical in the larger counseling framework, not as a specialty area but as an integral element of all human interaction" (p. 212). Therefore, it is not enough for counselor education programs to only offer a course in multicultural issues or diversity. Ethical counselor education programs infuse multiculturalism into all courses and workshops. Examine Case Illustration 12-6 and the examples of how programs may infuse multiculturalism and diversity into courses and workshops across the curriculum.

CASE ILLUSTRATION 12-6

During her Assessment and Testing course, a faculty member includes lectures and discussions about biases some tests may show toward certain populations.

(Continued)

(Continued)

During his course related to addictions and crisis intervention, a faculty member is sure to discuss how addictions may be viewed in various cultures and how understanding various cultures may affect the treatment modality used in certain situations.

During her course related to marriage and family counseling, a faculty member discusses family structures and how family structures differ by culture. The faculty member is sure to address various ways of working with families from varied cultures.

ACA Standard F.7.d. (2014) Integration of Study and Practice: In traditional, hybrid, and/or online formats, counselor educators establish education and training programs that integrate academic study and supervised practice.

Learning to be a skilled counselor takes more than sitting and listening to lectures and podcasts about how to be a counselor. Likewise, becoming a counselor involves more than practicing basic attending skills. The combination of classroom academic study and applying those learned skills during supervised practice is vital to becoming a well-rounded, competent professional counselor. As such, most counselor preparation programs combine lecture classes (e.g., Counseling Theories, Introduction to School and Clinical Mental Health Counseling, Diagnosis, Human Development, etc.) with supervised experience or field placement courses (e.g., practicum or internship).

ACA Standard F.7.e. (2014) Teaching Ethics: Throughout the program, counselor educators ensure that students are aware of the ethical responsibilities and standards of the profession and the ethical responsibilities of students to the profession. Counselor educators infuse ethical considerations throughout the curriculum.

Following the basic ethical guidelines of the code of ethics (ACA, 2014), counselor preparation programs are "required" only to infuse ethical considerations throughout the curriculum rather than offer a full course on ethics. Review Case Illustration 12-7 and how infusing ethical considerations throughout a program's course work may not be enough.

CASE ILLUSTRATION 12-7

Rhyder is a counseling student in the final semester of his graduate work. During this time he is also studying to take his state's professional counselor exam. While studying, Rhyder begins to feel underprepared in the area of ethics and sets up a meeting with his graduate advisor to discuss his concerns. During the meeting, Rhyder's advisor explains that even though the program does not offer a course specifically related to ethics, ethics is infused throughout the course work and discussed in every class as required by the ACA Code of Ethics. Rhyder understands but also expresses concerns stating that each course seemed to cover ethics during one to two class meetings and always covered the same areas of ethics (e.g., don't date or sleep with your clients, confidentiality, informed consent, and don't impose your own values on clients). Rhyder further explains how even though ethics was infused into every course, he feels as though it was covered only at the surface level because it was not the main focus of the course.

Is Rhyder's counselor education program operating ethically according to Standard F.7.e.?

How could Rhyder's counselor education program possibly address this situation to better prepare students?

The first question in Case Illustration 12-7 asks if the counselor education program is acting in an ethical manner. Yes, the program is following the wording of the ACA Code of Ethics (i.e., they are infusing ethics into the curriculum). However, the authors argue that the spirit of the standard is focused on all students having a solid understanding of the code, and thus ethics should be covered more than simply at the surface level. When ethics is "infused" throughout a program, many of the standards may be covered in a general sense, but finer intricacies are often left out. For example, students may know to avoid imposing values onto clients but not understand their own values or how impositions can occur in the subtlest of ways. Students may understand the potential dangers of counseling friends or family members but not realize the implications for counselors who might be the only mental health professional in a geographic region.

The second question queries how Rhyder's counselor education program might be able to address Rhyder's concerns and better prepare students. To avoid this situation continually occurring, the faculty in Rhyder's program could address the concern in various ways. Two possible solutions include (1) offering a course specifically addressing ethics and add it to the list of required courses, and (2) having the faculty teaching various courses coordinate and discuss the areas of the code of ethics they plan to infuse into their curriculums. Choosing one of these options may help insure all areas of the code of ethics are covered, and duplicate information can be avoided.

ACA Standard F.7.b. (2014) Innovative Theories and Techniques: Counselor educators promote the use of techniques, procedures, and modalities that are grounded in theory and/or have an empirical or scientific foundation. When counselor educators discuss developing or innovative techniques, procedures, and modalities, they explain the potential risks, benefits, and ethical considerations of using such techniques, procedures, and modalities.

Simply stated, counselor educators are truthful and honest about techniques and treatment modalities. Educators are sure to identify techniques grounded in theory and those still developing.

ACA Standard F.7.i. (2014) Field Placements: Counselor educators develop clear policies and provide direct assistance within their training programs regarding appropriate field placement and other clinical experiences. Counselor educators provide clearly stated roles and responsibilities for the student or supervisee, the site supervisor, and the program supervisor. They confirm that site supervisors are qualified to provide supervision in the formats in which services are provided and inform site supervisors of their professional and ethical responsibilities in this role.

Standard F.7.i. coincides with and reiterates Standard F.8.a. (Program Information and Orientation), discussed at the beginning of Chapter 12. Counselor education programs inform students of expectations related to field placements, notifying them of acceptable field placements, student roles during field placement, and supervisor roles during field placement. This information may often be provided to students in the form of a practicum or internship manual or through a syllabus provided at the beginning of the course. Additionally, counselor educators monitor and provide support to field supervisors to provide the highest-quality supervision to students. Providing orientations, conducting field placement visits throughout the semester, and sharing professional development opportunities to field supervisors are a few ways in which faculty members may inform field placement supervisors of their roles and monitor effectiveness.

Responsibilities of Counselor Educators

The axioms "those who can, do, and those who can't, teach" and working in an "ivory tower" are sometimes used to refer to faculty or those who work in higher education. Those terms infer counselor educators are out of touch and lack the practical skills needed to work in the field. Ethically, this should not be the case for counselor education programs. Consider the standards related to characteristics of counselor educators and ways in which counselor educators conduct their classes.

ACA Standard F.7.a. (2014) Counselor Educators: Counselor educators who are responsible for developing, implementing, and supervising educational programs are skilled as teachers and practitioners. They are knowledgeable regarding the ethical, legal, and regulatory aspects of the profession; are skilled in applying that knowledge; and make students and supervisees aware of their responsibilities. Whether in traditional, hybrid, and/or online formats, counselor educators conduct counselor education and training programs in an ethical manner and serve as role models for professional behaviors.

ACA Standard F.7.b. (2014) Counselor Educator Competence: Counselors who function as counselor educators or supervisors provide instruction within their areas of knowledge and competence and provide instruction based on current information and knowledge available in the profession. When using technology to deliver instruction, counselor educators develop competence in the use of the technology.

As noted for many other standards, Ethical Standards F.7.a. and F.7.b. include several components. (1) Counselor educators are skilled as teachers and practitioners. (2) Counselor educators pass their experiences and expertise along to their students and are considered role models for their students. Simply put, counselor educators should be experts in teaching, experts in the practice of counseling, and role models in terms of displaying professional and ethical behaviors. Consider whether you believe the faculty members depicted in Case Illustration 12-8 are acting ethically.

CASE ILLUSTRATION 12-8

Scenario 1

Michael, a newly hired assistant professor, expresses interest to his department chair in teaching practicum and counseling skills his first semester. Michael graduated from his doctoral program just three months prior to being hired as a faculty member. Prior to and during his doctoral program, Michael spent most of his time gaining experience in teaching and research. His only clinical experience was during his master's and doctoral practicum and internship courses.

Do you believe Michael is acting ethically according to Standard F.7.a.?

Scenario 2

Dr. Z is an experienced counselor educator with more than 10 years of experience. She is heavily involved in the community surrounding the university in which she teaches, has her own private practice, and is a proficient researcher. Due to her extremely busy schedule, Dr. Z often finds herself running late for classes. Even though she always sends an e-mail to her students letting them know she is on her way, she routinely arrives to her classes 15 to 20 minutes late. Furthermore, on most class days Dr. Z typically ends class 45 minutes to an hour early. Dr. Z's classes are usually held in the late afternoon, and she does not feel comfortable driving in the dark. She also rationalizes her decision as a way to increase her teaching evaluation scores because "students never complain about getting out of class early."

Is Dr. Z acting ethically according to Standard F.7.a.?

In the first scenario presented in Case Illustration 12-8, Michael is a counselor educator who has very limited experience in clinical practice and is scheduled to teach two clinical classes. While it is difficult to say for sure whether Michael is (or is not) acting ethically, there are some things Michael would want to consider prior to teaching clinical classes. Similar to professional counselors working in a school, community, or other setting, Michael would want to engage in an ethical decision-making process. He would want to reflect on his own clinical competency and whether or not he feels competent to teach clinical classes when he does not have extensive clinical experience.

In the second scenario Dr. Z is extremely busy and often arrives late to class. She also typically ends her classes early due to her fear of driving after dark. Dr. Z would most likely be considered to be acting unethically according to Standard F.7.a.; counselor educators must "serve as role models for professional behaviors." By showing up late and ending class early, Dr. Z is not modeling appropriate professional behaviors. For example, if a student routinely arrived late for scheduled counseling sessions and ended all sessions early, he/she would likely be confronted on their unprofessional behaviors. Similarly, Dr. Z should follow the guidelines of the course schedule, starting classes on time and ending classes at the appropriate time.

Similar to the standards discussed (F.7.a. and F.7.b.), ACA Ethics Standards F.7.f. (Use of Case Examples), F.7.g. (Student-to-Student Supervision and Instruction), and F.8.c. (Self-Growth Experiences) pertain to ethics and counselor educators. However, rather than focusing on characteristics of the faculty, these standards give more emphasis to teaching strategies used by counselor educators.

ACA Standard F.7.f. (2014) Use of Case Examples: The use of client, student, or supervisee information for the purposes of case examples in a lecture or classroom setting is permissible only when (a) the client, student, or supervisee has reviewed the material and agreed to its presentation or (b) the information has been sufficiently modified to obscure identity.

This standard reiterates ethical requirements for professional counselors and counselor educators to maintain the confidentiality of clients and supervisees (i.e., ACA Ethical Standard B.1.c.) It is the authors' experience when using case examples in class that counselor educators will most often modify the information used in the case example to protect the anonymity of the client or supervisee rather than seek out approval. See Text Box 12-3 for information from the APA related to this issue. Review Case Illustration 12-9 to see an example of how a faculty member might modify information to protect the anonymity of a client.

CASE ILLUSTRATION 12-9

Dr. Nelson has a private practice along with his teaching responsibilities at the local university. During today's class, Dr. Nelson talks about suicide and how to work with potentially suicidal clients. During his lecture he uses an example of one of his current clients who he recently had to assess for suicidal ideation. Dr. Nelson's client is named Rick and is a 41-year-old male who recently retired from the Air Force. Rick is married and has two young children. When discussing the case example in class, Dr. Nelson obscures the identity of his client by describing his client (not using a name) as a middle-aged man who is going through a career change.

Has Dr. Nelson acted ethically according to Standard F.7.f.?

By leaving off some identifiers (e.g., name and family status) and generalizing others (e.g., 41 becomes middle aged, and retired from the Air Force changes to career change), Dr. Nelson is able to give a brief summary of the client for his case example without providing any information threatening the confidentiality of the actual client. Therefore, Dr. Nelson would likely be seen as acting ethically.

ACA Standard F.7.g. (2014) Student-to-Student Supervision and Instruction: When students function in the role of counselor educators or supervisors, they understand that they have the same ethical obligations as counselor educators, trainers, and supervisors. Counselor educators make every effort to ensure that the rights of students are not compromised when their peers lead experiential counseling activities in traditional, hybrid, and/or online formats.

A common component among all doctoral programs in counselor education is the requirement that all doctoral students gain some experience in teaching or co-teaching master's-level courses. This requirement helps to prepare doctoral students for careers in counselor education and teaching courses on their own. Likewise, in many master's-level courses students are required to deliver presentations or lead the class in learning activities as part of a class assignment. In these situations, it is paramount students (master's or doctoral level) prepare and deliver their material in a way adhering to the ethical responsibilities of a counselor educator. Concomitantly, it is the counselor educator's (instructor of record) responsibility to assure the rights of students, clients, and supervisees are not violated. Consider Case Illustration 12-10 in which Ronnie delivers a presentation to his class.

CASE ILLUSTRATION 12-10

Ronnie, a master's student in a clinical mental health counseling program, delivered a presentation to his Couples and Families course related to gender roles and diverse families. During the course of his presentation, Ronnie described a couple he worked with at his practicum site. Ronnie described the couple in great detail without obscuring any of their identifying information. Additionally, he used some questionable language including a few homophobic slurs in his presentation.

Who is responsible for Ronnie's unethical behavior?

In Case Illustration 12-10, Ronnie is not acting ethically according several ethical standards (i.e., F.7.g. and F.7.a.). According to F.7.g., if Ronnie is functioning in the role of a counselor educator (delivering a presentation and leading an experiential activity), he is responsible for conducting himself in accordance with ethical standards for counselor educators (i.e., serve as a role model for professional behavior). However, in this situation, it is not only Ronnie who should be held accountable. The faculty member teaching Ronnie's class is also responsible for Ronnie's behavior and "making sure the rights of students are not compromised when their peers lead counseling activities" (ACA, 2014, p. 14). In the situation presented it would be appropriate for the counselor educator to intervene with Ronnie and take appropriate action to ensure no students were physically or emotionally harmed.

ACA Standard F.8.c. (2014) Self-Growth Experiences: Self-growth is an expected component of counselor education. Counselor educators are mindful of ethical principles when they require students to engage in self-growth experiences. Counselor educators and supervisors inform students that they have a right to decide what information will be shared or withheld in class.

TEXT BOX 12-3

American Psychological Association

APA Standard 7.04 (2010) Student Disclosure of Personal Information: Psychologists do not require students or supervisees to disclose personal information in course- or program-related activities, either orally or in writing, regarding sexual history, history of abuse and neglect, psychological treatment, and relationship with parents, peers, and spouses or significant others except if (1) the program or training facility has clearly identified this requirement in its admissions and program materials or (2) the information is necessary to evaluate or obtain assistance for students whose personal problems could reasonably be judged to be preventing them from performing their training or professionally related activities in a competent manner or posing a threat to the students or others.

Counselor educators must be mindful to remind students to be comfortable in what they share during self-growth activities For example, a counselor educator reminds his group class they will all be expected to both lead and be a part of a process group during the semester. Additionally, the faculty member encourages his students to be active in the group discussion but to only share information they are comfortable sharing. The faculty member then reiterates the group experience is a learning one and not actual group therapy for the class.

Roles and Relationships Between Counselor Educators and Students

Similar to the requirement that professional counselors avoid sexual and/or romantic relationships with clients, counselor educators are prohibited from sexual or romantic interactions with current students (ACA, 2014). In addition to this ethical requirement, most institutions of higher education have local policies prohibiting such interactions as well (Ford, 2006). Faculty members have inherent power over students (i.e., determining student grades or writing recommendation letters for students to further their education or gain employment) and therefore should be cognizant of the impact of nonacademic relationships (Welfel, 2010). Ethical standards, such as those listed next, using definitive terminology (i.e., "prohibited" and "do not"), may be seen as more common sense and easier to determine the rightness or wrongness of actions.

ACA Standard F.10.a. (2014) Sexual or Romantic Relationships: Counselor educators are prohibited from sexual or romantic interactions or relationships with students currently enrolled in a counseling or related program and over whom they have power and authority. This prohibition applies to both in-person and electronic interactions or relationships.

ACA Standard F.10.b. (2014) Sexual Harassment: Counselor educators do not condone or subject students to sexual harassment.

ACA Standard F.10.e. (2014) Counseling Services: Counselor educators do not serve as counselors to students currently enrolled in a counseling or related program and over whom they have power and authority.

However, standards using less definitive language (i.e., counselor educators "are aware," avoid non-academic relationships in "which there is risk") offer more room for interpretation. Being "aware" of a power differential and assessing whether or not there is "risk" is left up to the counselor educator to determine. Depending on morals, values, beliefs, and/or life experiences, awareness and risk may have different meanings. Therefore there is increased importance on self-awareness and understanding motivation when deciding how to act. Without taking all possible actions and outcomes into account, some seemingly innocuous actions have the potential to become ethical concerns. See Text Box 12-4 for additional information from the APA and AAMFT.

ACA Standard F.10.c. (2014) Relationships With Former Students: Counselor educators are aware of the power differential in the relationship between faculty and students. Faculty members discuss with former students potential risks when they consider engaging in social, sexual, or other intimate relationships.

TEXT BOX 12-4

American Psychological Association

APA Standard 7.05 (2010) Mandatory Individual or Group Therapy: (a) When individual or group therapy is a program or course requirement, psychologists responsible for that program allow students in undergraduate and graduate programs the option of selecting such therapy from practitioners unaffiliated with the program. (b) Faculty who are or are likely to be responsible for evaluating students' academic performance do not themselves provide that therapy.

APA Standard 7.07 (2010) Sexual Relationships With Students and Supervisees: Psychologists do not engage in sexual relationships with students or supervisees who are in their department, agency, or training center or over whom psychologists have or are likely to have evaluative authority.

American Association for Marriage and Family Therapists

AAMFT Standard 4.2 (2015) Therapy With Students or Supervisees: Marriage and family therapists do not provide therapy to current students or supervisees.

AAMFT Standard 4.3 (2015) Sexual Intimacy With Students or Supervisees: Marriage and family therapists do not engage in sexual intimacy with students or supervisees during the evaluative or training relationship between the therapist and student or supervisee.

(Continued)

(Continued)

AAMFT Standard 4.6 (2015) Existing Relationships With Students or Supervisees: Marriage and family therapists are aware of their influential positions with respect to supervisees, and they avoid exploiting the trust and dependency of such persons. Supervisors, therefore, make every effort to avoid conditions and multiple relationships with supervisees that could impair professional judgment or increase the risk of exploitation. Examples of such relationships include, but are not limited to, business or close personal relationships with supervisees or the supervisee's immediate family. When the risk of impairment or exploitation exists due to conditions or multiple roles, supervisors document the appropriate precautions taken.

Sexual and/or romantic relationships between faculty and current students are clearly unethical. However, what about in situations when the relationship is between a faculty member and a past student? Consider Case Illustration 12-11 in which Dr. A and Jacob develop a romantic relationship.

CASE ILLUSTRATION 12-11

At church one Sunday, Dr. A is approached by Jacob. Jacob is an elementary school teacher who has decided to go back to school to earn his degree in clinical mental health counseling. Jacob recognizes Dr. A from the faculty webpage and decides to introduce himself. The two talk shortly and then go their separate ways. Over the course of the next few years, Jacob takes a few classes Dr. A teaches, and the two see each other on a regular basis at church activities. Their conversations are typically very short (Dr. A is very careful to maintain appropriate boundaries with her students) even though the two clearly have a great deal in common (i.e., similar in age, both are divorced, and both enjoy sports and outdoor activities). After Jacob graduates, Dr. A is less concerned about her interactions with Jacob because he is no longer considered "one of her students." The two enjoy each other's company a great deal and have gone out for coffee a few times. On a few occasions the topic of a more serious relationship has come up.

As a recent graduate, how might Jacob's relationship with Dr. A help his ability to get a job in professional counseling? Similarly, how might it hurt his ability if their relationship ends negatively?

As a recent graduate, and someone who is looking to earn licensure, how might Jacob's relationship with Dr. A benefit him in the licensure process? Similarly, how might it hinder Jacob in the licensure process if his relationship with Dr. A were to end negatively?

In Case Illustration 12-11, Dr. A and Jacob developed a romantic relationship after he completed his degree. Therefore Jacob was no longer considered a student of Dr. A. Still, according to Standard F.10.c., Dr. A should be aware of the power differential in the relationship and initiate conversation with Jacob about potential risks.

Both questions in Case Illustration 12-11 ask about potential risks and benefits Jacob's relationship with Dr. A might have on his licensure and overall career. Above and beyond the personal relationship with Dr. A, having a strong relationship with her may benefit Jacob in attaining licensure, gaining employment, or even extending his opportunities for involvement in professional organizations. For example, because Dr. A is a faculty member, she may likely have many professional contacts in the community who might be willing to give Jacob special consideration due to his relationship with her. On the contrary, if the relationship were to deteriorate or end in a negative fashion, the breakup will most likely negatively affect Jacob in those same areas. Because she has the power (related to professional counseling) in this situation, it is Dr. A's responsibility to not only acknowledge her power but also initiate conversations with Jacob related to the potential risks of the power differential if they were to continue the relationship. In addition to simply having the conversations with Jacob, the authors recommend Dr. A document all conversations.

The following standards concern relationships between counselor educators and current students that are not intimate or sexual in nature.

ACA Standard F.10.d. (2014) Nonacademic Relationships: Counselor educators avoid nonacademic relationships with students in which there is a risk of potential harm to the student or which may compromise the training experience or grades assigned. In addition, counselor educators do not accept any form of professional services, fees, commissions, reimbursement, or remuneration from a site for student or supervisor placement.

ACA Standard F.10.f. (2014) Extending Educator-Student Boundaries: Counselor educators are aware of the power differential in the relationship between faculty and students. If they believe that a nonprofessional relationship with a student may be potentially beneficial to the student, they take precautions similar to those taken by counselors when working with clients. Examples of potentially beneficial interactions or relationships include, but are not limited to, attending a formal ceremony; conducting hospital visits; providing support during a stressful event; or maintaining mutual membership in a professional association, organization, or community. Counselor educators discuss with students the rationale for such interactions, the potential benefits and drawbacks, and the anticipated consequences for the student. Educators clarify the specific nature and limitations of the additional roles they will have with the student prior to engaging in a nonprofessional relationship. Nonprofessional relationships with students should be time limited and/or context specific and initiated with student consent.

Again, there is some vague terminology (i.e., "risk of potential harm," "aware of power differential," "potentially beneficial to the student") leaving room for interpretation. Consider the situations presented in Case Illustration 12-12 and whether you believe the interactions would be ethical or unethical according to Standards F.10.d. and F.10.f.

CASE ILLUSTRATION 12-12

A faculty member routinely goes out to have drinks with students after class.

A faculty member announces to his class that he is in need of a babysitter for his two children and wonders if anyone in the class would be willing to babysit. Additionally, the faculty member mentions that because he is in great need at the last minute, he is willing to give any volunteers two points on the final exam in addition to regular babysitter fees.

A student realizes that his professor uses many golf references and analogies during his lecture. After class, the student talks to the professor and asks if he would like to go play golf sometime.

In most cases the first situation presented in Case Illustration 12-12 would probably be seen as inappropriate or "compromising the training experience," especially if the interactions occurred on a regular occasion. However, the argument could be made that there is nothing wrong with going out with a few students at the end of a semester to celebrate a successful term. In any case, it is the counselor educator's responsibility to thoroughly consider the benefits and consequences of doing so, including the faculty members' motivation for going out with his/her students.

In the second situation the counselor educator is in great need of a babysitter. While possibly a successful way to recruit a babysitter, this would most likely be considered unethical and an abuse of the inherent power differential between faculty and students.

In the third situation a student approaches his professor and asks to play golf sometime. Although there may be arguments as to how this may benefit the student, this would most likely be considered an inappropriate extension of boundaries and could possibly compromise the training experience.

Conclusion

Chapter 12 covered ethical standards related to counselor education programs. For those students who have hopes of pursuing a doctoral degree and a career in counselor education, this material provides a base knowledge for the future. For master's-level students who are interested in school or clinical mental health counseling and have no desire to pursue a doctoral degree or a career in counselor education, this material is equally important. Informed consent, as discussed throughout this text, is paramount to all areas of professional counseling. Students may find themselves on the receiving end of unethical practices and must know how to respond or if to respond. Use the information learned in chapter to address the ethical dilemma and corresponding discussion questions presented in Case Exercise 12-1. Consider whether or not you believe the faculty member is acting ethically and how you might respond if put in a similar situation.

CASE EXERCISE 12-1

Dr. Reesen is a counselor educator and typically teaches the practicum class every semester as one of his assigned classes. Dr. Reesen is a skilled practitioner and is generally well liked by his students. One of Dr. Reesen's favorite things about the practicum class is that it is typically a small class (10–12 students), and he feels as though he is able to get to know the students on a more personal level. Every semester, prior to the first night of class, Dr. Reesen e-mails his practicum students and invites them over to his house for a barbeque dinner on the first night of class. In his e-mail he reminds everyone that while attendance is not mandatory, he does think it is a good way to meet classmates and highly encourages everyone to attend if they intend to earn full class participation points. He feels it is a good way for everyone to get to know each other and for his students to get a chance to relax before the hectic semester begins. Dr. Reesen provides all of the food; he just asks students bring their own choice of drinks (i.e., beer, wine, lemonade, or soft drinks).

At the end of every semester, Dr. Reesen again throws a "completion party" at his house during the last week of classes. He again provides all of the food and requests his students bring drinks. Additionally, he requests everyone bring their final practicum time logs and documentation forms to turn in at the party.

Do you see any potential ethical concerns in Dr. Reesen's actions?

As a student, how might you address any potential concerns? Use an ethical decision-making model to determine if and how you might act in this situation.

Identify the problem.

Review relevant ethical codes and laws.

Understand your own morals, values, and beliefs and how they might influence your interpretation of the code of ethics and laws.

Identify possible courses of action.

Identify benefits and consequences of possible courses of action.

Consult with others.

Decide on a course of action and implement.

Keystones

- Counselor education programs must provide informed consent to students related to program expectations throughout the educational training program.
- Ethical counselor education programs provide ongoing feedback to students.
- Counselor education programs must assist students in determining appropriate remediation strategies.

- Counselor education programs are able to require students to attend counseling to address issues affecting the student's professional competency.
- Counselor education programs must provide assistance to students who are seeking counseling services.
- Ethical counselor education programs infuse diversity issues into all required course work.
- Ethical counselor education programs require students to combine academic understanding and supervised practice.
- Counselor education programs must infuse ethics into the curriculum.
- Counselor educators must be competent in the areas in which they teach and serve as role models for professional and ethical behavior.
- Counselor educators understand the power differential between students and faculty and consider all potential risks and benefits prior to entering into a nonacademic relationship with former students.
- Sexual or romantic relationships between faculty and current students are prohibited.
- Counselor educators are cognizant of power differentials and consider potential risks and benefits prior to extending educator-student boundaries.

Additional Resources

Kiselica, M. S., & Ramsey, M. L. (2001). Multicultural counselor education: Historical perspectives and future dimensions. In D. C. Locke, J. E. Myers, & E. L. Herr (Eds.), *Handbook of counseling* (pp. 443–451). Thousand Oaks, CA: Sage.
Vaccaro, N., & Lambie, G. W. (2007). Computer-based counselor-in-training supervision: Ethical and practical implications for counselor educators and supervisors. *Counselor Education & Supervision, 47,* 46–57.

References

American Association for Marriage and Family Therapy. (2015). *Code of ethics.* Retrieved from https://www.aamft.org/iMIS15/AAMFT/Content/legal_ethics/code_of_ethics.aspx
American Counseling Association. (2014). *Code of ethics.* Alexandria, VA: Author.
American Psychological Association. (2010). American Psychological Association ethical principles of psychologists and code of conduct. Retrieved from http://www.apa.org/ethics/code/principles.pdf
Bobby, C. L. (2013). The evolution of specialties in the CACREP standards: CACREP's role in unifying the profession. *Journal of Counseling and Development: JCD, 91*(1), 35–43. Retrieved from http://search.proquest.com/docview/1293091340?accountid=7122
Cottone, R. R., & Tarvydas, V. M. (2007). *Counseling ethics and decision making* (3rd ed.). Upper Saddle River, NJ: Pearson Merrill Prentice-Hall.
Ford, G. G. (2006). *Ethical reasoning for mental health professionals.* Thousand Oaks, CA: Sage.
Remley, T. P., & Herlihy, B. (2014). *Ethical, legal, and professional issues in counseling* (4th ed.). Upper Saddle River, NJ: Pearson.
Schweiger, W. K., Henderson, D. A., & Clawson, T. W. (2007). *Counselor preparation: Programs, faculty, trends.* Retrieved from http://www.eblib.com
Welfel, E. R. (2010). *Ethics in counseling & psychotherapy: Standards, research, and emerging issues.* Belmont, CA: Brooks/Cole.

13

Ethics in Supervision

Often, it's not about becoming a new person, but becoming the person you were meant to be, and already are, but don't know how to be.

—Heath L. Buckmaster

S upervision takes place in many contexts. Students completing their degrees in counselor education will often have "site supervisors" offering mentorship and guidance at a particular training site. Counselor educators also wear a "supervisor hat" many times while teaching courses. Away from training institutions and after students graduate, many states require counselor interns to receive "clinical supervision" prior to becoming fully licensed. Finally, in school and clinical mental health settings, counselors may be asked to "supervise" others as a part of their job title or responsibilities. Although counselor supervisors work in many different settings, they all have common ethical obligations to which they must adhere.

Lack of appropriate supervision is one of the most common concerns brought before licensure and regulatory boards. Supervisors are not only responsible for their own actions as supervisors but are also liable for the actions of their supervisees (Cikanek, Veach, Braun, 2004). Similar to the counselor/client relationship and faculty/student relationship, ethical guidelines exist related to the supervisor/supervisee relationship. In Chapter 13 the authors discuss supervisor competency, informed consent, confidentiality, rights and responsibilities of supervisors and supervisees, and liability related to supervision. Comparable to the previous chapter concerning counselor education, Chapter 13 serves to educate students about ethical considerations for supervisors and possibly what to look for and expect as a practicum or internship student and/or supervisee heading toward licensure. Ethical dilemmas and case illustrations presented here will encourage students to evaluate various aspects of supervision. Specifically, after reading Chapter 13, students will be able to accomplish the following:

1. Explain the importance of supervisor competency.

2. Explain the importance of supervisors providing informed consent to supervisees.

3. Name the ethical responsibilities supervisors have in ensuring supervisees' and clients' rights are protected.

4. Discuss the importance of monitoring oneself for signs of impairment.

5. Define supervisors' ethical duties to act as gatekeepers for the counseling profession.

6. Define ethical standards related to relationships between supervisors and supervisees.

7. Understand ethical standards related to providing supervision to friends and family members.

8. Explain the importance of using a decision-making model when deciding whether or not to extend supervisor boundaries.

Supervisor Competency

Counselor supervisors are a central component of counselor training, and it is critical that counselor supervisors are trained and competent to act in supervisory roles. State licensure boards often have their own supervisor standards and may often have their own requirements for becoming an approved supervisor and credentialed to supervise those seeking state licensure. However, there are many professional counselors in supervisory roles who may not have or seek out the credentials of state licensure boards (e.g., a clinical supervisor of a nonprofit clinic, counselor educators and faculty members teaching practicum and internship courses, and/or school counselors in leadership and supervisory roles). In those situations and others, the ACA has identified several standards to address minimum competency standards for counselor supervisors.

ACA Standard F.2.a. (2014) Supervision Preparation: Prior to offering supervision services, counselors are trained in supervision methods and techniques. Counselors who offer supervision services regularly pursue continuing education activities, including both counseling and supervision topics and skills.

Counselor supervisors may acquire the training required in Standard F.2.a. in various ways. Counselor educators often are afforded the ability to gain supervisory experience during their doctoral programs acting as peer supervisors (Trepal & Hammer, 2014). Other supervisors may receive training at state, regional, or national conferences. For example, the Texas Counseling Association provides a "supervision track" at the association's annual Professional Growth Conference. However the necessary training is acquired, it is recommended by Corey, Corey, and Callanan (2011) and Ford (2006) that counselor supervisors:

Be skilled counselors themselves.

Have an understanding of ethical and professional responsibilities.

Understand and utilize supervision models.

Be competent in case conceptualization.

Be able to evaluate counselors and provide appropriate feedback.

Continue to stay atop the rapidly changing field of professional counseling.

Logically speaking, professional counselors who seek out or are placed in supervisory roles should be exceptional counselors themselves. Consider Case Illustration 13-1 and whether or not Keith fulfills the minimum standards for being a counselor supervisor.

CASE ILLUSTRATION 13-1

Keith is a licensed professional counselor, has a small private practice, and is also a full-time doctoral student at a local university. Keith decided to pursue his doctorate after working as a private practice clinician for 13 years. Keith is toward the end of his doctoral program and is in the final stages of completing his dissertation. Starting to think ahead and plan for his future after he successfully defends his dissertation and completes his degree in counselor education and supervision, Keith wonders if he is properly prepared to pursue his licensed professional counselor supervisor credential through his state licensure board. Reflecting on his doctoral course work, Keith knows he has taken several courses in supervision models and has even spent a semester supervising master's-level practicum students. Additionally, Keith always attends several counseling conferences each year and always makes a point to attend a few educational sessions related to counselor supervision.

Has Keith fulfilled the ethical requirements for counselor supervisory competency?

In Case Illustration 13-1, it is impossible to tell for sure if Keith will be a competent supervisor, but he has fulfilled the minimum requirements set by the ACA Code of Ethics (2014). Keith has taken many courses related to supervisory methods and techniques; he has more than 10 years of experience counseling and routinely pursues continuing education opportunities related to supervision.

Although Keith meets the minimum expectations, it's still critical for Keith to exercise self-awareness, evaluate his own competence as a clinician, and understand his motivation for offering licensure supervision to others. For example, if Keith believes he struggles in working with certain client populations or clinical work overall, he would want to seek assistance and address his own counselor competence prior to supervising others. Similarly, if while reflecting on his motivation to offer supervision Keith were to realize he was solely motivated by the financial aspect (i.e., Keith is only doing it for the money), he would want to closely monitor himself and be sure the financial gains never compromise the quality of the supervision he provides.

ACA Standard F.2.b. (2014) Multicultural Issues and Diversity in Supervision: Counseling supervisors are aware of and address the role of multiculturalism and diversity in the supervisory relationship.

Simply stated, counselor supervisors are sensitive to diversity and multicultural issues that may come up in the supervisory relationship and address issues when they do arise.

ACA Standard F.2.c. (2014) Online Supervision: When using technology in supervision, counselor supervisors are competent in the use of those technologies. Supervisors take the necessary precautions to protect the confidentiality of all information transmitted through any electronic means.

If or when counselor supervisors use technology as part of the supervision process, supervisors are knowledgeable about the technological resources they use. Additionally, if counselor supervisors are supervising counselors and counselors-in-training who utilize technology in their counselor practice, it is the supervisor's responsibility to be competent in the technology their supervisees use. Additional information related to technology and supervision is included in Chapter 9. Related to Ethical Standard F.2.c., consider the discussion between Gary and his clinical supervisor Dr. Lyssa presented in Case Illustration 13-2.

CASE ILLUSTRATION 13-2

Gary has been under the supervision of Dr. Lyssa for almost a year and has completed approximately 600 of the 3,000 supervised hours his state requires before he is able to become fully licensed. The two meet every week for an hour-long supervision session. Originally the meetings were easy for Gary to attend, but he has recently moved to a new home that is a much longer distance from Dr. Lyssa's office. After thinking about how to shorten his commute, Gary decided to approach Dr. Lyssa about using technology (i.e., Skype) to conduct their supervisory sessions. Dr. Lyssa was a bit hesitant, primarily due to her limited technological expertise. Still, Dr. Lyssa agreed to distance supervision after Gary agreed to download everything onto her computer and "get everything set up properly."

Is Dr. Lyssa acting ethically in providing distance supervision to Gary?

In response to the question posed in Case Illustration 13-2, no; Dr. Lyssa is not acting in an ethical manner. According to ACA Ethical Standard F.2.c., Dr. Lyssa must be competent to use technologies prior to using them for supervision. Dr. Lyssa is clearly not competent and therefore would clearly be guilty of unethical practice. Additionally, Dr. Lyssa would want to consult her state's licensure board to determine whether or not the licensure board allows distance supervision as a viable method when supervising counseling interns. If Dr. Lyssa's state board does not allow distance supervision or has specific procedures for conducting such supervision, Dr. Lyssa would be held responsible and be open to disciplinary action if she does not follow the stated guidelines.

Informed Consent

Whether it's a student entering into the practicum or internship course or a newly graduated student seeking out supervision as part of the licensure process, the first step in any supervisory relationship is informed consent. Similar to the counselor/client relationship and the teacher/student relationship, supervisees have the right to know what supervisors expect. The ACA Code of Ethics (2014) discusses this process in two separate standards.

ACA Standard F.4.a. (2014) Informed Consent for Supervision: Supervisors are responsible for incorporating into their supervision the principles of informed consent and participation. Supervisors inform supervisees of the policies and procedures to which supervisors are to adhere and the mechanisms for due process appeal of individual supervisors actions. The issues unique to the use of distance supervision are to be included in the documentation as necessary.

ACA Standard F.1.c. (2014) Informed Consent and Client Rights: Supervisors make supervisees aware of client rights, including the protection of client privacy and confidentiality in the counseling relationship. Supervisees provide clients with professional disclosure information and inform them of how the supervision process influences the limits of confidentiality. Supervisees make clients aware of who will have access to records of the counseling relationship and how these records will be stored, transmitted, or otherwise reviewed.

The first of these two ethical standards speaks to supervisors' ethical responsibility to inform potential supervisees of what is expected. In Chapter 5 the authors described the "who," "what," and "when" related to the informed consent process that counselors must review with clients. What follows are the same topics related to the informed consent process between supervisor and supervisee.

Who

The "who" is the individual providing the supervision. Supervisors should provide background information to potential supervisees (i.e., Who are you? What are your qualifications? What experience do you bring to the relationship that might be helpful to supervisees?).

What

The "what" is what happens during supervision. Most students have never experienced clinical supervision prior to the practicum or internship courses, and those seeking supervision as a part of the licensure process may also be unsure as to what to expect.

The supervisor must share what is expected. What should the supervisee share? What should the supervisee expect to learn during supervision? Does the supervisee need to bring anything with him/her to supervision? In accordance with Standard F.4.b., supervisors also must make supervisees aware of procedures for contacting the supervisor in case of emergencies or crisis situations (ACA, 2014).

When

The "when" is when supervision occurs. What days and/or times will the supervisee be expected to meet for supervision? Similarly, how long will the supervision session last? Is there a cost for supervision, and if so, what is the cost?

These three areas are typically covered in an informed consent document given to the supervisee by the supervisor. See the example of a supervisory agreement form or informed consent contract presented in Case Illustration 13-3.

CASE ILLUSTRATION 13-3

Dr. Cove agrees to provide clinical supervision to George Sontera, a licensed professional counselor intern. Dr. Cove earned his PhD in counselor education and supervision and is a licensed professional counselor and board approved supervisor. Dr. Cove's experience includes working with adolescents and adults. Dr. Cove agrees to keep his license and supervisory status current and in good standing for the remainder of this supervisory relationship.

The supervisory sessions will consist of a one-hour face-to-face meeting. It is expected that both parties be in attendance and on time for all supervisory sessions. In the event that a member of this supervisory relationship is unable to attend a session, it is that person's responsibility to contact the other party with a minimum of 24-hour notice and reschedule the appointment. All of the supervisory sessions will be held at Dr. Cove's office located at 1111 Broadway, Suite 1, San Antonio, TX. Dr. Cove's fee for supervision is $75 per hour visit. Mr. Sontera is responsible for paying those fees (cash or personal check) at the conclusion of every supervisory session.

Dr. Cove believes supervision is a vital component to becoming an effective licensed professional counselor. Therefore, it is expected that the supervisee, George Sontera, will openly engage in case consultation and discussions. He will be expected to come to supervisory meetings prepared and ready to discuss theoretical orientation, diagnosis, and ethical concerns for each of his cases in addition to other counseling-related topics. Additionally, Mr. Sontera is expected to follow all ethical guidelines set forth by the ACA, all pertinent laws of the state of Texas, and adhere to the policies and procedures of his clinical training site.

It is the supervisor's (Dr. Cove's) responsibility to model appropriate and ethical behavior and to monitor, provide feedback, and evaluate the supervisee (George Sontera). Dr. Cove will provide verbal feedback during the course of each supervisory meeting and will provide written feedback at the midpoint and conclusion of the supervisory relationship.

By signing below, both parties agree to the conditions and expectations outlined here.

_____ Date: _____
Dr. Cove, PhD, LPC

_____ Date: _____
George Sontera

The consent form provided in Case Illustration 13-3 illustrates one example and may vary depending on the supervisor's preferences and the state in which he/she practices. Overall the informed consent process between supervisor and supervisee should be an ongoing conversation and can be adapted and edited when agreed upon by both parties. Supervisees must also engage in an informed consent process with clients. While it is the supervisees responsibility to review information with clients (i.e., how the supervision process affects limits of confidentiality), the ACA Code of Ethics (2014) is clear in stating that it is the supervisor's responsibility to "make supervisees aware of client rights, including the protection of client privacy and confidentiality in the counseling relationship" (ACA, 2014, p. 13), meaning that supervisors must be sure to educate their supervisees on how to best protect their clients' confidentiality. Consider the supervisor/supervisee interaction depicted in Case Illustration 13-4 and subsequent interaction between supervised counselor and client.

CASE ILLUSTRATION 13-4

Example 1

Supervisor: During our supervision session today, I would like for us to talk about the informed consent process you are required to cover at the beginning of the initial session with every client.

Supervisee: What information do I need to include?

Supervisor: At the beginning of your first visit with every client (initial session) you must go through an informed consent process. During the process, you must include information about client privacy and confidentiality and how confidentiality and privacy are affected by our supervisory relationship. Please be sure to let all your clients know you are being supervised and you will be sharing session notes and

(Continued)

(Continued)

other information with me as a part of supervision. Also, please include my contact information on your consent form in case any clients would like to contact me with complaints or grievances.

Example 2

Counselor: Hello, welcome to counseling today. How are you doing?

Client: I'm doing alright, thank you.

Counselor: Before we get started, I wanted to go over a few forms and make sure I answer any and all of your questions about counseling. The first form I have is about informed consent. It lets you know what to expect during our sessions. The form includes information about my professional background and beliefs about the counseling process. It also lets you know that sessions are one hour in length and all the services are free of charge. The next section concerns confidentiality and limits of confidentiality. As you may know from your past counseling experiences, everything we talk about during session is confidential but with a few exceptions (i.e., if you let me know you are going to hurt yourself or someone else or if I suspect child abuse or abuse of a vulnerable adult). As I mentioned over the phone when we first scheduled this appointment, I am a licensed professional counselor intern. One of the requirements of my licensure board is that all interns receive supervision from a board-approved counselor supervisor. My supervisor's name is Dr. Bailey Cove. I meet with him on a weekly basis, and he provides me with feedback and suggestions on how to improve my clinical practice. On occasion, I may share some of the information we discuss in session with Dr. Cove. The information I share with him during our supervision sessions is kept confidential by both Dr. Cove and myself. You can see on the consent form that I have included Dr. Cove's contact information in the event you would like to contact him. Do you have any questions about what I have covered?

In Case Illustration 13-4, two examples are given related to the informed consent process involving counselor supervisors, counselors, and clients. In Example 1 of case illustration 13-4 the reader is able to see an example of how a supervisor may discuss informed consent with a supervisee as required by Standard F.1.c. (ACA, 2014). In addition to discussing the informed consent process, supervisors may also want to role-play with supervisees. Role-playing informed consent practices with supervisees may help in calming nerves prior to meeting with actual clients. In Example 2 the counselor intern follows through on the expectations of his supervisor and shares pertinent supervisory information with clients.

Responsibilities of Supervisors

In addition to the informed consent process and ensuring supervisees review informed consent and limits of confidentiality with clients, supervisors take on many other responsibilities upon entering a supervisory relationship. In short, supervisors may be held accountable for all of their supervisees' actions. The ACA Code of Ethics (2014) again identifies minimal standards for counselor supervisors in assuring supervisees act in a professional manner while also encouraging supervisees to adhere to certain standards. Text Box 13-1 provides information from the AAMFT about these issues.

ACA Standard F.4.c. (2014) Standards for Supervisees: Supervisors make their supervisees aware of professional and ethical standards and legal responsibilities.

ACA Standard F.5.a. (2014) Ethical Responsibilities: Students and supervisees have a responsibility to understand and follow the ACA Code of Ethics. Students and supervisees have the same obligation to clients as those required of professional counselors.

These two standards oblige counselor supervisors to do three things. Supervisors must first inform supervisees about the existence of ethical standards and legal obligations. Second, supervisors are responsible for making sure supervisees fully understand legal and ethical obligations. ACA Ethical Standard F.5.a. specifically states students and supervisees are to be held to the same obligations as fully licensed counselors (i.e., ignorance is no excuse). Third, supervisors are responsible for ensuring supervisees follow ethical and legal expectations.

ACA Standard F.5.b. (2014) Impairment: Students and supervisees monitor themselves for signs of impairment from their own physical, mental, or emotional problems and refrain from offering or providing professional services when such impairment is likely to harm a client or others. They notify their faculty and/or supervisors and seek assistance for problems that reach the level of professional impairment, and if necessary, they limit, suspend, or terminate their professional responsibilities until it is determined that they may safely resume their work.

According to Standard F.5.b. students and supervisees monitor themselves for signs of impairment and notify faculty or other supervisors if they believe the impairment will negatively impact their ability to work with clients. Counselors are also responsible for monitoring supervisees and students. Additionally, supervisors must also monitor supervisees and be alert for signs of impairment.

ACA Standard F.5.c. (2014) Professional Disclosure: Before providing counseling services, students and supervisees disclose their status as supervisees and explain how this status affects the limits of confidentiality. Supervisors ensure that clients are aware of the services rendered and the qualifications of the students or supervisees rendering those services. Students and supervisees obtain client permission before they use any information concerning the counseling relationship in the training process.

TEXT BOX 13-1

American Association for Marriage and Family Therapists

AAMFT Standard 4.4 (2015) Oversight of Supervisee Competence: Marriage and family thera-pists do not permit students or supervisees to perform or to hold themselves out as competent to perform professional services beyond their training, level of experience, and competence.

AAMFT Standard 4.5 (2015) Oversight of Supervisee Professionalism: Marriage and family therapists take reasonable measures to ensure that services provided by supervisees are professional.

Similar to the interaction in Example 2 of Case Illustration 13-4, supervisees inform clients of their supervisory status and how supervision affects limits of confidentiality. Understanding these standards, please consider Case Illustration 13-5 and how Bill interacts with his supervisees.

CASE ILLUSTRATION 13-5

Bill is a licensed professional counselor and has been working at a state-funded counseling agency for almost nine years. Due to his tenure at the agency, work ethic, and rapport with other staff members, he has recently been promoted to clinical coordinator. Along with a significant pay raise, Bill's new responsibilities include supervising the clinical work of the other three licensed professional counselors on staff. Additionally, the agency works closely with a local university and typically has two or three student counselors completing their hours. Bill's new job description includes supervising those interns as well.

In addition to his work responsibilities, Bill is a single father of two and feels strongly about being an active and involved parent. As a result, he often finds himself neglecting specifics of his work responsibilities, so he is able to spend more time with his children. Bill does his best to balance his work responsibilities with his family life. When work and home life conflict, Bill always leans more toward spending time with his family. He lives by the motto "Work so you can live rather than live so you can work."

Each semester when new interns start at the agency, Bill begins his first supervisory session by handing out a copy of the ACA Code of Ethics to each supervisee and telling them to "read it, know it, and use it." Additionally, he tells all supervisees to "take care of yourself, so you don't get burned out. If you think you are starting to get burned out, make sure you let me know." Finally, as Bill reviews confidentiality, he reminds his supervisees, "Don't forget to tell your clients that you are a student counselor and you are being supervised by me. They need to know that I will be talking with you about information they share during sessions."

> *In this scenario, Bill is an extremely busy person with multiple responsibilities both at work and home. If Bill only provides this information to his supervisees at the beginning of the supervisory relationship and no other times, is he being ethical in terms of fulfilling the requirements of ACA Ethical Code Standards F.4.c., F.5.a., F.5.b., and/or F.5.c.?*

In Case Illustration 13-5, Bill must work efficiently to manage his multiple responsibilities. As such, he is short and concise when covering ethical obligations with his new supervisees. The question in Case Illustration 13-5 asks if Bill is acting ethically when he is this short and concise. Arguments may be made for both the positive and negative. Arguments supporting Bill's behaviors as ethical and sufficient are that he followed the letter of the code of ethics as it is written. Bill provided information to his supervisees to make them aware of ethical responsibilities; he encouraged them to monitor themselves for signs of impairment and directed them to disclose their status as student counselors to clients. On the contrary, arguments supporting Bill's actions as unethical are that he did the bare minimum in providing adequate supervision. Bill provided his supervisees with information but did not follow the spirit of the code of ethics.

Corey, Corey, and Callanan (2011) identify supervisors as responsible for monitoring supervisee's "ongoing personal and professional development" (p. 371). Therefore, it is the authors' belief even though Bill followed the basic words written into the ACA Code of Ethics (2014), Bill did not follow the spirit of the code. Bill used minimal standards rather than striving toward aspirational ethics. Although Bill has many responsibilities and seems to be trying to maximize the time he is able to spend with his children, he is still in the position of a counselor supervisor and must perform appropriately. To adhere to the ethical standards highlighted in this scenario, Bill would want to follow up at various times with his supervisees throughout the semester. He would want to ensure his supervisees are acting ethically by discussing supervision and how it affects confidentiality with clients. Furthermore, supervisees should engage in their own process to continuously monitor their own risk of impairment.

Concomitant to the previous discussion, one of the most vital roles of a counselor supervisor is that of gatekeeper (Hutchens, Block, & Young, 2013). In general, gatekeepers are responsible for controlling access. Counselor supervisors who act as gatekeepers to the counseling profession control supervisee's access to becoming a professional counselor. Simply stated, counselor supervisors, along with state licensure boards and counselor education programs, are responsible for determining who meets the threshold for becoming a professional counselor. The ACA Code of Ethics (2014) Standards F.6.a. and F.6.b. provide guidance to counselor supervisors specific to gatekeeping.

> Supervisors document and provide supervisees with ongoing feedback regarding their performance and schedule periodic formal evaluative sessions throughout the supervisory relationship. (ACA, 2014, p. 13)

Through initial and ongoing evaluation, supervisors are aware of supervisee limitations that might impede performance. Supervisors assist supervisees in securing remedial assistance when needed. They recommend dismissal from training programs, applied counseling settings, and state or voluntary professional credentialing processes when those supervisees are unable to demonstrate that they can provide competent professional services to a range of diverse clients. Supervisors seek consultation and document their decisions to dismiss or refer supervisees for assistance. They ensure that supervisees are aware of options available to them to address such decision. (ACA, 2014, p.13)

Understanding these standards, please consider Case illustration 13-6 and how Carol interacts with her supervisees.

CASE ILLUSTRATION 13-6

Carol is a licensed professional counselor and an approved supervisor in her state. She routinely supervises licensed professional counselor interns in addition to her small private practice. Carol has been supervising Freeman for almost three years, and Freeman is near completion of the state-required 3,000 supervised counseling hours he must acquire prior to receiving a license to practice independently. Over the course of the supervision, Carol has had some concerns about Freeman's counseling skills and his ability to integrate theory into his practice. Carol has documented all of her concerns in her "supervision notes" but has never shared her full concerns with Freeman. She doesn't want to come across as negative or judgmental. She remains hopeful the general discussions they have about theory during supervision sessions will get him to start using theory.

Several weeks later when Freeman completes his 3,000 hours, he brings a copy of his licensure endorsement form to supervision for Carol to sign. Carol shares with him that although he has finished the 3,000 hours, she does not feel comfortable signing his endorsement form and presents him with documentation related to her concerns. She then tells Freeman she had hoped he would "get it" on his own and through the weekly supervision sessions. Carol also shares her belief that Freeman has not quite raised his skills to an acceptable level. She indicates she would like to continue to meet with him for an additional three months before she would feel comfortable signing his form. The three months will give them a chance to really concentrate on integrating theory into his practice

Is Carol acting ethically in regard to Standards F.6.a. and F.6.b.?

What might Carol have done differently to align her supervision more with Standards F.6.a. and F.6.b.?

The first question in Case Illustration 13-6 inquires about the ethicality of Carol's actions. Carol would most likely be seen as acting in an unethical manner. She did document her concerns and offer to assist Freeman in remediating (i.e., request Freeman meet with her for an additional three months to improve on integrating theory into his practice), but she left out the critical component of passing along her concerns to Freeman on an ongoing basis. Even though the scenario points out that Carol engaged Freeman in "general discussions" about theory, it seems as though he did not fully understand her concerns. It is the supervisor's responsibility to be clear in providing feedback about concerns and expectations.

The second question asks how Carol might have acted differently to align her supervision more with ethical standards. Carol should have shared her concerns with Freeman and let him know of her expectations rather than waiting to share it with him upon the completion of his hours. In providing Freeman with ongoing feedback, Carol would have given Freeman the chance to adjust his behaviors earlier. Clear and honest communication is a must between supervisors and supervisees. As a counselor supervisor, Carol is ethically required to avoid endorsement of supervisees who "are unable to demonstrate that they can provide competent professional services" (ACA, 2014, p. 13). Still, the term "competent" is open to interpretation, and various supervisors may interpret it differently. It is the supervisor's (i.e., Carol's) responsibility to communicate with her supervisee her interpretation of "competent services."

Relationships Between Supervisors and Supervisees

Power differentials exist between supervisors and supervisees, and it is the supervisor's duty to be aware of such differentials and ensure the supervisor/supervisee professional relationship is not compromised by nonprofessional relationships (Gu, Veach, Eubanks, LeRoy, & Callanan, 2010). The authors believe most student counselors, counselor interns, and counselor supervisors would agree any sexual or romantic relationship between a supervisor and supervisee would be inappropriate. Still, similar to addressing sexual and romantic relationships with current clients, the ACA Code of Ethics specifically addresses relationships between supervisors and supervisees. See Text Box 13-2 for where to find information on APA and AAMFT standards related to this area.

ACA Standard F.3.b. (2014) Sexual Relationships: Sexual or romantic interactions or relationships with current supervisees are prohibited. This prohibition applies to both in-person and electronic interactions or relationships.

TEXT BOX 13-2

American Psychological Association

See Chapter 12 (Text Box 12-4) and Standard 7.07 (Sexual Relationships With Students and Supervisees).

American Association for Marriage and Family Therapists

See Chapter 12 (Text Box 12-4) and Standard 4.3 (Sexual Intimacy With Students or Supervisees).

As stated previously, supervisors possess inherent power over supervisees; therefore, sexual or romantic relationships are to be absolutely avoided. Similar to counselor/client relationships and counselor educator/student relationships, supervisors are held accountable for modeling appropriate boundaries and assuring exploitation of power does not take place (Žorga, 2002). Concomitantly, counselor supervisors "do not condone or subject supervisees to sexual harassment" (ACA, 2014, p. 13).

Similar to the prohibition of sexual or intimate relationships with supervisees, the ACA Code of Ethics (2014) directs counselor supervisors to avoid entering into supervisory relationships with those whom they are unable to stay objective.

ACA Standard F.3.d. (2014) Friends or Family Members: Supervisors are prohibited from engaging in supervisory relationships with individuals with whom they have an inability to remain objective.

Although the standard is titled "Friends or Family Members," the critical component of this standard is those "with whom they have an inability to remain objective." The burden is on the counselor supervisor to engage in an ethical decision-making process and determine whether he/she is able to objectively supervise. Consider Case Illustration 13-7 in which Dr. M is asked to provide licensure supervision to a neighborhood friend.

CASE ILLUSTRATION 13-7

Dr. M is a full-time counselor educator and has a small private practice where he visits with clients on weekends. Additionally, he is a board-approved counselor supervisor in his state. Maggie, an acquaintance of Dr. M (i.e., families live in the same neighborhood, and their children play together frequently), finished her degree in clinical mental health four years ago but decided not to pursue licensure after graduation due to other interests. Recently, Maggie has become more interested in pursuing licensure and has been talking to Dr. M at various neighborhood gatherings about the process. Although Dr. M knows very little about Maggie personally, he sees her as a genuine, nice person who cares about others and would most likely be a very effective counselor. Because Maggie is aware of Dr. M's status as a counselor supervisor and is unfamiliar with any other board-approved supervisors in the area, she asks him if he would be willing to supervise her.

Maggie is neither a family member nor a friend (he considers her more of an acquaintance). Therefore, would it be ethical for Dr. M to supervise Maggie?

The situation presented in Case Illustration 13-7 involves Maggie and Dr. M. Maggie asks Dr. M if he would be willing to supervise her while she completes the necessary supervised experience hours needed to become fully licensed. Counselor supervisors are able to choose who they supervise. The authors recommend supervisors and supervisees approach the supervisory relationship much like a job interview. Supervisees are able to interview potential supervisors as a way to make sure the supervisor's experience, personality, and expectations are a good match. Likewise, supervisors are able to interview supervisees and determine whether or not to enter into a supervisory relationship. In the scenario presented in Case illustration 13-7, and many others, the authors stress answering "would it be ethical for Dr. M to supervise Maggie" rather than "should Dr. M supervise Maggie." In Case Illustration 13-7, Dr. M has a choice whether or not he wants to supervise Maggie. If Dr. M is busy with other obligations or does not want to supervise her for any other reason, he is legally and ethically able to deny her request to enter into a supervisory relationship. The question of ethicality applies if or when Dr. M wants to supervise Maggie. If Dr. M doesn't want to supervise Maggie, he can simply say no. However, if he is leaning toward saying yes, then he must engage in an ethical decision-making process to determine the ethicality of entering into this potential supervisory relationship. What follows is an example of an ethical decision-making model Dr. M might use.

Identify the Problem

The problem or dilemma presented in Case Illustration 13-7 is that Dr. M has been asked to supervise Maggie, who is an acquaintance of his and the mother of one his child's friends. He is leaning toward saying yes but first wants to determine whether it would be ethical for him to do so.

Review Relevant Ethical Codes and Laws

There are no relevant laws potentially affecting Dr. M's decision. The relevant ethical code is Standard F.3.d.: "Supervisors are prohibited from engaging in supervisory relationships with individuals with whom they have an inability to remain objective (ACA, 2014, p. 13).

Understand Your Own Morals, Values and Beliefs and How They Might Influence Your Interpretation of the Code of Ethics and Laws

In this situation, it would be important for Dr. M to understand why he is leaning toward saying yes to supervision. What is his motivation? If he says yes, is he interpreting the standard too liberally? If he says no, is he being too strict?

Identify Possible Courses of Action

Dr. M can say yes and supervise Maggie.

Dr. M can say no and offer Maggie some other options for supervision.

Identify Benefits and
Consequences of Possible Courses of Action

If Dr. M says yes, things may go well, and Maggie may earn her license with no complications. If he says yes, the two may encounter some difficulties if Maggie does not agree with Dr. M's feedback or supervision practices. If conflict does arise, it might negatively affect the relationship Dr. M's family has with Maggie's family.

If Dr. M says no, things may go well, and Maggie may be happy finding another supervisor. If he says no, it could also impact their relationship as acquaintances and impact future interactions between the two.

Consult With Others

Dr. M should consult with a few colleagues, asking them about their thoughts and feelings about the ethicality of his situation. Dr. M might also want to consult with his state licensure board and consider any advice offered.

Decide on a Course of Action and Implement

In this situation it would most likely be considered ethical if Dr. M decided to supervise Maggie's licensure process as he is able to stay objective in providing feedback. However, prior to beginning supervision, Dr. M would need to review his supervision contract with Maggie (as discussed earlier in this chapter). Additionally, Dr. M must discuss any potential risks and benefits their particular supervisory relationship may pose (see Standard F.3.a., which follows).

In previous editions of the ACA Code of Ethics terms such as "dual relationships" and "potentially beneficial interactions" were used. In the most recent edition (2014), the term "extending conventional supervisory relationships" was chosen to describe the process in which a counselor must participate prior to initiating a nonprofessional relationship with a supervisee.

ACA Standard F.3.a. (2014) Extending Conventional Supervisory Relationships: Counseling supervisors clearly define and maintain ethical professional, personal, and social relationships with their supervisees. Supervisors consider the risks and benefits of extending current supervisory relationships in any form beyond conventional parameters. In extending these boundaries, supervisors take appropriate professional precautions to ensure that judgment is not impaired and that no harm occurs.

Applying Case Illustration 13-7 (Dr. M and Maggie) to this standard, Dr. M has several obligations prior to initiating a supervisory relationship with Maggie. First, Dr. M must clearly define the roles of each person in the relationship. Second, Dr. M must discuss potential benefits and risks that might arise. Dr. M and Maggie will be involved in multiple relationships (children are friends, they are acquaintances, and they have a potential supervisory relationship), and it is Dr. M's responsibility to initiate conversation about possible conflicts before they occur. Review the conversation between Dr. M and

Maggie in Case Illustration 13-8 as an example of how Dr. M might address the issues previously discussed.

CASE ILLUSTRATION 13-8

Maggie, I would be happy to supervise your licensure process, but before we get started, I want to make sure we are both on the same page about our roles and responsibilities. I think it's important that we talk about this first, so there is no miscommunication. I believe it is important during our supervision sessions that we talk only about supervision and counseling-related concerns. Likewise, I feel it is important that we talk only about supervision and counseling-related concerns during supervision and avoid discussing those topics during neighborhood activities or other gatherings.

Maggie, I also want to talk about some other potential difficult situations. Acting as your supervisor requires me to give you feedback related to your counseling skills. At times, feedback may be positive, and at other times it may be very critical. As a supervisor, one of my responsibilities is to mentor you, provide you feedback (both positive and negative), and also act as a gatekeeper to the profession. If you ever have questions or disagree with the feedback I have, I hope you will feel comfortable sharing your concerns with me during supervision. I don't want our supervisory relationship to negatively affect any other relationships we have (community or family relationships).

In Case Illustration 13-8, Dr. M initiates a conversation with Maggie to prevent any potential consequences. By setting firm boundaries and expectations at the beginning of the relationship, Dr. M is able to vanquish potential conflicts. In addition to sharing his concerns with Maggie, Dr. M would also want to engage Maggie in a discussion about any concerns she may have. Finally, upon entering into a formal supervisory relationship with Maggie, Dr. M would want to be sure to review his informed consent form at the onset.

Although supervisors have inherent power over their supervisees, either member is able to terminate the supervisory relationship as long as they give appropriate notice to the other member. The ACA Code of Ethics includes guidance related to termination of supervisory relationships in Standard F.4.d.

ACA Standard F.4.d. (2014) Termination of the Supervisory Relationship: Supervisors or supervisees have the right to terminate the supervisory relationship with adequate notice. Reasons for considering termination are discussed, and both parties work to resolve differences. When termination is warranted, supervisors make appropriate referrals to possible alternative supervisors.

Termination can occur in either positive or negative situations. In either case, ethical guidelines require that supervisors and supervisees discuss the termination and work to resolve differences as a part of terminating the relationship. Consider the scenario presented in Case Illustration 13-9 and how Sebastian terminates his supervisory relationship with Camilla.

CASE ILLUSTRATION 13-9

Camilla is a licensed professional counselor intern and has worked over the past eight months as an intern at a local nonprofit agency. The internship was a great find, and Camilla feels lucky to have found a place so close to her home where she can earn her licensure hours and receive free supervision. The relatively small nonprofit has only a few full-time employees and depends heavily on the volunteer work counselor interns provide. Millie, the agency's clinical director is the only board-approved supervisor working there, and she typically provides supervision to all the interns. Camilla and Millie have similar interests, and the two seem to have built a strong working relationship. Camilla appreciates Millie's style of providing detailed feedback.

Over the past two months, Camilla has started to notice concerning behaviors from her clinical supervisor. During Camilla's supervision sessions, Millie sometimes dozes off or loses her train of thought and has become very fidgety. After discussing the behaviors with other interns at the agency, Camilla realizes she is not the only one concerned about the behaviors. Camilla and other interns have become increasingly concerned about not only the quality of the supervision they are receiving but also the quality of services Millie is providing to her own clients. Understanding her ethical obligation to discuss concerns with her supervisor, Camilla broaches the subject with Millie at her next supervisory session. Upon hearing Camilla's concerns Millie becomes defensive and denies any wrongdoing on her part.

After careful consideration, Camilla decides to seek licensure supervision from another supervisor. Although her current site is close to her home and offers free supervision, Camilla now lacks trust in her supervisor and wants to move on. Camilla schedules a time to meet with Millie to notify her about terminating the relationship. During the meeting Millie is again defensive about the situation and refuses to sign any of Camilla's documentation time logs. Furthermore, Millie asks Camilla to leave the premises immediately and is told the police will be called if she refuses.

Did Camilla act in an ethical manner?

Did Millie act in an ethical manner?

Ethically speaking, how should Camilla move forward with this situation?

The first question in Case Illustration 13-9 asks if Camilla, the supervisee, acted in an ethical manner. Yes, Camilla acted appropriately in all of her interactions with Millie. Camilla believed her clinical supervisor was violating an ethical standard (i.e., Camilla thought Millie was impaired and thus violating Ethical Standard C.2.g. [Impairment]). As a result, Camilla then tried to address the issue with Millie in accordance with Standard I.2.a. (Informal Resolution).

ACA Standard I.2.a. (2014) Informal Resolution: When counselors have reason to believe that another counselor is violating or has violated an ethical standard and substantial harm has not occurred, they attempt to first resolve the issue informally with the other counselor if feasible, provided such action does not violate confidentiality rights that may be involved.

The second question asks whether or not Millie acted appropriately in her response to Camilla's concerns. No, Millie did not act appropriately according to a few ethical standards. First, Millie did not model appropriate professional behavior and did not respect Camilla's right to terminate the supervisory relationship as stated in Ethical Standard F.4.d. Second, after Camilla expressed her concerns, Millie became defensive and asked her to leave the premises. In doing so, she was penalizing Camilla for exposing an "inappropriate employer policy" as described in Standard D.1.i. (Protection From Punitive Action).

ACA Standard D.1.i. (2014) Protection From Punitive Action: Counselors do not harass a colleague or employee or dismiss an employee who has acted in a responsible and ethical manner to expose inappropriate employer policies or practices.

Finally, the third question inquires as to how Camilla might move forward with this situation. Camilla has accrued many hours over the first several months of her internship and would certainly want to know how to account for those hours because Millie refused to sign her time logs. Additionally, Camilla would want to follow through on any and all ethical responsibilities she might have of further reporting Millie's behaviors. Camilla would first want to consult with a past mentor or faculty member or call her state licensure board as directed by Ethical Standard I.2.c. (Consultation).

ACA Standard I.2.c. (2014) Consultation: When uncertain about whether a particular situation or course of action may be in violation of the ACA Code of Ethics, counselors consult with other counselors who are knowledgeable about ethics and the ACA Code of Ethics, with colleagues, or with appropriate authorities, such as the ACA Ethics and Professional Standards Department.

After consulting, Camilla would likely be able to determine how to go about finding another licensure supervisor and how to receive credit for the hours she already accrued. Camilla may also be encouraged to report Millie's ethical violations as directed by Ethical Standard I.2.b. (Reporting Ethical Violations).

ACA Standard I.2.b. (2014) Reporting Ethical Violations: If an apparent violation has substantially harmed or is likely to substantially harm a person or organization and is not appropriate for informal resolution or is not resolved properly, counselors take further action depending on the situation. Such action may include referral to state or national committees on professional ethics, voluntary national certification bodies, state licensing boards, or appropriate institutional authorities. The confidentiality rights of clients should be considered in all actions. This standard does not apply when counselors have been retained to review the work of another counselor whose professional conduct is in question (e.g., consultation or expert testimony).

Conclusion

Counselor supervisors are gatekeepers to the profession. They educate, mentor, and train future professional counselors. As such, they have immense power over their supervisees. Because supervisors may be held accountable for their supervisee's actions, they must monitor the actions of supervisees as well as their own. ACA ethical guidelines offer assistance to counselor supervisors by denoting the types of information to be included in informed consent between supervisors and supervisees, how to maintain appropriate professional boundaries with supervisees, and the types of feedback supervisors should provide throughout the supervisory relationship. Use the information learned in Chapter 13 to respond to the ethical dilemma and corresponding discussion questions presented in Case Exercise 13-1.

CASE EXERCISE 13-1

Dr. Byron teaches in the department of counseling at a local university. He has been teaching for approximately 15 years at the university and typically teaches clinical courses (practicum and internship). As part of his class, he always discusses the licensure process and educates his students about the steps needed to gain licensure. In his discussions, he always shares that he is one of many state-approved supervisors in the area and is open to supervising students during their licensure process (after they graduate of course). He explains his views of supervision and even passes out copies of his own supervision contract when discussing the topic during his class. At the end of his course, he always invites students to contact him if they would be interested in having him supervise their licensure process.

As a result, Dr. Byron typically has two to three of his previous students contact him each year inquiring about his supervision. Because they were previous students, he does not feel the need to go over a supervision contract with them again (they already know his style and expectations). Instead he briefly describes expectations and then discusses his pricing for supervision. He says his "individual supervision" rate is $75 an hour. However, the "group rate" is only $100 an hour. If supervisees are able to find another person to "join them as a supervisee of Dr. Boyd," then the two can split the cost, meaning each would only pay $50 a week instead of $75.

Do you believe Dr. Boyd's supervision practices are ethical? Why, or why not?

If you believe they are unethical, what might he be able to do to more align his practices with the ACA Code of Ethics?

How might ACA Ethical Standard C.3.d. (Recruiting Through Employment) apply to this situation?

If you believe Dr. Boyd's practices are unethical, what are your obligations in reporting his behaviors?

Keystones

- Counselor supervision takes place in many contexts.
- Lack of appropriate supervision is one of the most common issues brought before licensure boards.
- Counselor supervisors must have knowledge of supervision techniques and case conceptualization, continually pursue continuing education, and be skilled counselors themselves.
- Counselor supervisors must discuss diversity and multicultural issues with supervisees.
- When using technology-assisted supervision, supervisors must be competent in understanding and using the technologies prior to implementing them into supervision.
- Supervisors must provide supervisees with informed consent, including information about supervisor expectations.
- Supervisors make supervisees aware of client rights and how supervision may affect limits of confidentiality.
- Supervisors educate supervisees about ethical expectations.
- Supervisors and supervisees monitor their effectiveness and watch for signs of impairment.
- Supervisees are honest in disclosing their supervisee status to clients prior to entering into a counseling relationship.
- Supervisors provide ongoing feedback to supervisees and assist supervisees in locating remedial assistance when necessary.
- Sexual and romantic interactions between supervisors and supervisees is prohibited.
- Counselor supervisors avoid entering into a supervisory relationship with friends, family members, or anyone with whom they are unable to remain objective.
- Counselor supervisors consider the risks and benefits and document their decision-making process prior to extending conventional supervisory boundaries.
- Both supervisors and supervisees may terminate the supervisory relationship with proper notice.

Additional Resources

Cruikshanks, D. R. (2000). An investigation of factors affecting sexual boundary violations in counseling supervision (Order No. AAI9973330). *Dissertation Abstracts International Section A: Humanities and Social Sciences*, 1750. Retrieved from http://search.proquest.com/docview/619561851?accountid=7122

Deaver, S. P., & Shiflett, C. (2011). Art-based supervision techniques. *The Clinical Supervisor, 30*(2), 257–276. doi:http://dx.doi.org/10.1080/07325223.2011.619456

Mastoras, S. M., & Andrews, J. J. W. (2011). The supervisee experience of group supervision: Implications for research and practice. *Training and Education in Professional Psychology, 5*(2), 102–111. doi:http://dx.doi.org/10.1037/a0023567

Tsong, Y., & Goodyear, R. K. (2014). Assessing supervision's clinical and multicultural impacts: The supervision outcome scale's psychometric properties. *Training and Education in Professional Psychology, 8*(3), doi:http://dx.doi.org/10.1037/tep0000049

References

American Association for Marriage and Family Therapy. (2015). Code of ethics. Retrieved from https://www.aamft.org/iMIS15/AAMFT/Content/legal_ethics/code_of_ethics.aspx

American Counseling Association. (2014). *Code of ethics.* Alexandria, VA: Author.

Cikanek, K., Veach, P., & Braun, C. (2004). Advanced doctoral students' knowledge and understanding of clinical supervisor ethical responsibilities. *The Clinical Supervisor, 23*(1), 191–196.

Corey, G., Corey, M. S., & Callanan, P. (2011). *Issues and ethics in the helping professions* (8th ed.). Belmont, CA: Brooks/Cole, Cengage Learning.

Ford, G. G. (2006). *Ethical reasoning for mental health professionals.* Thousand Oaks, CA: Sage.

Gu, L., Veach, P., Eubanks, S., LeRoy, B., & Callanan, N. (2010). Boundary issues and multiple relationships in genetic counseling supervision: Supervisor, non-supervisor, and student perspectives. *Journal of Genetic Counseling, 20*(1), 35–48.

Hutchens, N., Block, J., & Young, M. (2013). Counselor educators' gatekeeping responsibilities and students' first amendment rights. *Counselor Ed & Supervision, 52*, 82–95. doi:10.1002/j.1556-6978.2013.00030.x

Trepal, H. C., & Hammer, T. R. (2014). Critical incidents in supervision training: Doctoral students' perspectives. *Journal of Professional Counseling, Practice, Theory, & Research, 41*(1), 29–41. Retrieved from http://search.proquest.com/docview/1534305288?accountid=7122

Žorga, S. (2002). Professional supervision as a mean of learning and development of counselors. *International Journal for the Advancement of Counselling, 24*, 261–274.

14

Ethics in Research and Publications

Do research. Feed your talent. Research not only wins the war on cliché, it's the key to victory over fear and its cousin, depression.

—Robert McKee

hapter 14 concerning ethics in research and publication was left to the end because it serves to educate students on an area of the ACA Code of Ethics in which they may not have much experience (i.e., master's-level counseling students may likely have little or no experience in conducting research and/or writing manuscripts for publication). In Chapter 14 the authors discuss ethical obligations related to research and publication. Readers will gain a greater understanding of research processes and, as a result, be ethically prepared for engaging in their own research or working with others as a research assistant. Readers will also be provided information about publication and the ethics involved in writing and publishing materials. Specifically, after reading Chapter 14, readers will be able to accomplish the following:

1. Discuss the importance of conducting research in adherence to ethical standards and state and federal laws.

2. Explain the purpose and function of Institutional Review Boards (IRBs).

3. Name counselor responsibilities in protecting participants' welfare throughout the research process.

4. Explain ethical obligations of principle investigators.

5. Explain information to be included in informed consent between researcher and participants.

6. Define ethical standards pertaining to researcher and participant relationships.

7. Explain the importance of being truthful and honest when reporting research findings.

8. Discuss plagiarism and ethical standards prohibiting plagiarism.

9. Explain the importance of authorship when writing manuscripts and acknowledging manuscript contributors.

10. Explain the manuscript submission process and ethics pertaining to submitting manuscripts for publication.

Researcher Responsibilities

Prior to engaging in any type of research, one must first understand the responsibilities accompanying the title of "researcher." To aid professional counselors and counselors in training in conducting ethical research, the ACA Code of Ethics (2014) has six standards addressing the responsibilities of researchers. For related APA and AMMFT standards, see Text Box 14-1. In the six standards, readers will notice most are fairly straightforward (i.e., dos and don'ts); however, there is still some opportunity for interpretation by counselors.

ACA Standard G.1.a. (2014) Conducting Research: Counselors plan, design, conduct, and report research in a manner that is consistent with pertinent ethical principles, federal and state laws, host institutional regulations, and scientific standards governing research.

TEXT BOX 14-1

American Psychological Association

APA Standard 8.01 (2010) Institutional Approval: When institutional approval is required, psychologists provide accurate information about their research proposals and obtain approval prior to conducting the research. They conduct the research in accordance with the approved research protocol.

American Association for Marriage and Family Therapists

AAMFT Standard 5.1 (2015) Institutional Approval: When institutional approval is required, marriage and family therapists submit accurate information about their research proposals and obtain appropriate approval prior to conducting the research.

When conducting research, professional counselors, counselor educators, and counselors in training must all follow state and federal laws. Additionally, they must follow all agency, organization, and/or company policies. Consider Case Illustration 14-1 as an example of how Standard G.1.a. might apply to an actual situation.

CASE ILLUSTRATION 14-1

Dr. John is a counselor educator who works at an institution of higher education. The university in which Dr. John teaches recently implemented a new policy prohibiting faculty from conducting research using university students as participants. When the policy was first announced, Dr. John was in the process of designing a qualitative research study in which he was planning on interviewing graduate students about disordered eating habits and body image concerns. Dr. John received approval from the university's IRB at the end of the spring semester in hopes of starting his interviews during the following fall semester. One week prior to the first scheduled interview, Dr. John (as well as every other faculty member at the university) received an e-mail reviewing new university policies. Among the new policies was a prohibition on using students as participants in research. Knowing he had already contacted and set up interview appointments with all participants and he had already received approval from his university IRB, John decided to continue with his research. Dr. John rationalized his decision to ignore the new policy by believing the new policy only affected future research projects and not current ones.

Did Dr. John act ethically by carrying on with his research?

In response to the question in Case Illustration 14-1, no; Dr. John did not act in an ethical manner. If he were uncertain about the meaning of the policy and whether it affected current or only future projects, he should have verified the meaning of the policy before simply carrying on.

Similar to the expectation that information will be kept confidential in a counseling session, research participants should be able to expect the same rights to confidentiality. Ethical Standard G.1.b. specifically addresses this issue.

ACA Standard G.1.b. (2014) Confidentiality in Research: Counselors are responsible for understanding and adhering to state, federal, agency, or institutional policies or applicable guidelines regarding confidentiality in their research.

It is also the researcher's responsibility to understand policies and procedures related to confidentiality prior to beginning his/her research protocol. State laws vary by state and organizations and agencies are able to create their own operational procedures (within state and federal regulations). Researchers are encouraged to be knowledgeable of such laws and policies. Ignorance is not a viable defense for inappropriate breach of confidentiality.

Institutional Review Boards

IRBs were first developed in the late 1970s and early 1980s and came out of *The Belmont Report*. *The Belmont Report* was focused on protecting human rights in research and the ethical principles of beneficence and justice. Any institution receiving federal funding is required to have an IRB, which is tasked with reviewing research proposals and ensuring the rights of human subjects in research (Ford, 2006). Simply stated, IRBs ensure research conducted by employees of specific institutions meet federal requirements. Still, some researchers may not work at large institutions or may not have access to IRBs.

The authors believe there is some belief among professional counselors that only counselor educators or those who work in research facilities conduct research. In actuality it is quite opposite; conducting research and publishing the findings is encouraged for all professional counselors regardless of their work settings. The introduction to Section G of the ACA Code of Ethics (2014) even encourages all professional counselors to "contribute to the knowledge base of the profession and promote a clearer understanding of the conditions that lead to a healthy and more just society" (p. 15).

It may be more convenient for professors or researchers to design, implement, and disseminate results due to their identified job responsibilities, but all counselors are encouraged to share their knowledge. IRBs provide guidance and monitor the quality of research. They act as regulatory boards in making sure research abides by all federal and state laws and that it is in line with local policies and procedures. Standard G.1.c. speaks to counselors who conduct research outside of large institutions. If counselors are conducting research independently and do not have access to IRBs, they are still responsible for adhering to all federal and state laws and relevant ethic principles.

ACA Standard G.1.c. (2014) Independent Researchers: When counselors conduct independent research and do not have access to an institutional review board, they are bound to the same ethical principles and federal and state laws pertaining to the review of their plan, design, conduct, and reporting of research.

Examine Case Illustration 14-2 and the various examples of ways in which counselors may conduct research either with or without the assistance of an IRB.

CASE ILLUSTRATION 14-2

Example 1

A counselor educator is interested in conducting research focused on homeless adolescents and their access to mental health services. Prior to beginning her research, the counselor educator must submit her research design to her university's IRB to make sure her research design, data collection, and data analysis procedures meet university and legal standards.

Example 2

A school counselor wishes to conduct research on the effectiveness of some of his parent deployment groups. He has spent the past two years writing and adapting the curriculum and now wants to share his work with others. After conducting his research on the effectiveness of his groups, he hopes to publish the results in a regional journal. Prior to collecting data, the school counselor must submit his research proposal to the school district's IRB for clearance.

Example 3

A professional counselor working in private practice wishes to conduct research on new techniques he is using to work with clients who self-injure. Because the professional counselor does not have access to an IRB, he is responsible for making sure the rights of participants are fully protected and data collection, analysis, and reporting procedures follow all ethic principles in addition to state and federal laws.

Examples 1 and 2 in Case Illustration 14-2 present counselors working within a larger system likely to have an IRB. In the first example the university would likely have an office dedicated to institutional research. The counselor educator would need only to contact the office and follow their guidance (i.e., complete the necessary paperwork and other requirements set forth by the university). The second example is very similar to the first, except the counselor works within a school district instead of a university. Still, the district would likely have a research compliance department and policies for conducting research within the district. The third example depicts a counselor working in private practice without the assistance of an IRB. Therefore the counselor would need to follow federal and state laws related to research (as directed by Ethical Standard G.1.c. To locate guidelines, the counselor would want to either look up applicable state and federal laws on his own or contact his state licensure board or professional counseling association for assistance in locating guidelines.

Participant Safety

Ethical Standards G.1.d. and G.1.e. both highlight the importance of participant safety. See Text Box 14-2 for safety standards for AAMFT members.

ACA Standard G.1.d. (2014) Deviation From Standard Practice: Counselors seek consultation and observe stringent safeguards to protect the rights of research participants when research indicates that a deviation from standard or acceptable practices may be necessary.

ACA Standard G.1.e. (2014) Precautions to Avoid Injury: Counselors who conduct research are responsible for their participants' welfare throughout the research process and should take reasonable precautions to avoid causing emotional, physical, or social harm to participants.

TEXT BOX 14-2

American Psychological Association

The APA does not address research participant protection in the 2010 code of ethics.

American Association for Marriage and Family Therapists

AAMFT Standard (2015) 5.2 Protection of Research Participants: Marriage and family therapists are responsible for making careful examinations of ethical acceptability in planning research. To the extent that services to research participants may be compromised by participation in research, marriage and family therapists seek the ethical advice of qualified professionals not directly involved in the investigation and observe safeguards to protect the rights of research participants.

Researchers must always consider the safety and well-being of participants ahead of the necessity for research. Reiterating the first standard in the ACA Code of Ethics (2014; i.e., Standard A.1.a., the primary responsibility of counselors is to respect the dignity and promote the welfare of clients), researchers must promote the well-being of their participants. Similar to the vulnerability of clients, research participants are vulnerable to researchers, and in volunteering to participate, they put their trust in researchers that no harm will come to them. Although the responsibility of participant safety falls on the shoulders of all members of the research team, the principle researcher bears the primary responsibility.

ACA Standard G.1.f. (2014) Principal Researcher Responsibility: The ultimate responsibility for ethical research practice lies with the principal researcher. All others involved in the research activities share ethical obligations and responsibility for their own actions.

In research, the principle or primary researcher receives the majority of the credit for the work. Along with the accolades, the principle researcher also takes on much of the burden of work and responsibility. All members of the research team are responsible for their own actions; however, the principle researcher is the one primarily responsible for making sure the entire project is conducted in an ethical manner.

Later in this chapter the authors discuss rights of research participants. The primary right participants have is the right to informed consent. Simply stated, this is the right to understand everything there is to know about the research to make an informed decision whether or not to participate. Because participants have a right to informed consent, it is the researcher's responsibility to provide said consent. Understanding this and knowing there are many individuals involved in research, researchers must take into consideration various concerns when providing informed consent. See the following list of considerations when providing information to participants.

Voluntary Participation

Participation in research is voluntary to all participants, and all are able to choose whether or not they would like to participate. When counselors decide to conduct research involving clients as participants, they take special precautions. Counselors have inherent power over their clients, and many clients may feel obligated to participate in research if presented the opportunity to do so by his/her counselor. Ethical Standard G.2.c. is clear about requiring counselors to fully articulate the voluntary nature of research when presenting opportunities to clients. See Text Box 14-3 for related standards for the APA and AAMFT.

ACA Standard G.2.c. (2014) Client Participation: Counselors conducting research involving clients make clear in the informed consent process that clients are free to choose whether to participate in research activities. Counselors take necessary precautions to protect clients from adverse consequences of declining or withdrawing from participation.

Similar to Standard G.2.c., Ethical Standard G.2.b. requires counselor educators and supervisors to take necessary precautions to protect students and supervisees.

ACA Standard G.2.b. (2014) Student and Supervisee Participation: Researchers who involve students or supervisees in research make clear to them that the decision regarding participation in research activities does not affect their academic standing or supervisory relationship. Students or supervisees who choose not to participate in research are provided with an appropriate alternative to fulfill their academic or clinical requirement.

TEXT BOX 14-3

American Psychological Association

APA Standard 8.04 (2010): Client or Patient, Student, and Subordinate Research Participants: (a) When psychologists conduct research with clients or patients, students, or subordinates as participants, psychologists take steps to protect the prospective participants from adverse consequences of declining or withdrawing from participation. (b) When research participation is a course requirement or an opportunity for extra credit, the prospective participant is given the choice of equitable alternative activities.

American Association for Marriage and Family Therapists

AAMFT Standard 5.4 (2015) Right to Decline or Withdraw Participation: Marriage and family therapists respect each participant's freedom to decline participation in or to withdraw from a research study at any time. This obligation requires special thought and consideration when investigators or other members of the research team are in positions of authority or influence over participants. Marriage and family therapists, therefore, make every effort to avoid multiple relationships with research participants that could impair professional judgement or increase the risk of exploitation. When offering inducements for research participation, marriage and family therapists make reasonable efforts to avoid offering inappropriate or excessive inducements when such inducements are likely to coerce participation.

Consider Case Illustration 14-3 to see how Dr. M recruits students to participate in his research.

CASE ILLUSTRATION 14-3

Dr. M is a counselor educator and is teaching ethics this semester, which he hopes will help him with a new research project concerning graduate students' ethical reasoning. On the first day of class, Dr. M describes his research and encourages all his students to participate. There is little to no chance any harm or discomfort will come to participants, and as an extra incentive for filing out three surveys (beginning, middle, and end of semester), Dr. M is willing to give those who participate three points on their final grade.

Is Dr. M acting in an ethical manner according to Standard G.2.b. Student and Supervisee Participation?

What might Dr. M want to do or take into consideration to assure he is acting ethically?

Case Illustration 14-3 presents a case in which Dr. M encourages his students to participate in his research. Students will likely not be harmed in any way due to their participation. Dr. M also offers to compensate participants with three extra points on their final exam. The first question asks if Dr. M is acting ethically according to Standard G.2.b.

While it is difficult to determine the ethicality of Dr. M's actions from this brief description, there are some areas that cause initial concern.

To assure he is acting in an ethical manner, Dr. M might want to consider the following actions. First, rather than simply describing the research, Dr. M would want to provide students an informed consent document, so each could read the requirements of the project and understand their participation fully. Dr. M could either provide students with a separate document or include the informed consent in his course syllabus. Next, Dr. M discusses the three point incentive for students who participate but does not discuss an alternate activity providing those who do not wish to participate with a similar opportunity to earn extra credit points. Dr. M would want to have such an activity to offer nonparticipants. In choosing an activity, Dr. M would want to be sure to choose one requiring approximately the same amount of effort and time participants would spend completing the research participation requirements. He would want to avoid making the alternative activity excessively burdensome (e.g., the alternative activity for nonparticipants being a 20-page research paper). Finally, Dr. M would want to be absolutely clear to his students that participation in the research, or lack of participation, in no way affected students' academic standing.

Persons Not Able to Give Consent

In many instances the individuals asked to participate in research may not be able to legally give consent on their own (e.g., research involving children or minors). Ethical Standard G.2.e. addresses such situations.

ACA Standard G.2.e. (2014) When a research participant is not capable of giving informed consent, counselors provide an appropriate explanation to, obtain agreement for participation from, and obtain and appropriate consent of a legally authorized person.

Similar to Standard A.2.d. (Inability to Give Consent) requiring professional counselors to gain assent from those unable to give legal consent prior to beginning a counseling relationship, researchers are obligated to get participants to assent to participation even when a legally authorized person must consent for their participation.

Commitments to Participants

When researchers make promises or commit to research participants, they are sure to follow through on those commitments as encouraged by Standard G.2.f.

ACA Standard G.2.f. (2014) Commitments to Participants: Counselors take reasonable measures to honor all commitments to research participants.

Consider Case Illustration 14-4 as Johnny commits to providing his research participants findings from his study.

CASE ILLUSTRATION 14-4

Johnny is a doctoral student in counselor education. As part of a pilot study for his dissertation, he is conducting qualitative research and interviewing parents on best practices for raising healthy children. Johnny recruits 10 parents to participate in his pilot study. During the informed consent process, several parents appear genuinely interested in knowing the findings from Johnny's pilot study. During the interview portion, Johnny agrees to share results with the families once all data analysis is completed. After the interviews are completed, Johnny analyzes the data and submits a manuscript for publication. While analyzing the data and completing the manuscript, Johnny is also extremely busy trying to keep up with his doctoral studies. As a result he forgets about his promise to his participants until nearly a year later. Because it has been such a long time, Johnny decides to forget about it and does not send any information to his participants.

Did Johnny act appropriately according to ACA Standard G.2.f?

In response to the question posed in Case Illustration 14-4, no; Johnny did not act in accordance to Standard G.2.f. No matter how long it has been since the initial research was completed, Johnny must still make reasonable efforts to provide the results to his participants.

Confidentiality of Information

Researchers working within organizations having IRBs will likely be required to follow institutional procedures ensuring confidentiality. However, it is the responsibility of the researcher to ensure information is kept confidential as stated in Standard G.2.d. Read about confidentiality for AAMFT in Text Box 14-4.

ACA Standard G.2.d. (2014) Confidentiality of Information: Information obtained about research participants during the course of research is confidential. Procedures are implemented to protect confidentiality.

TEXT BOX 14-4

American Psychological Association

The APA does not specifically address confidentiality of research data in the 2010 APA Code of Ethics.

American Association for Marriage and Family Therapists

AAMFT Standard 5.5 (2015) Confidentiality of Research Data: Information obtained about a research participant during the course of an investigation is confidential unless there is a waiver previously obtained in writing. When the possibility exists that others, including family members, may obtain access to such information, this possibility, together with the plan for protecting confidentiality, is explained as part of the procedure for obtaining informed consent.

Deception

Some research projects may require the use of deception to maintain the integrity of the data collected. In such situations counselors must consult Ethical Standard G.2.g. for guidance on how to inform participants of deceptive measures taken. Text Box 14-5 describes the use of deception in the APA.

ACA Standard G.2.g. (2014) Explanations After Data Collection: After data are collected, counselors provide participants with full clarification of the nature of the study to remove any misconceptions participants might have regarding the research. Where scientific or human values justify delaying or withholding information, counselors take reasonable measures to avoid causing harm.

TEXT BOX 14-5

American Psychological Association

APA Standard 8.07 (2010) Deception in Research: (a) Psychologists do not conduct a study involving deception unless they have determined that the use of deceptive techniques is justified by the study's significant prospective scientific, education, or applied value and that effective, nondeceptive alternative procedures are not feasible. (b) Psychologists do not deceive prospective participants about research that is reasonably expected to cause physical pain or severe emotional distress. (c) Psychologists explain that deception is an integral feature of the design and conduct of an experiment to participants as early as is feasible, preferably at the conclusion of their participation, but no later than at the conclusion of the data collection, and permit participants to withdraw their data.

APA standard 8.08 (2010) Debriefing: (a) Psychologists provide a prompt opportunity for participants to obtain appropriate information about the nature, results, and conclusions of the research, and they take reasonable steps to correct any misconceptions that participants may have of which the psychologists are aware. (b) If scientific or humane values justify delaying or withholding this information, psychologists take reasonable measures to reduce the risk of harm. (c) When psychologists become aware that research procedures have harmed a participant, they take reasonable steps to minimize the harm.

American Association for Marriage and Family Therapists

The AAMFT does not specifically address the use of deception or debriefing clients in the 2015 AAMFT Code of Ethics.

Review Case Illustration 14-5 and how a counselor uses deception when researching waiting room etiquette.

CASE ILLUSTRATION 14-5

A researcher studying waiting room behaviors advertises her study to potential participants as a study geared toward learning about individuals' learning styles. Participants are invited to an office building and directed to wait in the waiting room until the researcher is ready for them. Unknown to participants, there is a camera in the waiting room area filming all of their behaviors. Participants are all exposed to various waiting times and stimuli. After participants are made to wait for their set length of time and their behaviors have been recorded, they are called back to another room in the office. At that time they are informed of the actual purpose of the study and provided with a thorough debriefing.

Was the counselor acting ethically by using deception during her research project?

Case Illustration 14-5 describes a counselor conducting research on waiting room behaviors. The counselor uses some deception techniques in her study. The question in Case Illustration 14-5 asks if the counselor was ethical in her use of deception. Yes, the counselor was ethical. If she were to have informed participants ahead of time that their waiting room behaviors were going to be filmed and evaluated, each participant may have been more guarded. The participants would not have acted as they usually would. Minor deception was needed to collect the data. After the data was collected the researcher informed each participant of the true focus of the research as directed by Ethical Standard G.2.g.

Records Custodian

Researchers, like clinicians, must be prepared for unforeseen accidents or events. Standard G.2.i. requires researchers to set up procedures for such incidents.

ACA Standard G.2.i. (2014) Research Records Custodian: As appropriate, researchers prepare and disseminate to an identified colleague or records custodian a plan for the transfer of research data in the case of their incapacitation, retirement, or death.

Rights of Research Participants

All individuals who volunteer to participate in research activities expose themselves to some risk of harm. Although there is seldom a risk of physical harm in counseling research, the risk of psychological harm is often elevated (e.g., stress, anxiety, and discomfort) (Remley & Herlihy, 2014). Therefore the primary right of research participants is the right to informed consent. Similar to the informed consent necessary prior to the beginning of a counselor/client relationship, informed consent allows research participants to understand what they are getting themselves into at the outset. The ACA Code of Ethics (2014) identifies nine specific components of informed consent for research participants.

1. Counselors are truthful and accurate in explaining the procedures and the purpose of the research project. The explanations and procedures are also explained in a manner that is easily understood by potential participants.

2. Counselors specifically address any procedures or practices that are new or experimental.

3. Counselors discuss any areas in which participants may be at risk for harm or discomfort. Counselors also discuss the power differentials between researchers and participants.

4. Counselors describe any potential benefits that participants may realize in relation to their participation in the research.

5. Counselors share any alternative activities that may benefit participants outside of the research procedures (i.e., counselor educators who may be recruiting their students to participate in research notify them of alternative activities where they may get the same benefit as they would get by participating in the research).

6. Counselors answer any questions potential participants may have related to the research.

7. Counselors describe confidentiality and any limitations to confidentiality.

8. Counselors describe how the results of the research will be disseminated.

9. Counselors inform potential participants that they are able to withdraw from the study at any time. In the case of student, supervisee, or client participation, counselors explain that they may withdraw at any time without the risk of any negative effects on their other relationships with the counselor or institution conducting the research.

Understanding these nine requirements, review Case Illustration 14-6 as an example of how those requirements are integrated into an informed consent document.

CASE ILLUSTRATION 14-6

You are being asked to participate in a research study. This form provides you with information about the study. You will also receive a copy of this form to keep for your reference. The principle investigator or his representative will provide you with any additional information needed and answer any questions you may have. Read the information that follows, and ask questions about anything you do not understand before you decide whether or not to take part. Your participation is entirely voluntary, and you can refuse to participate or withdraw at any time without penalty or loss of benefits to which you are otherwise entitled.

What is the purpose of the study?

We are asking you to take part in a study of self-injurious behavior. We want to learn how individuals begin self-injuring, how they describe the meaning of self-injury, and what has been helpful to them in their attempts to discontinue self-injury. We are asking you to take part in this study because you have previously performed and/or are currently performing self-injury.

What will be done if you agree to take part in this research study?

Interviews are expected to last anywhere from 45 minutes to an hour. The interviews will take place at a mutually agreed-upon place and time. The interviews will entail questions regarding the participants' self-injury. The interview will be audio recorded to later transcribe the information.

What are the possible discomforts and risks?

Participants will be asked to describe some of their self-injurious behaviors. There is a possibility that recollections and descriptions may cause some discomfort and/or stress to the participant. The stress and discomfort to the participants, however, is anticipated to be at low levels. The interview will be conducted by Dr. John, a licensed professional counselor who

(Continued)

(Continued)

specializes in the treatment of individuals who self-injure, or by Ms. Jane, a licensed professional counselor intern. Dr. John or Ms. Jane will address any discomfort or stress arising during the interview.

What are the possible direct benefits to the participant for taking part in this research?

Although there are no specific benefits addressed to each participant, by responding to some of the interview questions, participants may possibly gain a greater understanding of his/her own self-injurious behaviors and how they contribute to their own lives. We do not guarantee you will benefit from participation.

What are the possible benefits to society from this research?

The knowledge gained from this study may contribute to our understanding of self-injurious behaviors and what is useful to individuals who want to cease self-injury.

Will there be any compensation for participation?

Yes. Participants will receive a $20 Visa gift card.

If you do not want to take part in this study, what other options are available to you?

Your participation in this study is entirely voluntary. You are free to refuse to be in the study or to withdraw from the study at any time. Your refusal will not influence current or future relationships with the university.

How will your privacy and the confidentiality of your research records be protected?

All information provided will remain confidential. Your name will not be recorded with your data to protect your right to privacy. Your research records will not be released without your consent unless required by law or a court order. Your records may be viewed by the IRB, but the confidentiality of your records will be protected to the extent permitted by law. The data resulting from your participation may be used in publications and/or presentations, but your identity will not be disclosed.

The interview session will be audio taped for research purposes, but your identity will not be recorded. The recordings will be kept in a secure place and will only be heard by the investigator and his research associates. Recordings will be erased after they have been transcribed.

How can you withdraw from this research study, and who should you call if you have questions?

If you wish to stop your participation for any reason, please contact the principle investigator, Dr. John, PhD, LPC-S, at (555) 555-1111, or tell research personnel. Throughout the study, the researchers will notify you of new information that may become available and that might affect your decision to remain in the study.

If you have questions now, you may ask the principle investigator (or representative staff). If you have questions later, you may contact principle investigator Dr. John, PhD, LPC-S, at (555) 555-1111.

In addition, if you have questions about your rights as a research subject, or if you have complaints, concerns, or questions about the research, you may contact the university's Institutional Review Board at (555) 555-2222.

Your participation in this study is entirely voluntary. You are free to refuse to be in the study or to withdraw at any time. Your refusal will not influence current or future relationships with the university.

You have been informed about this study's purpose, procedures, possible benefits, and risks. You have been given the opportunity to ask questions before you sign, and you have been told that you can ask other questions at any time.

You voluntarily agree to participate in this study. By signing this form, you are not waiving any of your legal rights.

You will be given a copy of this form to keep.

_____

Printed Name of Subject

_____

Signature of Subject/Date

_____

Printed Name of Person Obtaining Consent

_____

Signature of Person Obtaining Consent/Date

Researcher and Participant Relationships

It is the author's opinion that extending boundaries with research participants is seldom encountered, and coincidently there are seldom occasions when extending researcher and participant boundaries would be appropriate. In cases where researchers believe an extension of boundaries may be beneficial to participants, researchers are careful to thoroughly consider the risks and benefits of such an extension. Similar to Standard

A.6.b., Standard F.3.a. and Standard F.10.f. related to extending counselor/client boundaries, extending supervisor/supervisee boundaries, and student/counselor educator boundaries, researchers document their reasoning for the extension and all potential benefits and risks prior to extending. If any harm comes to the participant, researchers must show and document ways in which he/she attempted to remedy the harm.

ACA Standard G.3.a. (2014) Extending Researcher/Participant Boundaries: Researchers consider the risks and benefits of extending current research relationships beyond conventional parameters. When a non-research interaction between the researcher and the research participant may be potentially beneficial, the researcher must document, prior to the interaction (when feasible), the rationale for such an interaction, the potential benefit, and anticipated consequences for the research participant. Such interactions should be initiated with appropriate consent of the research participant. Where unintentional harm occurs to the research participant, the researcher must show evidence of an attempt to remedy such harm.

While some extensions may be potentially beneficial to research participants, sexual and/or romantic relationships are prohibited with current research participants as stated in Standard G.3.b.

ACA Standard G.3.b. (2014) Relationships With Research Participants: Sexual or romantic counselor/research participant interactions or relationships with current research participants are prohibited. This prohibition applies to both in-person and electronic interactions or relationships.

Concomitantly, Standard G.3.c. (Sexual Harassment and Research Participants) prohibits researchers from subjecting participants to sexual harassment.

Overall, the authors believe researchers should maintain strict boundaries with participants. Blurred boundaries have the potential to not only affect the welfare of the participants but also affect the outcomes of the research. Counselors must work to stay objective when counseling clients, supervising counselors in training, and conducting research.

Reporting Results

After all data has been collected and analyzed, research results are most often reported in some form. Sometimes researchers choose to report their findings in the form of a book or journal manuscript, and in other instances the reporting is specifically directed toward the entity sponsoring the research. For example, a nonprofit counseling agency may hire a local counselor educator to evaluate the effectiveness of the agency's summer small-group camp. The results of the evaluation would be sent directly to the nonprofit agency.

In any case, the ACA provides counseling researchers with guidelines to ensure the ethicality of reports. Summaries of APA and AAMFT guidelines are in Text Box 14-6. First and foremost, counselors are accurate in all aspects of their research as directed by Standard G.4.a.

ACA Standard G.4.a. (2014) Accurate Results: Counselors plan, conduct, and report research accurately. Counselors do not engage in misleading or fraudulent research, distort data, misrepresent data, or deliberately bias their results. They describe the extent to which results are applicable for diverse populations.

TEXT BOX 14-6

American Psychological Association

APA Standard 8.10 (2010) Reporting Research Results: (a) Psychologists do not fabricate data. (b) If psychologists discover significant errors in their published data, they take reasonable steps to correct such errors in a correction, retraction, erratum, or other appropriate publication means.

American Association for Marriage and Family Therapists

AAMFT Standard 5.6 (2015) Publication: Marriage and family therapists do not fabricate research results. Marriage and family therapists disclose potential conflicts of interest and take authorship credit only for work they have performed or to which they have contributed. Publication credits accurately reflect the relative contributions of the individual involved.

AAMFT Standard 5.9 (2015) Accuracy in Publication: Marriage and family therapists who are authors of books or other materials published or distributed by an organization take reasonable precautions to ensure that the published materials are accurate and factual.

This guideline requires counselors to be knowledgeable of the research methodologies, data collection, and data analysis and reporting. Consider the actions of Drs. Sully and Moore in Case Illustration 14-7.

CASE ILLUSTRATION 14-7

Dr. Sully and Dr. Moore are both professors at a local university. Due to their standing in the community and their reputations related to program evaluation, they are hired by a local juvenile detention center to evaluate the effectiveness of the center's life skills training. During the negotiations, Dr. Sully and Dr. Moore are informed that the company that runs the detention center has many other satellite centers around the state. If this partnership is successful, the company will most likely want to hire Drs. Sully and Moore to evaluate the other programs as well. In their data analysis the two professors find the life skills training has not been affective. However, in completing the data analysis, the two also realize if they were to manipulate the data a small amount, they would be able to report back to the center that the life skills training did show positive results. The two understand that no one at the center has a clear understanding of the statistical analysis they used and would certainly not question their methodology. Drs. Moore and Sully also realize if they share unfavorable results with the center, they are not likely to be hired again in the future and may miss out on future financial opportunities with this company.

Would it be ethical for Dr. Sully and Dr. Moore to manipulate the data?

Case Illustration 14-7 describes Drs. Sully and Moore and their evaluation of a detention center's life skills program. The professors' evaluation shows the life skills program is ineffective; however, the two faculty members could produce positive results by minimally manipulating the data. Regardless of the financial benefits or drawbacks or the extent to which the two professors would need to manipulate the data, it would be considered unethical and should not be done according to Standards G.4.a. Additionally, Ethical Standard G.4.b. focuses directly on Drs. Moore and Sully's dilemma and requires them to report unfavorable results.

ACA Standard G.4.b. (2014) Obligation to Report Unfavorable Results: Counselors report the results of any research of professional value. Results that reflect unfavorably on institutions, programs, services, prevailing opinions, or vested interests are not withheld.

Case Illustration 14-7 again highlights the importance of counselor self-awareness. The authors discussed motivation in Chapter 1 and how the conflict between egoistic and altruistic actions often causes ethical dilemmas. The conflict between the egoistic and altruistic could cause a dilemma for Drs. Sully and Moore in Case Illustration 14-7. The illustration states no one at the agency understood the statistical data analysis the two faculty members used and therefore would not know if the analysis was done correctly or not. If Drs. Moore and Sully were more egoistically motivated (motivated by the financial benefits of evaluating the program), they may be more tempted to manipulate the data. If the two were more altruistically motivated (motivated by providing accurate information to the detention center), they would likely be less tempted to manipulate the information.

Publications

It is the authors' experience when discussing ethics related to research and publication that many times students will lose interest and focus because they see research and publication as something in which only professors and doctoral students participate. Those having interest in furthering their academic training past the master's level may have more interest than those who are not. Still, publication may affect all graduate students at some time (e.g., publishing a best practices article in a state journal as a practicing clinician or participating on a research team as a graduate assistant), and thus it is critical that all counselors and counselors in training understand ethical guidelines related to publication and specifically the eight standards related to publication in the ACA Code of Ethics (2014).

Using Case Examples When Sharing Research Results

ACA Standard G.5.a. (2014) Use of Case Examples: The use of participants', clients', students', or supervisees' information for the purpose of case examples in a presentation or publication is permissible only when (a) participants, clients, students, or supervisees have reviewed the material and agreed to its presentation or publication or (b) the information has been sufficiently modified to obscure identity.

When using examples in one's writing, it is critical to either modify or change the information enough so those reading or hearing the information are not able to determine about whom you are speaking or get the written permission of the individual to be included. Review Case Illustration 14-8 to see how Dr. Sally incorporates case examples into a research manuscript.

CASE ILLUSTRATION 14-8

Dr. Sally conducts qualitative research. This past semester she interviewed mothers whose husbands were in the armed forces and currently deployed. As part of the informed consent process, Dr. Sally informed her participants she planned on incorporating the interviews into a presentation. Dr. Sally further explained the presentation would be delivered at her state counseling association's annual conference. After hearing about Dr. Sally's plans, all but one of the participants consented to allowing Dr. Sally to use their first names and demographic information in the presentation. The one participant refusing consent asked Dr. Sally to use a pseudonym instead of her real name and also asked her to avoid using any of the demographic information provided.

How should Dr. Sally move forward in preparing her presentation?

Case Illustration 14-8 describes Dr. Sally and her research with military spouses. Dr. Sally has received permission from all but one of her participants to use their information in her presentation. For the participants who consented, Dr. Sally is able to use their first names and demographic information. Still, Dr. Sally would want to be cognizant of the information she includes and only include as much identifying information as needed. For the one participant who declined consent, Dr. Sally might want to ask the participant to choose her own pseudonym and verify the types of information she is able to include and which should be left out. The main goal of Standard G.5.a. is to protect participant confidentiality unless given written permission.

Plagiarism

Plagiarism seems like a commonsense ethical standard, yet it still remains a concern. Therefore ACA Ethical Standard G.5.b. reminds counselors to avoid plagiarism (for guidelines from the APA and AAMFT, see Text Box 14-7).

ACA Standard G.5.b. (2014) Plagiarism: Counselors do not plagiarize; that is, they do not present another person's work as their own.

TEXT BOX 14-7

American Psychological Association

APA Standard 8.11 (2010) Plagiarism: Psychologists do not present portions of another's work or data as their own, even if the other work or data source is cited occasionally.

American Association for Marriage and Family Therapists

AAMFT Standard 5.8 (2015) Plagiarism: Marriage and family therapists who are the authors of books or other materials that are published or distributed do not plagiarize or fail to cite persons to whom credit for original ideas or work is due.

Counselors must take special care to acknowledge and give credit to all authors who participate in research and publication. Counselors are also careful to only use others' information with the owner's consent, are sure to give credit to original authors, and make sure all audiences understand who is responsible for creating materials. For those who do not have writing experience or have previously used other writing styles, writing and properly citing materials may be a challenge at first. However, as with all other aspects of ethics, ignorance is not a valid excuse. In regard to plagiarism, it is the counselor's and counselor in training's responsibility to understand how to properly cite material and seek training or guidance when unfamiliar with proper guidelines.

Authorship

The degree to which an individual contributed to the publication of a manuscript is indicated by where their name falls in the list of authors. Typically, those who contribute the most are listed as the primary or first author. Their names are listed first on the list. Subsequent contributors are listed after the first author. Depending on the manuscript, some may have only one author (i.e., a single author publication), and others may have multiple authors (i.e., a coauthored manuscript). Similar guidelines are used in APA and AAMFT (see Text Box 14-8).

ACA Standard G.5.c. (2014) Contributors: Counselors give credit through joint authorship, acknowledgment, footnote statement, or other appropriate means to those who have contributed significantly to research or concept development in accordance with such contributions. The principal contributor is listed first, and minor technical or professional contributions are acknowledged in notes or introductory statements.

TEXT BOX 14-8

American Psychological Association

APA Standard 8.12 (2010) Publication Credit: (a) Psychologists take responsibility and credit, including authorship credit, only for work they have actually performed or to which they have substantially contributed. (b) Principal authorship and other publication credits accurately reflect the relative scientific or professional contributions of the individuals involved, regardless of their relative status. Mere possession of an institutional position, such as department chair, does not justify authorship credit. Minor contributions to the research or to the writing for publications are acknowledged appropriately, such as in footnotes or in an introductory statement. (c) Except under exceptional circumstances, a student is listed as principal author on any multiple-authored article that is substantially based on the student's doctoral dissertation. Faculty advisors discuss publication credit with students as early as feasible and throughout the research and publication process as appropriate.

American Association for Marriage and Family Therapists

AAMFT Standard 5.7 (2015) Authorship of Student Work: Marriage and family therapists do not accept or require authorship credit for a publication based from student's research, unless the marriage and family therapist made a substantial contribution beyond being a faculty advisor or research committee member. Coauthorship on student research should be determined in accordance with principles of fairness and justice.

Consider Case Illustration 14-9 and the ethicality of Dr. Q's behaviors related to authorship.

CASE ILLUSTRATION 14-9

Dr. Q is a tenured faculty member at a small counselor education program. She is a prolific writer and has been teaching at the same institution for almost 20 years. Over her tenure, Dr. Q has chaired many doctoral dissertations and master's theses. Many students request her as a dissertation chair due to her national notoriety and reputation for having many of her students land jobs in other respected counselor education programs.

(Continued)

(Continued)

When doctoral students approach Dr. Q about chairing their dissertation, she is very straightforward about her expectations. She requires her doctoral students to conduct their dissertation research in one of her main research interest areas. Upon graduation and completing their doctoral degrees, Dr. Q further expects her students to include her as a second author when publishing their dissertations and any future research in that area. As Dr. Q's students graduate, get hired to teach in other counselor education programs, and complete their own research, Dr. Q's list of publications increases as her past doctoral students publish their own materials. As a result, Dr. Q receives many accolades for her prolific writing skills.

Is Dr. Q acting ethically by requiring her doctoral students to always include her as a second author on their own publications?

Dr. Q's behaviors in Case Illustration 14-9 would most likely be seen as unethical according to Standard G.5.c. Moreover, Dr. Q could be seen as exploiting the power she has as a counselor educator. Even though Dr. Q may have contributed to the first manuscript (i.e., dissertation) and acted as a contributor by editing and offering feedback, she in no way participates in her students' future research and therefore should not be included as an author.

As a way to avoid the exploitation described in Case Illustration 14-9, authors should always discuss joint authorship projects prior to beginning the project. At the onset of all writing endeavors, all those involved should discuss authorship expectations in accordance with Ethical Standard G.5.e.

ACA Standard G.5.e. (2014) Agreement of Contributors: Counselors who conduct joint research with colleagues or students or supervisors establish agreements in advance regarding allocation or tasks, publication credit, and types of acknowledgment that will be received.

In Case Illustration 14-9, Dr. Q abused her power by requiring her doctoral students to include her on every publication. In doing so Dr. Q. was receiving credit for contributing to manuscripts she did not contribute to at all. In some cases counselor educators may use student work, without the student's knowledge, to further their own research. Doing so is a violation of the ACA Code of Ethics according to Ethical Standard G.5.f.

ACA Standard G.5.f. (2014) Student Research: Manuscripts or professional presentations in any medium that are substantially based on a student's course papers, projects, dissertations, or theses are used only with the student's permission and list the student as lead author.

Review Case Illustration 14-10 as an example of how a counselor educator might use student work to promote his/her own research agenda.

CASE ILLUSTRATION 14-10

Dr. T is a faculty member in a counselor education program and traditionally teaches a doctoral-level research methods course. As one of the assignments each semester, Dr. T requires his students to write a research paper. As a part of the assignment, students are expected to write a literature review and research methods section. Although they are not forced to pick specific topics, students are encouraged to pick their topics from a list that Dr. T provides. Each of the topics listed also happens to be a topic that Dr. T focuses on for his own research. After papers are completed, turned in, and graded each semester, Dr. T gives the stack of papers to his graduate assistants, who are coincidentally also students in the counseling program in which Dr. T teaches. Dr. T directs his graduate assistants to go through the papers and look for ones that "stand out and are written better than the others." After Dr. T approves the topics and papers separated by his graduate assistants, he directs them to complete IRB applications, so he may get approval to complete the studies on his own. Each year, Dr. T is usually able to complete at least one study from the previous year's research papers and get the results published in a state or national journal.

This year Linda, a graduate student in the counseling program, is working as Dr. T's graduate assistant. As she is completing the tasks Dr. T has asked of her, she hesitantly asks Dr. T about the ethicality of his actions. Dr. T laughs a bit and says that because students have turned the papers in as assignments, the writing technically doesn't belong to them anymore. He also rationalizes that because he is only taking parts of what his students wrote, rewriting it, and doing the actual research on his own that he doesn't need to include his students on the list of authors.

Linda feels uneasy about Dr. T's actions, especially as she might be held liable because she participated in the activities as part of her graduate assistant work. However she is worried about confronting Dr. T again or reporting him to anyone else due to her fear of how it may affect her standing in the program. She also fears that she may lose her graduate assistant position if she does not follow Dr. T's instructions.

Are Dr. T's actions ethical according to Ethical Standard G.5.f.?

What should Linda do with her knowledge about Dr. T's actions?

In Case Illustration 14-10, Dr. T uses the work of his graduate students to build his own research agenda. Even though Dr. T writes a considerable amount of the overall manuscript, he is basing his writing on his students' course papers and thus would be in violation of Ethical Standard G.5.f. The second question is perhaps more difficult. Linda is in a vulnerable position. She is a graduate student and likely susceptible to the evaluation of Dr. T. At the same time, Linda is a counselor in training and required to adhere to the ACA Code of Ethics. Ethical Standard I.2.a. requires Linda to attempt to resolve her dilemma with Dr. T. If she does not believe Dr. T will respond to her concerns, Linda is then obligated to report his behaviors to a state licensure board or professional ethics committee. Linda would likely also want to report the behaviors to the department chair of the program in which she is enrolled.

Manuscript Submissions

Professional counselors wishing to have manuscripts published in professional counseling journals must submit them for review. All publication outlets supported by the ACA and the vast majority of other publication outlets all conduct a blind review of submitted manuscripts. Blind review means that manuscripts are de-identified (author names and identifiers are removed) and sent out to reviewers to determine their appropriateness for publication. When submitting manuscripts for review, counselors must be sure to submit their manuscripts to only one journal at a time (as directed by Ethical Standard G.5.g.).

ACA Standard G.5.g. (2014) Duplicate Submissions: Counselors submit manuscripts for consideration to only one journal at a time. Manuscripts that are published in whole or in substantial part in one journal or published work are not submitted for publication to another publisher without acknowledgment and permission from the original publisher.

If authors wish to submit a manuscript to another journal, they must either wait until the manuscript is rejected by the journal it was originally submitted to or withdraw the manuscript from consideration. Once the article is withdrawn, it may be ethically submitted to another journal for consideration.

Manuscript Reviews

In contrast to the previous ethical standard directed toward counselors submitting manuscripts for review, Ethical Standard G.5.h. pertains to counselors who act as reviewers for journal publications. (See Text Box 14.9 for APA's guidelines regarding reviews.) Counselors who review manuscripts are to review objectively, provide feedback to editors in a timely manner, and only review manuscripts within their scope of competency.

ACA Standard G.5.h. (2014) Professional Review: Counselors who review material submitted for publication, research, or other scholarly purposes respect the confidentiality and proprietary rights of those who submitted it. Counselors make publication decisions based on valid and defensible standards. Counselors review article submissions in a timely manner and based on their scope and competency in research methodologies. Counselors who serve as reviewers at the request of editors or publishers make every effort to only review materials that are within their scope of competency and avoid personal biases.

TEXT BOX 14-9

American Psychological Association

APA Standard 8.15 (2010) Reviewers: Psychologists who review material submitted for presentation, publication, grant, or research proposal review respect the confidentiality of and the proprietary rights in such information of those who submitted it.

Conclusion

Research and publication may be intimidating for some graduate students, and others may have high aspirations of sharing their research with professional counselors around the world. Whichever category you belong to, it is critical that you have some knowledge of ethical standards related to research and publication. Those conducting research must understand the necessity of providing informed consent to, protecting the safety of, and maintaining appropriate boundaries with research participants. Individuals must also understand the intricacies related to manuscript authorship and submitting articles for publication. Without proper knowledge, students and counselors in training leave themselves open to exploitation by those who may be more familiar with the process. Use the information learned in this chapter to address the ethical dilemma and corresponding discussion questions presented in Case Exercise 14-1.

CASE EXERCISE 14-1

Dr. J teaches in the counselor education department at a large, public university. He has been teaching at the same university for the past 10 years and has built up a reputation as a well-respected member of the university and surrounding community. Master's students in Dr. J's program are usually required to complete a master's thesis as part of their degree requirements, even though many do not ever go on to pursue a doctoral degree or even publish the results of their theses. Because the thesis papers usually sit idle and are never published by the students, Dr. J has begun to collect the papers after his students graduate. Dr. J typically waits two to three years after his students have graduated and then revisits their master's thesis papers. He reviews those he remembers to be well done, makes some small edits (i.e., updates the citations and corrects any typos or grammatical mistakes), and submits them to various journal publications as his own work.

While reading through the journal published by her state counseling association, Ria, one of Dr. J's previous students, is perplexed to see her master's thesis paper published in the journal. Ria knows she never submitted her thesis for publication and feels taken advantage of by Dr. J.

What would you do if you were in Ria's position?

What, if any, ethical obligations does Ria have as she knows Dr. J did not write the manuscript in the journal?

Keystones

- All professional counselors are encouraged to participate in and support research whenever possible.
- Counselors implement research projects in accordance with federal and state laws.

- IRBs were first established in the 1970s and were designed to protect human rights in research.
- Even though all research team members are responsible for ethical conduct, the principle researcher bears the ultimate responsibility for assuring all research activities are carried out legally and ethically.
- Counselors ensure participants know participation in research is always voluntary, and participants may withdraw at any time without repercussions.
- When students and supervisees are involved or recruited as research participants, counselors are sure to remind them that participation in the project does not affect their standing in the program or supervisory relationship in any way. Counselors also provide alternative methods for students to acquire any academic incentive provided to those participating in the research.
- When conducting research with participants who are unable to give legal consent, researchers get consent from legally authorized persons and gain assent from the participants.
- Researchers fulfill all commitments made to research participants.
- Researchers protect the confidentiality of participants.
- When deception is needed, researchers debrief participants immediately after data is collected and provide participants with full clarification.
- Sexual and romantic relationships between researchers and participants are prohibited.
- When considering extending researcher/participant boundaries, counselors consider all potential risks and benefits to the participant and document any concerns.
- Researchers must report results accurately and avoid biasing results or manipulating data to provide more favorable results.
- Counselors report results for all research having professional value even if the results are unfavorable.
- Plagiarism is prohibited.
- Counselors give credit to all persons contributing to a manuscript based on the amount of work contributed to the project.
- When submitting a manuscript for publication review, counselors submit manuscripts to only one journal at a time.
- When counselors act as a reviewer for journal outlets, they are sure to review in an objective manner, provide timely feedback, and only review manuscripts within their range of competency.

Additional Resources

Abrahams, H. (2007). Ethics in counselling research fieldwork. *Counselling and Psychotherapy Research, 7*(4), 240–244. doi:10.1080/14733140701707068

Hébert, J. R., Satariano, W. A., Friedman, D. B., Armstead, C. A., Greiner, A., Felder, T. M., & Braun, K. L. (2015). Fulfilling ethical responsibility: Moving beyond the minimal standards of protecting human subjects from research harm. *Progress in Community Health Partnerships: Research, Education, and Action, 9,* 41–50.

Kocet, M. M., & Herlihy, B. J. (2014). Addressing value-based conflicts within the counseling relationship: A decision-making model. *Journal of Counseling & Development, 92,* 180–186. doi:10.1002/j.1556-6676.2014.00146.x

Rosenthal, R. (1994). Science and ethics in conducting, analyzing, and reporting psychological research. *Psychological Science, 5,* 127–133.

Sales, B. D., & Lavin, M. (2000). Identifying conflicts of interest and resolving ethical dilemmas. In B. D. Sales & S. Folkman (Eds.), *Ethics in research with human participants* (pp. 109–128). Washington, DC: American Psychological Association.

Silva, P. D. (1999). Ethics in counselling and psychotherapy: Standards, research and emerging issues. *Sexual and Marital Therapy, 14*(3), 341.

References

American Association for Marriage and Family Therapy. (2015). *Code of ethics.* Retrieved from https://www.aamft.org/iMIS15/AAMFT/Content/legal_ethics/code_of_ethics.aspx

American Counseling Association. (2014). *Code of ethics.* Alexandria, VA: Author.

American Psychological Association. (2010). *American Psychological Association ethical principles of psychologists and code of conduct.* Retrieved from http://www.apa.org/ethics/code/principles.pdf

Ford, G. G. (2006). *Ethical reasoning for mental health professionals.* Thousand Oaks, CA: Sage.

Remley, T. P., & Herlihy, B. (2014). *Ethical, legal, and professional issues in counseling* (4th ed.). Upper Saddle River, NJ: Pearson.

Appendix A: American Counseling Association Code of Ethics

Mission

> The mission of the American Counseling Association is to enhance the quality of life in society by promoting the development of professional counselors, advancing the counseling profession, and using the profession and practice of counseling to promote respect for human dignity and diversity.
>

Contents

American Counseling Association (2014). ACA Code of Ethics. Alexandria, VA.

Section D

Relationships With Other Professionals

Section E

Evaluation, Assessment, and Interpretation

Section F

Supervision, Training, and Teaching

Section G

Research and Publication

Section H

Distance Counseling, Technology, and Social Media

Section I

Resolving Ethical Issues

Glossary of Terms

Index

ACA Code of Ethics Preamble

The American Counseling Association (ACA) is an educational, scientific, and professional organization whose members work in a variety of settings and serve in multiple capacities. Counseling is a professional relationship that empowers diverse individuals, families, and groups to accomplish mental health, wellness, education, and career goals.

Professional values are an important way of living out an ethical commitment. The following are core professional values of the counseling profession:

1. enhancing human development throughout the life span;

2. honoring diversity and embracing a multicultural approach in support of the worth, dignity, potential, and uniqueness of people within their social and cultural contexts;

3. promoting social justice;

4. safeguarding the integrity of the counselor–client relationship; and

5. practicing in a competent and ethical manner.

These professional values provide a conceptual basis for the ethical principles enumerated below. These principles are the foundation for ethical behavior and decision making. The fundamental principles of professional ethical behavior are

- *autonomy*, or fostering the right to control the direction of one's life;
- *nonmaleficence*, or avoiding actions that cause harm;

- *beneficence,* or working for the good of the individual and society by promoting mental health and well-being;
- *justice,* or treating individuals equitably and fostering fairness and equality;
- *fidelity,* or honoring commitments and keeping promises, including fulfilling one's responsibilities of trust in professional relationships; and
- *veracity,* or dealing truthfully with individuals with whom counselors come into professional contact.

ACA Code of Ethics Purpose

The *ACA Code of Ethics* serves six main purposes:

1. The *Code* sets forth the ethical obligations of ACA members and provides guidance intended to inform the ethical practice of professional counselors.

2. The *Code* identifies ethical considerations relevant to professional counselors and counselors-in-training.

3. The *Code* enables the association to clarify for current and prospective members, and for those served by members, the nature of the ethical responsibilities held in common by its members.

4. The *Code* serves as an ethical guide designed to assist members in constructing a course of action that best serves those utilizing counseling services and establishes expectations of conduct with a primary emphasis on the role of the professional counselor.

5. The *Code* helps to support the mission of ACA.

6. The standards contained in this *Code* serve as the basis for processing inquiries and ethics complaints concerning ACA members.

The *ACA Code of Ethics* contains nine main sections that address the following areas:

Section A: The Counseling Relationship

Section B: Confidentiality and Privacy

Section C: Professional Responsibility

Section D: Relationships With Other Professionals

Section E: Evaluation, Assessment, and Interpretation

Section F: Supervision, Training, and Teaching

Section G: Research and Publication

Section H: Distance Counseling, Technology, and Social Media

Section I: Resolving Ethical Issues

Each section of the *ACA Code of Ethics* begins with an introduction. The introduction to each section describes the ethical behavior and responsibility to which counselors aspire. The introductions help set the tone for each particular section and provide a starting point that invites reflection on the ethical standards contained in each part of the *ACA Code of Ethics*. The standards outline professional responsibilities and provide direction for fulfilling those ethical responsibilities.

When counselors are faced with ethical dilemmas that are difficult to resolve, they are expected to engage in a carefully considered ethical decision-making process, consulting available resources as needed. Counselors acknowledge that resolving ethical issues is a process; ethical reasoning includes consideration of professional values, professional ethical principles, and ethical standards.

Counselors' actions should be consistent with the spirit as well as the letter of these ethical standards. No specific ethical decision-making model is always most effective, so counselors are expected to use a credible model of decision making that can bear public scrutiny of its application. Through a chosen ethical decision-making process and evaluation of the context of the situation, counselors work collaboratively with clients to make decisions that promote clients' growth and development. A breach of the standards and principles provided herein does not necessarily constitute legal liability or violation of the law; such action is established in legal and judicial proceedings.

The glossary at the end of the *Code* provides a concise description of some of the terms used in the *ACA Code of Ethics*.

SECTION A: THE COUNSELING RELATIONSHIP

Introduction

Counselors facilitate client growth and development in ways that foster the interest and welfare of clients and promote formation of healthy relationships. Trust is the cornerstone of the counseling relationship, and counselors have the responsibility to respect and safeguard the client's right to privacy and confidentiality. Counselors actively attempt to understand the diverse cultural backgrounds of the clients they serve. Counselors also explore their own cultural identities and how these affect their values and beliefs about the counseling process. Additionally, counselors are encouraged to contribute to society by devoting a portion of their professional activities for little or no financial return (*pro bono publico*).

A.1. Client Welfare

A.1.a. Primary Responsibility

The primary responsibility of counselors is to respect the dignity and promote the welfare of clients.

A.1.b. Records and Documentation

Counselors create, safeguard, and maintain documentation necessary for rendering professional services. Regardless of the medium, counselors include sufficient and timely documentation to facilitate the delivery and continuity of services. Counselors take reasonable steps to ensure that documentation accurately reflects client progress and services provided. If amendments are made to records and documentation, counselors take steps to properly note the amendments according to agency or institutional policies.

A.1.c. Counseling Plans

Counselors and their clients work jointly in devising counseling plans that offer reasonable promise of success and are consistent with the abilities, temperament, developmental level, and circumstances of clients. Counselors and clients regularly review and revise counseling plans to assess their continued viability and effectiveness, respecting clients' freedom of choice.

A.1.d. Support Network Involvement

Counselors recognize that support networks hold various meanings in the lives of clients and consider enlisting the support, understanding, and involvement of others (e.g., religious/spiritual/ community leaders, family members, friends) as positive resources, when appropriate, with client consent.

A.2. Informed Consent in the Counseling Relationship

A.2.a. Informed Consent

Clients have the freedom to choose whether to enter into or remain in a counseling relationship and need adequate information about the counseling process and the counselor. Counselors have an obligation to review in writing and verbally with clients the rights and responsibilities of both counselors and clients. Informed consent is an ongoing part of the counseling process, and counselors appropriately document discussions of informed consent throughout the counseling relationship.

A.2.b. Types of Information Needed

Counselors explicitly explain to clients the nature of all services provided. They inform clients about issues such as, but not limited to, the following: the purposes, goals, techniques, procedures, limitations, potential risks, and benefits of services; the counselor's qualifications, credentials, relevant experience, and approach to counseling; continuation of services upon the incapacitation or death of the counselor; the role of technology; and other pertinent information. Counselors take steps to ensure that clients understand the implications of diagnosis and the intended use of tests and reports. Additionally, counselors inform clients about fees and billing arrangements, including procedures for nonpayment of fees. Clients have the right to confidentiality and to be provided with an explanation of its limits (including how supervisors and/or treatment or interdisciplinary team professionals are involved), to obtain clear information about their records, to participate in the ongoing counseling plans, and to refuse any services or modality changes and to be advised of the consequences of such refusal.

A.2.c. Developmental and Cultural Sensitivity

Counselors communicate information in ways that are both developmentally and culturally appropriate. Counselors use clear and understandable language when discussing issues related to informed consent. When clients have difficulty understanding the language that counselors use, counselors provide necessary services (e.g., arranging for a qualified interpreter or translator) to ensure comprehension by clients. In collaboration with clients, counselors consider cultural implications of informed consent procedures and, where possible, counselors adjust their practices accordingly.

A.2.d. Inability to Give Consent

When counseling minors, incapacitated adults, or other persons unable to give voluntary consent, counselors seek the assent of clients to services and include them in decision making as appropriate. Counselors recognize the need to balance the ethical rights of clients to make choices, their capacity to give consent or assent to receive services, and parental or familial legal rights and responsibilities to protect these clients and make decisions on their behalf.

A.2.e. Mandated Clients

Counselors discuss the required limitations to confidentiality when working with clients who have been mandated for counseling services. Counselors also explain what type of information and with whom that information is shared prior to the beginning of counseling. The client may choose to refuse services. In this case, counselors will, to the best of their ability, discuss with the client the potential consequences of refusing counseling services.

A.3. Clients Served by Others

When counselors learn that their clients are in a professional relationship with other mental health professionals, they request release from clients to inform the other professionals and strive to establish positive and collaborative professional relationships.

A.4. Avoiding Harm and Imposing Values

A.4.a. Avoiding Harm

Counselors act to avoid harming their clients, trainees, and research participants and to minimize or to remedy unavoidable or unanticipated harm.

A.4.b. Personal Values

Counselors are aware of—and avoid imposing—their own values, attitudes, beliefs, and behaviors. Counselors respect the diversity of clients, trainees, and research participants and seek training in areas in which they are at risk of imposing their values onto clients, especially when the counselor's values are inconsistent with the client's goals or are discriminatory in nature.

A.5. Prohibited Noncounseling Roles and Relationships

A.5.a. Sexual and/or Romantic Relationships Prohibited

Sexual and/or romantic counselor–client interactions or relationships with current clients, their romantic partners, or their family members are prohibited. This prohibition applies to both in-person and electronic interactions or relationships.

A.5.b. Previous Sexual and/or Romantic Relationships

Counselors are prohibited from engaging in counseling relationships with persons with whom they have had a previous sexual and/or romantic relationship.

A.5.c. Sexual and/or Romantic Relationships With Former Clients

Sexual and/or romantic counselor–client interactions or relationships with former clients, their romantic partners, or their family members are prohibited for a period of 5 years following the last professional contact. This prohibition applies to both in-person and electronic interactions or relationships. Counselors, before engaging in sexual and/or romantic interactions or relationships with former clients, their romantic partners, or their family members, demonstrate forethought and document (in written form) whether the interaction or relationship can be viewed as exploitive in any way and/or whether there is still potential to harm the former client; in cases of potential exploitation and/or harm, the counselor avoids entering into such an interaction or relationship.

A.5.d. Friends or Family Members

Counselors are prohibited from engaging in counseling relationships with friends or family members with whom they have an inability to remain objective.

A.5.e. Personal Virtual Relationships With Current Clients

Counselors are prohibited from engaging in a personal virtual relationship with individuals with whom they have a current counseling relationship (e.g., through social and other media).

A.6. Managing and Maintaining Boundaries and Professional Relationships

A.6.a. Previous Relationships

Counselors consider the risks and benefits of accepting as clients those with whom they have had a previous relationship. These potential clients may include individuals with whom the counselor has had a casual, distant, or past relationship. Examples include mutual or past membership in a professional association, organization, or community. When counselors accept these clients, they take appropriate professional precautions such as informed consent, consultation, supervision, and documentation to ensure that judgment is not impaired and no exploitation occurs.

A.6.b. Extending Counseling Boundaries

Counselors consider the risks and benefits of extending current counseling relationships beyond conventional parameters. Examples include attending a client's formal ceremony (e.g., a wedding/commitment ceremony or graduation), purchasing a service or product provided by a client (excepting unrestricted bartering), and visiting a client's ill family member in the hospital. In extending these boundaries, counselors take appropriate professional precautions such as informed consent, consultation, supervision, and documentation to ensure that judgment is not impaired and no harm occurs.

A.6.c. Documenting Boundary Extensions

If counselors extend boundaries as described in A.6.a. and A.6.b., they must officially document, prior to the interaction (when feasible), the rationale for such an interaction, the potential benefit, and anticipated consequences for the client or former client and other individuals significantly involved with the client or former client. When unintentional harm occurs to the client or former client, or to an individual significantly involved with the client or former client, the counselor must show evidence of an attempt to remedy such harm.

A.6.d. Role Changes in the Professional Relationship

When counselors change a role from the original or most recent contracted relationship, they obtain informed consent from the client and explain the client's right to refuse services related to the change. Examples of role changes include, but are not limited to

1. changing from individual to relationship or family counseling, or vice versa;

2. changing from an evaluative role to a therapeutic role, or vice versa; and

3. changing from a counselor to a mediator role, or vice versa.

Clients must be fully informed of any anticipated consequences (e.g., financial, legal, personal, therapeutic) of counselor role changes.

A.6.e. Nonprofessional Interactions or Relationships (Other Than Sexual or Romantic Interactions or Relationships)

Counselors avoid entering into non-professional relationships with former clients, their romantic partners, or their family members when the interaction is potentially harmful to the client. This applies to both in-person and electronic interactions or relationships.

A.7. Roles and Relationships at Individual, Group, Institutional, and Societal Levels

A.7.a. Advocacy

When appropriate, counselors advocate at individual, group, institutional, and societal levels to address potential barriers and obstacles that inhibit access and/or the growth and development of clients.

A.7.b. Confidentiality and Advocacy

Counselors obtain client consent prior to engaging in advocacy efforts on behalf of an identifiable client to improve the provision of services and to work toward removal of systemic barriers or obstacles that inhibit client access, growth, and development.

A.8. Multiple Clients

When a counselor agrees to provide counseling services to two or more persons who have a relationship, the counselor clarifies at the outset which person or persons are clients and the nature of the relationships the counselor will have with each involved person. If it becomes apparent that the counselor may be called upon to perform potentially conflicting roles, the counselor will clarify, adjust, or withdraw from roles appropriately.

A.9. Group Work

A.9.a. Screening

Counselors screen prospective group counseling/therapy participants. To the extent possible, counselors select members whose needs and goals are compatible with the goals of the group, who will not impede the group process, and whose well-being will not be jeopardized by the group experience.

A.9.b. Protecting Clients

In a group setting, counselors take reasonable precautions to protect clients from physical, emotional, or psychological trauma.

A.10. Fees and Business Practices

A.10.a. Self-Referral

Counselors working in an organization (e.g., school, agency, institution) that provides counseling services do not refer clients to their private practice unless the policies of a particular organization make explicit provisions for self-referrals. In such instances, the clients must be informed of other options open to them should they seek private counseling services.

A.10.b. Unacceptable Business Practices

Counselors do not participate in fee splitting, nor do they give or receive commissions, rebates, or any other form of remuneration when referring clients for professional services.

A.10.c. Establishing Fees

In establishing fees for professional counseling services, counselors consider the financial status of clients and locality. If a counselor's usual fees create undue hardship for the client, the counselor may adjust fees, when legally permissible, or assist the client in locating comparable, affordable services.

A.10.d. Nonpayment of Fees

If counselors intend to use collection agencies or take legal measures to collect fees from clients who do not pay for services as agreed upon, they include such information in their informed consent documents and also inform clients in a timely fashion of intended actions and offer clients the opportunity to make payment.

A.10.e. Bartering

Counselors may barter only if the bartering does not result in exploitation or harm, if the client requests it, and if such arrangements are an accepted practice among professionals in the community. Counselors consider the cultural implications of bartering and discuss relevant concerns with clients and document such agreements in a clear written contract.

A.10.f. Receiving Gifts

Counselors understand the challenges of accepting gifts from clients and recognize that in some cultures, small gifts are a token of respect and gratitude. When determining whether to accept a gift from clients, counselors take into account the therapeutic relationship, the monetary value of the gift, the client's motivation for giving the gift, and the counselor's motivation for wanting to accept or decline the gift.

A.11. Termination and Referral

A.11.a. Competence Within Termination and Referral

If counselors lack the competence to be of professional assistance to clients, they avoid entering or continuing counseling relationships. Counselors are knowledgeable about culturally and clinically appropriate referral resources and suggest these alternatives. If clients decline the suggested referrals, counselors discontinue the relationship.

A.11.b. Values Within Termination and Referral

Counselors refrain from referring prospective and current clients based solely on the counselor's personally held values, attitudes, beliefs, and behaviors. Counselors respect the diversity of clients and seek training in areas in which they are at risk of imposing their values onto clients, especially when the counselor's values are inconsistent with the client's goals or are discriminatory in nature.

A.11.c. Appropriate Termination

Counselors terminate a counseling relationship when it becomes reasonably apparent that the client no longer needs assistance, is not likely to benefit, or is being harmed by continued counseling. Counselors may terminate counseling when in jeopardy of harm by the client or by another person with whom the client has a relationship, or when clients do not pay fees as agreed upon. Counselors provide pretermination counseling and recommend other service providers when necessary.

A.11.d. Appropriate Transfer of Services

When counselors transfer or refer clients to other practitioners, they ensure that appropriate clinical and administrative processes are completed and open communication is maintained with both clients and practitioners.

A.12. Abandonment and Client Neglect

Counselors do not abandon or neglect clients in counseling. Counselors assist in making appropriate arrangements for the continuation of treatment, when necessary, during interruptions such as vacations, illness, and following termination.

SECTION B: CONFIDENTIALITY AND PRIVACY

Introduction

Counselors recognize that trust is a cornerstone of the counseling relationship. Counselors aspire to earn the trust of clients by creating an ongoing partnership, establishing and upholding appropriate boundaries, and maintaining confidentiality. Counselors communicate the parameters of confidentiality in a culturally competent manner.

B.1. Respecting Client Rights

B.1.a. Multicultural/Diversity Considerations

Counselors maintain awareness and sensitivity regarding cultural meanings of confidentiality and privacy. Counselors respect differing views toward disclosure of information. Counselors hold ongoing discussions with clients as to how, when, and with whom information is to be shared.

B.1.b. Respect for Privacy

Counselors respect the privacy of prospective and current clients. Counselors request private information from clients only when it is beneficial to the counseling process.

B.1.c. Respect for Confidentiality

Counselors protect the confidential information of prospective and current clients. Counselors disclose information only with appropriate consent or with sound legal or ethical justification.

B.1.d. Explanation of Limitations

At initiation and throughout the counseling process, counselors inform clients of the limitations of confidentiality and seek to identify situations in which confidentiality must be breached.

B.2. Exceptions

B.2.a. Serious and Foreseeable Harm and Legal Requirements

The general requirement that counselors keep information confidential does not apply when disclosure is required to protect clients or identified others from serious and foreseeable harm or when legal requirements demand that confidential information must be revealed. Counselors consult with other professionals when in doubt as to the validity of an exception. Additional considerations apply when addressing end-of-life issues.

B.2.b. Confidentiality Regarding End-of-Life Decisions

Counselors who provide services to terminally ill individuals who are considering hastening their own deaths have the option to maintain confidentiality, depending on applicable laws and the specific circumstances of the situation and after seeking consultation or supervision from appropriate professional and legal parties.

B.2.c. Contagious, Life-Threatening Diseases

When clients disclose that they have a disease commonly known to be both communicable and life threatening, counselors may be justified in disclosing information to identifiable third parties, if the parties are known to be at serious and foreseeable risk of contracting the disease. Prior to making a disclosure, counselors assess the intent of clients to inform the third parties about their disease or to engage in any behaviors that may be harmful to an identifiable third party. Counselors adhere to relevant state laws concerning disclosure about disease status.

B.2.d. Court-Ordered Disclosure

When ordered by a court to release confidential or privileged information without a client's permission, counselors seek to obtain written, informed consent from the client or take steps to prohibit the disclosure or have it limited as narrowly as possible because of potential harm to the client or counseling relationship.

B.2.e. Minimal Disclosure

To the extent possible, clients are informed before confidential information is disclosed and are involved in the disclosure decision-making process. When circumstances require the disclosure of confidential information, only essential information is revealed.

B.3. Information Shared With Others

B.3.a. Subordinates

Counselors make every effort to ensure that privacy and confidentiality of clients are maintained by subordinates, including employees, supervisees, students, clerical assistants, and volunteers.

B.3.b. Interdisciplinary Teams

When services provided to the client involve participation by an interdisciplinary or treatment team, the client will be informed of the team's existence and composition, information being shared, and the purposes of sharing such information.

B.3.c. Confidential Settings

Counselors discuss confidential information only in settings in which they can reasonably ensure client privacy.

B.3.d. Third-Party Payers

Counselors disclose information to third-party payers only when clients have authorized such disclosure.

B.3.e. Transmitting Confidential Information

Counselors take precautions to ensure the confidentiality of all information transmitted through the use of any medium.

B.3.f. Deceased Clients

Counselors protect the confidentiality of deceased clients, consistent with legal requirements and the documented preferences of the client.

B.4. Groups and Families

B.4.a. Group Work

In group work, counselors clearly explain the importance and parameters of confidentiality for the specific group.

B.4.b. Couples and Family Counseling

In couples and family counseling, counselors clearly define who is considered "the client" and discuss expectations and limitations of confidentiality. Counselors seek agreement and document in writing such agreement among all involved parties regarding the confidentiality of information. In the absence of an agreement to the contrary, the couple or family is considered to be the client.

B.5. Clients Lacking Capacity to Give Informed Consent

B.5.a. Responsibility to Clients

When counseling minor clients or adult clients who lack the capacity to give voluntary, informed consent, counselors protect the confidentiality of information received—in any medium— in the counseling relationship as specified by federal and state laws, written policies, and applicable ethical standards.

B.5.b. Responsibility to Parents and Legal Guardians

Counselors inform parents and legal guardians about the role of counselors and the confidential nature of the counseling relationship, consistent with current legal and custodial arrangements. Counselors are sensitive to the cultural diversity of families and respect the inherent rights and responsibilities of parents/guardians regarding the welfare of their children/charges according to law. Counselors work to establish, as appropriate, collaborative relationships with parents/guardians to best serve clients.

B.5.c. Release of Confidential Information

When counseling minor clients or adult clients who lack the capacity to give voluntary consent to release confidential information, counselors seek permission from an appropriate third party to disclose information. In such instances, counselors inform clients consistent with their level of understanding and take appropriate measures to safeguard client confidentiality.

B.6. Records and Documentation

B.6.a. Creating and Maintaining Records and Documentation

Counselors create and maintain records and documentation necessary for rendering professional services.

B.6.b. Confidentiality of Records and Documentation

Counselors ensure that records and documentation kept in any medium are secure and that only authorized persons have access to them.

B.6.c. Permission to Record

Counselors obtain permission from clients prior to recording sessions through electronic or other means.

B.6.d. Permission to Observe

Counselors obtain permission from clients prior to allowing any person to observe counseling sessions, review session transcripts, or view recordings of sessions with supervisors, faculty, peers, or others within the training environment.

B.6.e. Client Access

Counselors provide reasonable access to records and copies of records when requested by competent clients. Counselors limit the access of clients to their records, or portions of their records, only when there is compelling evidence that such access would cause harm to the client. Counselors document the request of clients and the rationale for withholding some or all of the records in the files of clients. In situations involving multiple clients, counselors provide individual clients with only those parts of records that relate directly to them and do not include confidential information related to any other client.

B.6.f. Assistance With Records

When clients request access to their records, counselors provide assistance and consultation in interpreting counseling records.

B.6.g. Disclosure or Transfer

Unless exceptions to confidentiality exist, counselors obtain written permission from clients to disclose or transfer records to legitimate third parties. Steps are taken to ensure that receivers of counseling records are sensitive to their confidential nature.

B.6.h. Storage and Disposal After Termination

Counselors store records following termination of services to ensure reasonable future access, maintain records in accordance with federal and state laws and statutes such as licensure laws and policies governing records, and dispose of client records and other sensitive materials in a manner that protects client confidentiality. Counselors apply careful discretion and deliberation before destroying records that may be needed by a court of law, such as notes on child abuse, suicide, sexual harassment, or violence.

B.6.i. Reasonable Precautions

Counselors take reasonable precautions to protect client confidentiality in the event of the counselor's termination of practice, incapacity, or death and appoint a records custodian when identified as appropriate.

B.7. Case Consultation

B.7.a. Respect for Privacy

Information shared in a consulting relationship is discussed for professional purposes only. Written and oral reports present only data germane to the purposes of the consultation, and every effort is made to protect client identity and to avoid undue invasion of privacy.

B.7.b. Disclosure of Confidential Information

When consulting with colleagues, counselors do not disclose confidential information that reasonably could lead to the identification of a client or other person or organization with whom they have a confidential relationship unless they have obtained the prior consent of the person or organization or the disclosure cannot be avoided. They disclose information only to the extent necessary to achieve the purposes of the consultation.

SECTION C: PROFESSIONAL RESPONSIBILITY

Introduction

Counselors aspire to open, honest, and accurate communication in dealing with the public and other professionals. Counselors facilitate access to counseling services, and they practice in a nondiscriminatory manner within the boundaries of professional and personal competence; they also have a responsibility to abide by the *ACA Code of Ethics*. Counselors actively participate in local, state, and national associations that foster the development and improvement of counseling. Counselors are expected to advocate to promote changes at the individual, group, institutional, and societal levels that improve the quality of life for individuals and groups and remove potential barriers to the provision or access of appropriate services being offered. Counselors have a responsibility to the public to engage in counseling practices that are based on rigorous re-search methodologies. Counselors are encouraged to contribute to society by devoting a portion of their professional activity to services for which there is little or no financial return (*pro bono publico*). In addition, counselors engage in self-care activities to maintain and promote their own emotional, physical, mental, and spiritual well-being to best meet their professional responsibilities.

C.1. Knowledge of and Compliance With Standards

Counselors have a responsibility to read, understand, and follow the *ACA Code of Ethics* and adhere to applicable laws and regulations.

C.2. Professional Competence

C.2.a. Boundaries of Competence

Counselors practice only within the boundaries of their competence, based on their education, training, supervised experience, state and national professional credentials, and appropriate professional experience. Whereas multicultural counseling competency is required across all counseling specialties, counselors gain knowledge, personal awareness, sensitivity, dispositions, and skills pertinent to being a culturally competent counselor in working with a diverse client population.

C.2.b. New Specialty Areas of Practice

Counselors practice in specialty areas new to them only after appropriate education, training, and supervised experience. While developing skills in new specialty areas, counselors take steps to ensure the competence of their work and protect others from possible harm.

C.2.c. Qualified for Employment

Counselors accept employment only for positions for which they are qualified given their education, training, supervised experience, state and national professional credentials, and appropriate professional experience. Counselors hire for professional counseling positions only individuals who are qualified and competent for those positions.

C.2.d. Monitor Effectiveness

Counselors continually monitor their effectiveness as professionals and take steps to improve when necessary. Counselors take reasonable steps to seek peer supervision to evaluate their efficacy as counselors.

C.2.e. Consultations on Ethical Obligations

Counselors take reasonable steps to consult with other counselors, the ACA Ethics and Professional Standards Department, or related professionals when they have questions regarding their ethical obligations or professional practice.

C.2.f. Continuing Education

Counselors recognize the need for continuing education to acquire and maintain a reasonable level of awareness of current scientific and professional information in their fields of activity. Counselors maintain their competence in the skills they use, are open to new procedures, and remain informed regarding best practices for working with diverse populations.

C.2.g. Impairment

Counselors monitor themselves for signs of impairment from their own physical, mental, or emotional problems and refrain from offering or providing professional services when impaired. They seek assistance for problems that reach the level of professional impairment, and, if necessary, they limit, suspend, or terminate their professional responsibilities until it is determined that they may safely resume their work. Counselors assist colleagues or supervisors in recognizing their own professional impairment and provide consultation and assistance when warranted with colleagues or supervisors showing signs of impairment and intervene as appropriate to prevent imminent harm to clients.

C.2.h. Counselor Incapacitation, Death, Retirement, or Termination of Practice

Counselors prepare a plan for the transfer of clients and the dissemination of records to an identified colleague or records custodian in the case of the counselor's incapacitation, death, retirement, or termination of practice.

C.3. Advertising and Soliciting Clients

C.3.a. Accurate Advertising

When advertising or otherwise representing their services to the public, counselors identify their credentials in an accurate manner that is not false, misleading, deceptive, or fraudulent.

C.3.b. Testimonials

Counselors who use testimonials do not solicit them from current clients, former clients, or any other persons who may be vulnerable to undue influence. Counselors discuss with clients the implications of and obtain permission for the use of any testimonial.

C.3.c. Statements by Others

When feasible, counselors make reasonable efforts to ensure that statements made by others about them or about the counseling profession are accurate.

C.3.d. Recruiting Through Employment

Counselors do not use their places of employment or institutional affiliation to recruit clients, supervisors, or consultees for their private practices.

C.3.e. Products and Training Advertisements

Counselors who develop products related to their profession or conduct workshops or training events ensure that the advertisements concerning these products or events are accurate and disclose adequate information for consumers to make informed choices.

C.3.f. Promoting to Those Served

Counselors do not use counseling, teaching, training, or supervisory relationships to promote their products or training events in a manner that is deceptive or would exert undue influence on individuals who may be vulnerable. However, counselor educators may adopt textbooks they have authored for instructional purposes.

C.4. Professional Qualifications

C.4.a. Accurate Representation

Counselors claim or imply only professional qualifications actually completed and correct any known misrepresentations of their qualifications by others. Counselors truthfully represent the qualifications of their professional colleagues. Counselors clearly distinguish between paid and volunteer work experience and accurately describe their continuing education and specialized training.

C.4.b. Credentials

Counselors claim only licenses or certifications that are current and in good standing.

C.4.c. Educational Degrees

Counselors clearly differentiate between earned and honorary degrees.

C.4.d. Implying Doctoral-Level Competence

Counselors clearly state their highest earned degree in counseling or a closely related field. Counselors do not imply doctoral-level competence when possessing a master's degree in counseling or a related field by referring to themselves as "Dr." in a counseling context when their doctorate is not in counseling or a related field. Counselors do not use "ABD" (all but dissertation) or other such terms to imply competency.

C.4.e. Accreditation Status

Counselors accurately represent the accreditation status of their degree program and college/university.

C.4.f. Professional Membership

Counselors clearly differentiate between current, active memberships and former memberships in associations. Members of ACA must clearly differentiate between professional membership, which implies the possession of at least a master's degree in counseling, and regular membership, which is open to individuals whose interests and activities are consistent with those of ACA but are not qualified for professional membership.

C.5. Nondiscrimination

Counselors do not condone or engage in discrimination against prospective or current clients, students, employees, supervisees, or research participants based on age, culture, disability, ethnicity, race, religion/spirituality, gender, gender identity, sexual orientation, marital/ partnership status, language preference, socioeconomic status, immigration status, or any basis proscribed by law.

C.6. Public Responsibility

C.6.a. Sexual Harassment

Counselors do not engage in or condone sexual harassment. Sexual harassment can consist of a single intense or severe act, or multiple persistent or pervasive acts.

C.6.b. Reports to Third Parties

Counselors are accurate, honest, and objective in reporting their professional activities and judgments to appropriate third parties, including courts, health insurance companies, those who are the recipients of evaluation reports, and others.

C.6.c. Media Presentations

When counselors provide advice or comment by means of public lectures, demonstrations, radio or television programs, recordings, technology-based applications, printed articles, mailed material, or other media, they take reasonable precautions to ensure that

1. the statements are based on appropriate professional counseling literature and practice,

2. the statements are otherwise consistent with the *ACA Code of Ethics*, and

3. the recipients of the information are not encouraged to infer that a professional counseling relationship has been established.

C.6.d. Exploitation of Others

Counselors do not exploit others in their professional relationships.

C.6.e. Contributing to the Public Good (Pro Bono Publico)

Counselors make a reasonable effort to provide services to the public for which there is little or no financial return (e.g., speaking to groups, sharing professional information, offering reduced fees).

C.7. Treatment Modalities

C.7.a. Scientific Basis for Treatment

When providing services, counselors use techniques/procedures/modalities that are grounded in theory and/or have an empirical or scientific foundation.

C.7.b. Development and Innovation

When counselors use developing or innovative techniques/procedures/modalities, they explain the potential risks, benefits, and ethical considerations of using such techniques/procedures/modalities. Counselors work to minimize any potential risks or harm when using these techniques/procedures/modalities.

C.7.c. Harmful Practices

Counselors do not use techniques/procedures/modalities when substantial evidence suggests harm, even if such services are requested.

C.8. Responsibility to Other Professionals

C.8.a. Personal Public Statements

When making personal statements in a public context, counselors clarify that they are speaking from their personal perspectives and that they are not speaking on behalf of all counselors or the profession.

SECTION D: RELATIONSHIPS WITH OTHER PROFESSIONALS

Introduction

Professional counselors recognize that the quality of their interactions with colleagues can influence the quality of services provided to clients. They work to become knowledgeable about colleagues within and outside the field of counseling. Counselors develop positive working relationships and systems of communication with colleagues to enhance services to clients.

D.1. Relationships With Colleagues, Employers, and Employees

D.1.a. Different Approaches

Counselors are respectful of approaches that are grounded in theory and/or have an empirical or scientific foundation but may differ from their own. Counselors acknowledge the expertise of other professional groups and are respectful of their practices.

D.1.b. Forming Relationships

Counselors work to develop and strengthen relationships with colleagues from other disciplines to best serve clients.

D.1.c. Interdisciplinary Teamwork

Counselors who are members of interdisciplinary teams delivering multifaceted services to clients remain focused on how to best serve clients. They participate in and contribute to decisions that affect the well-being of clients by drawing on the perspectives, values, and experiences of the counseling profession and those of colleagues from other disciplines.

D.1.d. Establishing Professional and Ethical Obligations

Counselors who are members of interdisciplinary teams work together with team members to clarify professional and ethical obligations of the team as a whole and of its individual members. When a team decision raises ethical concerns, counselors first attempt to resolve the concern within the team. If they cannot reach resolution among team members, counselors pursue other avenues to address their concerns consistent with client well-being.

D.1.e. Confidentiality

When counselors are required by law, institutional policy, or extraordinary circumstances to serve in more than one role in judicial or administrative proceedings, they clarify role expectations and the parameters of confidentiality with their colleagues.

D.1.f. Personnel Selection and Assignment

When counselors are in a position requiring personnel selection and/or assigning of responsibilities to others, they select competent staff and assign responsibilities compatible with their skills and experiences.

D.1.g. Employer Policies

The acceptance of employment in an agency or institution implies that counselors are in agreement with its general policies and principles. Counselors strive to reach agreement with employers regarding acceptable standards of client care and professional conduct that allow for changes in institutional policy conducive to the growth and development of clients.

D.1.h. Negative Conditions

Counselors alert their employers of inappropriate policies and practices. They attempt to effect changes in such policies or procedures through constructive action within the organization. When such policies are potentially disruptive or damaging to clients or may limit the effectiveness of services provided and change cannot be affected, counselors take appropriate further action. Such action may include referral to appropriate certification, accreditation, or state licensure organizations, or voluntary termination of employment.

D.1.i. Protection From Punitive Action

Counselors do not harass a colleague or employee or dismiss an employee who has acted in a responsible and ethical manner to expose inappropriate employer policies or practices.

D.2. Provision of Consultation Services

D.2.a. Consultant Competency

Counselors take reasonable steps to ensure that they have the appropriate resources and competencies when providing consultation services. Counselors provide appropriate referral resources when requested or needed.

D.2.b. Informed Consent in Formal Consultation

When providing formal consultation services, counselors have an obligation to review, in writing and verbally, the rights and responsibilities of both counselors and consultees. Counselors use clear and understandable language to inform all parties involved about the purpose of the services to be provided, relevant costs, potential risks and benefits, and the limits of confidentiality.

SECTION E: EVALUATION, ASSESSMENT, AND INTERPRETATION

Introduction

Counselors use assessment as one component of the counseling process, taking into account the clients' personal and cultural context. Counselors promote the well-being of individual clients or groups of clients by developing and using appropriate educational, mental health, psychological, and career assessments.

E.1. General

E.1.a. Assessment

The primary purpose of educational, mental health, psychological, and career assessment is to gather information regarding the client for a variety of purposes, including, but not limited to, client decision making, treatment planning, and forensic proceedings. Assessment may include both qualitative and quantitative methodologies.

E.1.b. Client Welfare

Counselors do not misuse assessment results and interpretations, and they take reasonable steps to prevent others from misusing the information provided. They respect the client's right to know the results, the interpretations made, and the bases for counselors' conclusions and recommendations.

E.2. Competence to Use and Interpret Assessment Instruments

E.2.a. Limits of Competence

Counselors use only those testing and assessment services for which they have been trained and are competent. Counselors using technology-assisted test interpretations are trained in the construct being measured and the specific instrument being used prior to using its technology-based application. Counselors take reasonable measures to ensure the proper use of assessment techniques by persons under their supervision.

E.2.b. Appropriate Use

Counselors are responsible for the appropriate application, scoring, interpretation, and use of assessment instruments relevant to the needs of the client, whether they score and interpret such assessments themselves or use technology or other services.

E.2.c. Decisions Based on Results

Counselors responsible for decisions involving individuals or policies that are based on assessment results have a thorough understanding of psychometrics.

E.3. Informed Consent in Assessment

E.3.a. Explanation to Clients

Prior to assessment, counselors explain the nature and purposes of assessment and the specific use of results by potential recipients. The explanation will be given in terms and language that the client (or other legally authorized person on behalf of the client) can understand.

E.3.b. Recipients of Results

Counselors consider the client's and/or examinee's welfare, explicit understandings, and prior agreements in determining who receives the assessment results. Counselors include accurate and appropriate interpretations with any release of individual or group assessment results.

E.4. Release of Data to Qualified Personnel

Counselors release assessment data in which the client is identified only with the consent of the client or the client's legal representative. Such data are released only to persons recognized by counselors as qualified to interpret the data.

E.5. Diagnosis of Mental Disorders

E.5.a. Proper Diagnosis

Counselors take special care to provide proper diagnosis of mental disorders. Assessment techniques (including personal interviews) used to determine client care (e.g., locus of treatment, type of treatment, recommended follow-up) are carefully selected and appropriately used.

E.5.b. Cultural Sensitivity

Counselors recognize that culture affects the manner in which clients' problems are defined and experienced. Clients' socioeconomic and cultural experiences are considered when diagnosing mental disorders.

E.5.c. Historical and Social Prejudices in the Diagnosis of Pathology

Counselors recognize historical and social prejudices in the misdiagnosis and pathologizing of certain individuals and groups and strive to become aware of and address such biases in themselves or others.

E.5.d. Refraining From Diagnosis

Counselors may refrain from making and/or reporting a diagnosis if they believe that it would cause harm to the client or others. Counselors carefully consider both the positive and negative implications of a diagnosis.

E.6. Instrument Selection

E.6.a. Appropriateness of Instruments

Counselors carefully consider the validity, reliability, psychometric limitations, and appropriateness of instruments when selecting assessments and, when possible, use multiple forms of assessment, data, and/or instruments in forming conclusions, diagnoses, or recommendations.

E.6.b. Referral Information

If a client is referred to a third party for assessment, the counselor provides specific referral questions and sufficient objective data about the client to ensure that appropriate assessment instruments are utilized.

E.7. Conditions of Assessment Administration

E.7.a. Administration Conditions

Counselors administer assessments under the same conditions that were established in their standardization. When assessments are not administered under standard conditions, as may be necessary to accommodate clients with disabilities, or when unusual behavior or irregularities occur during the administration, those conditions are noted in interpretation, and the results may be designated as invalid or of questionable validity.

E.7.b. Provision of Favorable Conditions

Counselors provide an appropriate environment for the administration of assessments (e.g., privacy, comfort, freedom from distraction).

E.7.c. Technological Administration

Counselors ensure that technologically administered assessments function properly and provide clients with accurate results.

E.7.d. Unsupervised Assessments

Unless the assessment instrument is designed, intended, and validated for self-administration and/or scoring, counselors do not permit unsupervised use.

E.8. Multicultural Issues/Diversity in Assessment

Counselors select and use with caution assessment techniques normed on populations other than that of the client. Counselors recognize the effects of age, color, culture, disability, ethnic group, gender, race, language preference, religion, spirituality, sexual orientation, and socioeconomic status on test administration and interpretation, and they place test results in proper perspective with other relevant factors.

E.9. Scoring and Interpretation of Assessments

E.9.a. Reporting

When counselors report assessment results, they consider the client's personal and cultural background, the level of the client's understanding of the results, and the impact of the results on the client. In reporting assessment results, counselors indicate reservations that exist regarding validity or reliability due to circumstances of the assessment or inappropriateness of the norms for the person tested.

E.9.b. Instruments With Insufficient Empirical Data

Counselors exercise caution when interpreting the results of instruments not having sufficient empirical data to support respondent results. The specific purposes for the use of such instruments are stated explicitly to the examinee. Counselors qualify any conclusions, diagnoses, or recommendations made that are based on assessments or instruments with questionable validity or reliability.

E.9.c. Assessment Services

Counselors who provide assessment, scoring, and interpretation services to support the assessment process confirm the validity of such interpretations. They accurately describe the purpose, norms, validity, reliability, and applications of the procedures and any special qualifications applicable to their use. At all times, counselors maintain their ethical responsibility to those being assessed.

E.10. Assessment Security

Counselors maintain the integrity and security of tests and assessments consistent with legal and contractual obligations. Counselors do not appropriate, reproduce, or modify published assessments or parts thereof without acknowledgment and permission from the publisher.

E.11. Obsolete Assessment and Outdated Results

Counselors do not use data or results from assessments that are obsolete or outdated for the current purpose (e.g., noncurrent versions of assessments/instruments). Counselors make every effort to prevent the misuse of obsolete measures and assessment data by others.

E.12. Assessment Construction

Counselors use established scientific procedures, relevant standards, and current professional knowledge for assessment design in the development, publication, and utilization of assessment techniques.

E.13. Forensic Evaluation: Evaluation for Legal Proceedings

E.13.a. Primary Obligations

When providing forensic evaluations, the primary obligation of counselors is to produce objective findings that can be substantiated based on information and techniques appropriate to the evaluation, which may include examination of the individual and/or review of records. Counselors form professional opinions based on their professional knowledge and expertise that can be supported by the data gathered in evaluations. Counselors define the limits of their reports or testimony, especially when an examination of the individual has not been conducted.

E.13.b. Consent for Evaluation

Individuals being evaluated are informed in writing that the relationship is for the purposes of an evaluation and is not therapeutic in nature, and entities or individuals who will receive the evaluation report are identified. Counselors who perform forensic evaluations obtain written consent from those being evaluated or from their legal representative unless a court orders evaluations to be conducted without the written consent of the individuals being evaluated. When children or adults who lack the capacity to give voluntary consent are being evaluated, informed written consent is obtained from a parent or guardian.

E.13.c. Client Evaluation Prohibited

Counselors do not evaluate current or former clients, clients' romantic partners, or clients' family members for forensic purposes. Counselors do not counsel individuals they are evaluating.

E.13.d. Avoid Potentially Harmful Relationships

Counselors who provide forensic evaluations avoid potentially harmful professional or personal relationships with family members, romantic partners, and close friends of individuals they are evaluating or have evaluated in the past.

SECTION F: SUPERVISION, TRAINING, AND TEACHING

Introduction

Counselor supervisors, trainers, and educators aspire to foster meaningful and respectful professional relationships and to maintain appropriate boundaries with supervisees and students in both face-to-face and electronic formats. They have theoretical and pedagogical foundations for their work; have knowledge of supervision models; and aim to be fair, accurate, and honest in their assessments of counselors, students, and supervisees.

F.1. Counselor Supervision and Client Welfare

F.1.a. Client Welfare

A primary obligation of counseling supervisors is to monitor the services provided by supervisees. Counseling supervisors monitor client welfare and supervisee performance and professional development. To fulfill these obligations, supervisors meet regularly with supervisees to review the supervisees' work and help them become prepared to serve a range of diverse clients. Supervisees have a responsibility to understand and follow the *ACA Code of Ethics*.

F.1.b. Counselor Credentials

Counseling supervisors work to ensure that supervisees communicate their qualifications to render services to their clients.

F.1.c. Informed Consent and Client Rights

Supervisors make supervisees aware of client rights, including the protection of client privacy and confidentiality in the counseling relationship. Supervisees provide clients with professional disclosure information and inform them of how the supervision process influences the limits of confidentiality. Supervisees make clients aware of who will have access to records of the counseling relationship and how these records will be stored, transmitted, or otherwise reviewed.

F.2. Counselor Supervision Competence

F.2.a. Supervisor Preparation

Prior to offering supervision services, counselors are trained in supervision methods and techniques. Counselors who offer supervision services regularly pursue continuing education activities, including both counseling and supervision topics and skills.

F.2.b. Multicultural Issues/Diversity in Supervision

Counseling supervisors are aware of and address the role of multiculturalism/diversity in the supervisory relationship.

F.2.c. Online Supervision

When using technology in supervision, counselor supervisors are competent in the use of those technologies. Supervisors take the necessary precautions to protect the confidentiality of all information transmitted through any electronic means.

F.3. Supervisory Relationship

F.3.a. Extending Conventional Supervisory Relationships

Counseling supervisors clearly define and maintain ethical professional, personal, and social relationships with their supervisees. Supervisors consider the risks and benefits of extending current supervisory relationships in any form beyond conventional parameters. In extending these boundaries, supervisors take appropriate professional precautions to ensure that judgment is not impaired and that no harm occurs.

F.3.b. Sexual Relationships

Sexual or romantic interactions or relationships with current supervisees are prohibited. This prohibition applies to both in-person and electronic interactions or relationships.

F.3.c. Sexual Harassment

Counseling supervisors do not condone or subject supervisees to sexual harassment.

F.3.d. Friends or Family Members

Supervisors are prohibited from engaging in supervisory relationships with individuals with whom they have an inability to remain objective.

F.4. Supervisor Responsibilities

F.4.a. Informed Consent for Supervision

Supervisors are responsible for incorporating into their supervision the principles of informed consent and participation. Supervisors inform supervisees of the policies and procedures to which supervisors are to adhere and the mechanisms for due process appeal of individual supervisor actions. The issues unique to the use of distance supervision are to be included in the documentation as necessary.

F.4.b. Emergencies and Absences

Supervisors establish and communicate to supervisees procedures for contacting supervisors or, in their absence, alternative on-call supervisors to assist in handling crises.

F.4.c. Standards for Supervisees

Supervisors make their supervisees aware of professional and ethical standards and legal responsibilities.

F.4.d. Termination of the Supervisory Relationship

Supervisors or supervisees have the right to terminate the supervisory relationship with adequate notice. Reasons for considering termination are discussed, and both parties work to resolve differences. When termination is warranted, supervisors make appropriate referrals to possible alternative supervisors.

F.5. Student and Supervisee Responsibilities

F.5.a. Ethical Responsibilities

Students and supervisees have a responsibility to understand and follow the *ACA Code of Ethics*. Students and supervisees have the same obligation to clients as those required of professional counselors.

F.5.b. Impairment

Students and supervisees monitor themselves for signs of impairment from their own physical, mental, or emotional problems and refrain from offering or providing professional services when such impairment is likely to harm a client or others. They notify their faculty and/or supervisors and seek assistance for problems that reach the level of professional impairment, and, if necessary, they limit, suspend, or terminate their professional responsibilities until it is determined that they may safely resume their work.

F.5.c. Professional Disclosure

Before providing counseling services, students and supervisees disclose their status as supervisees and explain how this status affects the limits of confidentiality. Supervisors ensure that clients are aware of the services rendered and the qualifications of the students and supervisees rendering those services. Students and supervisees obtain client permission before they use any information concerning the counseling relationship in the training process.

F.6. Counseling Supervision Evaluation, Remediation, and Endorsement

F.6.a. Evaluation

Supervisors document and provide supervisees with ongoing feedback regarding their performance and schedule periodic formal evaluative sessions throughout the supervisory relationship.

F.6.b. Gatekeeping and Remediation

Through initial and ongoing evaluation, supervisors are aware of supervisee limitations that might impede performance. Supervisors assist supervisees in securing remedial assistance when needed. They recommend dismissal from training programs, applied counseling settings, and state or voluntary professional credentialing processes when those supervisees are unable to demonstrate that they can provide competent professional services to a range of diverse clients. Supervisors seek consultation and document their decisions to dismiss or refer supervisees for assistance. They ensure that supervisees are aware of options available to them to address such decisions.

F.6.c. Counseling for Supervisees

If supervisees request counseling, the supervisor assists the supervisee in identifying appropriate services. Supervisors do not provide counseling services to supervisees. Supervisors address interpersonal competencies in terms of the impact of these issues on clients, the supervisory relationship, and professional functioning.

F.6.d. Endorsements

Supervisors endorse supervisees for certification, licensure, employment, or completion of an academic or training program only when they believe that supervisees are qualified for the endorsement. Regardless of qualifications, supervisors do not endorse supervisees whom they believe to be impaired in any way that would interfere with the performance of the duties associated with the endorsement.

F.7. Responsibilities of Counselor Educators

F.7.a. Counselor Educators

Counselor educators who are responsible for developing, implementing, and supervising educational programs are skilled as teachers and practitioners. They are knowledgeable regarding the ethical, legal, and regulatory aspects of the profession; are skilled in applying that knowledge; and make students and supervisees aware of their responsibilities. Whether in traditional, hybrid, and/or online formats, counselor educators conduct counselor education and training programs in an ethical manner and serve as role models for professional behavior.

F.7.b. Counselor Educator Competence

Counselors who function as counselor educators or supervisors provide instruction within their areas of knowledge and competence and provide instruction based on current information and knowledge available in the profession. When using technology to deliver instruction, counselor educators develop competence in the use of the technology.

F.7.c. Infusing Multicultural Issues/Diversity

Counselor educators infuse material related to multiculturalism/diversity into all courses and workshops for the development of professional counselors.

F.7.d. Integration of Study and Practice

In traditional, hybrid, and/or online formats, counselor educators establish education and training programs that integrate academic study and supervised practice.

F.7.e. Teaching Ethics

Throughout the program, counselor educators ensure that students are aware of the ethical responsibilities and standards of the profession and the ethical responsibilities of students to the profession. Counselor educators infuse ethical considerations throughout the curriculum.

F.7.f. Use of Case Examples

The use of client, student, or supervisee information for the purposes of case examples in a lecture or classroom setting is permissible only when (a) the client, student, or supervisee has reviewed the material and agreed to its presentation or (b) the information has been sufficiently modified to obscure identity.

F.7.g. Student-to-Student Supervision and Instruction

When students function in the role of counselor educators or supervisors, they understand that they have the same ethical obligations as counselor educators, trainers, and supervisors. Counselor educators make every effort to ensure that the rights of students are not compromised when their peers lead experiential counseling activities in traditional, hybrid, and/or online formats (e.g., counseling groups, skills classes, clinical supervision).

F.7.h. Innovative Theories and Techniques

Counselor educators promote the use of techniques/procedures/modalities that are grounded in theory and/or have an empirical or scientific foundation. When counselor educators discuss developing or innovative techniques/procedures/modalities, they explain the potential risks, benefits, and ethical considerations of using such techniques/ procedures/modalities.

F.7.i. Field Placements

Counselor educators develop clear policies and provide direct assistance within their training programs regarding appropriate field placement and other clinical experiences. Counselor educators provide clearly stated roles and responsibilities for the student or supervisee, the site supervisor, and the program supervisor. They confirm that site supervisors are qualified to provide supervision in the formats in which services are provided and inform site supervisors of their professional and ethical responsibilities in this role.

F.8. Student Welfare

F.8.a. Program Information and Orientation

Counselor educators recognize that program orientation is a developmental process that begins upon students' initial contact with the counselor education program and continues throughout the educational and clinical training of students. Counselor education faculty provide prospective and current students with information about the counselor education program's expectations, including

1. the values and ethical principles of the profession;
2. the type and level of skill and knowledge acquisition required for successful completion of the training;
3. technology requirements;
4. program training goals, objectives, and mission, and subject matter to be covered;
5. bases for evaluation;
6. training components that encourage self-growth or self-disclosure as part of the training process;
7. the type of supervision settings and requirements of the sites for required clinical field experiences;
8. student and supervisor evaluation and dismissal policies and procedures; and
9. up-to-date employment prospects for graduates.

F.8.b. Student Career Advising

Counselor educators provide career advisement for their students and make them aware of opportunities in the field.

F.8.c. Self-Growth Experiences

Self-growth is an expected component of counselor education. Counselor educators are mindful of ethical principles when they require students to engage in self-growth experiences. Counselor educators and supervisors inform students that they have a right to decide what information will be shared or withheld in class.

F.8.d. Addressing Personal Concerns

Counselor educators may require students to address any personal concerns that have the potential to affect professional competency.

F.9. Evaluation and Remediation

F.9.a. Evaluation of Students

Counselor educators clearly state to students, prior to and throughout the training program, the levels of competency expected, appraisal methods, and timing of evaluations for both didactic and clinical competencies. Counselor educators provide students with ongoing feedback regarding their performance throughout the training program.

F.9.b. Limitations

Counselor educators, through ongoing evaluation, are aware of and address the inability of some students to achieve counseling competencies. Counselor educators do the following:

1. assist students in securing remedial assistance when needed,

2. seek professional consultation and document their decision to dismiss or refer students for assistance, and

3. ensure that students have recourse in a timely manner to address decisions requiring them to seek assistance or to dismiss them and provide students with due process according to institutional policies and procedures.

F.9.c. Counseling for Students

If students request counseling, or if counseling services are suggested as part of a remediation process, counselor educators assist students in identifying appropriate services.

F.10. Roles and Relationships
Between Counselor Educators and Students

F.10.a. Sexual or Romantic Relationships

Counselor educators are prohibited from sexual or romantic interactions or relationships with students currently enrolled in a counseling or related program and over whom they have power and authority. This prohibition applies to both in-person and electronic interactions or relationships.

F.10.b. Sexual Harassment

Counselor educators do not condone or subject students to sexual harassment.

F.10.c. Relationships With Former Students

Counselor educators are aware of the power differential in the relationship between faculty and students. Faculty members discuss with former students potential risks when they consider engaging in social, sexual, or other intimate relationships.

F.10.d. Nonacademic Relationships

Counselor educators avoid nonacademic relationships with students in which there is a risk of potential harm to the student or which may compromise the training experience or grades assigned. In addition, counselor educators do not accept any form of professional services, fees, commissions, reimbursement, or remuneration from a site for student or supervisor placement.

F.10.e. Counseling Services

Counselor educators do not serve as counselors to students currently enrolled in a counseling or related program and over whom they have power and authority.

F.10.f. Extending Educator–Student Boundaries

Counselor educators are aware of the power differential in the relationship between faculty and students. If they believe that a nonprofessional relationship with a student may be potentially beneficial to the student, they take precautions similar to those taken by counselors when working with clients. Examples of potentially beneficial interactions or relationships include, but are not limited to, attending a formal ceremony; conducting hospital visits; providing support during a stressful event; or maintaining mutual membership in a professional association, organization, or community. Counselor educators discuss with students the rationale for such interactions, the potential benefits and drawbacks, and the anticipated consequences for the student. Educators clarify the specific nature and limitations of the additional role(s) they will have with the student prior to engaging in a nonprofessional relationship. Nonprofessional relationships with students should be time limited and/or context specific and initiated with student consent.

F.11. Multicultural/Diversity Competence in Counselor Education and Training Programs

F.11.a. Faculty Diversity

Counselor educators are committed to recruiting and retaining a diverse faculty.

F.11.b. Student Diversity

Counselor educators actively attempt to recruit and retain a diverse student body. Counselor educators demonstrate commitment to multicultural/diversity competence by recognizing and valuing the diverse cultures and types of abilities that students bring to the training experience. Counselor educators provide appropriate accommodations that enhance and support diverse student well-being and academic performance.

F.11.c. Multicultural/Diversity Competence

Counselor educators actively infuse multicultural/diversity competency in their training and supervision practices. They actively train students to gain awareness, knowledge, and skills in the competencies of multicultural practice.

SECTION G: RESEARCH AND PUBLICATION

Introduction

Counselors who conduct research are encouraged to contribute to the knowledge base of the profession and promote a clearer understanding of the conditions that lead to a healthy and more just society. Counselors support the efforts of researchers by participating fully and willingly whenever possible. Counselors minimize bias and respect diversity in designing and implementing research.

G.1. Research Responsibilities

G.1.a. Conducting Research

Counselors plan, design, conduct, and report research in a manner that is consistent with pertinent ethical principles, federal and state laws, host institutional regulations, and scientific standards governing research.

G.1.b. Confidentiality in Research

Counselors are responsible for understanding and adhering to state, federal, agency, or institutional policies or applicable guidelines regarding confidentiality in their research practices.

G.1.c. Independent Researchers

When counselors conduct independent research and do not have access to an institutional review board, they are bound to the same ethical principles and federal and state laws pertaining to the review of their plan, design, conduct, and reporting of research.

G.1.d. Deviation From Standard Practice

Counselors seek consultation and observe stringent safeguards to protect the rights of research participants when research indicates that a deviation from standard or acceptable practices may be necessary.

G.1.e. Precautions to Avoid Injury

Counselors who conduct research are responsible for their participants' welfare throughout the research process and should take reasonable precautions to avoid causing emotional, physical, or social harm to participants.

G.1.f. Principal Researcher Responsibility

The ultimate responsibility for ethical research practice lies with the principal researcher. All others involved in the research activities share ethical obligations and responsibility for their own actions.

G.2. Rights of Research Participants

G.2.a. Informed Consent in Research

Individuals have the right to decline requests to become research participants. In seeking consent, counselors use language that

1. accurately explains the purpose and procedures to be followed;

2. identifies any procedures that are experimental or relatively untried;

3. describes any attendant discomforts, risks, and potential power differentials between researchers and participants;

4. describes any benefits or changes in individuals or organizations that might reasonably be expected;

5. discloses appropriate alternative procedures that would be advantageous for participants;

6. offers to answer any inquiries concerning the procedures;

7. describes any limitations on confidentiality;

8. describes the format and potential target audiences for the dissemination of research findings; and

9. instructs participants that they are free to withdraw their consent and discontinue participation in the project at any time, without penalty.

G.2.b. Student/Supervisee Participation

Researchers who involve students or supervisees in research make clear to them that the decision regarding participation in research activities does not affect their academic standing or supervisory relationship. Students or supervisees who choose not to participate in research are provided with an appropriate alternative to fulfill their academic or clinical requirements.

G.2.c. Client Participation

Counselors conducting research involving clients make clear in the informed consent process that clients are free to choose whether to participate in research activities. Counselors take necessary precautions to protect clients from adverse consequences of declining or withdrawing from participation.

G.2.d. Confidentiality of Information

Information obtained about research participants during the course of research is confidential. Procedures are implemented to protect confidentiality.

G.2.e. Persons Not Capable of Giving Informed Consent

When a research participant is not capable of giving informed consent, counselors provide an appropriate explanation to, obtain agreement for participation from, and obtain the appropriate consent of a legally authorized person.

G.2.f. Commitments to Participants

Counselors take reasonable measures to honor all commitments to research participants.

G.2.g. Explanations After Data Collection

After data are collected, counselors provide participants with full clarification of the nature of the study to remove any misconceptions participants might have regarding the research. Where scientific or human values justify delaying or withholding information, counselors take reasonable measures to avoid causing harm.

G.2.h. Informing Sponsors

Counselors inform sponsors, institutions, and publication channels regarding research procedures and outcomes. Counselors ensure that appropriate bodies and authorities are given pertinent information and acknowledgment.

G.2.i. Research Records Custodian

As appropriate, researchers prepare and disseminate to an identified colleague or records custodian a plan for the transfer of research data in the case of their incapacitation, retirement, or death.

G.3. Managing and Maintaining Boundaries

G.3.a. Extending Researcher–Participant Boundaries

Researchers consider the risks and benefits of extending current research relationships beyond conventional parameters. When a nonresearch interaction between the researcher and the research participant may be potentially beneficial, the researcher must document, prior to the interaction (when feasible), the rationale for such an interaction, the potential benefit, and anticipated consequences for the research participant. Such interactions should be initiated with appropriate consent of the research participant. Where unintentional harm occurs to the research participant, the researcher must show evidence of an attempt to remedy such harm.

G.3.b. Relationships With Research Participants

Sexual or romantic counselor–research participant interactions or relationships with current research participants are prohibited. This prohibition applies to both in-person and electronic interactions or relationships.

G.3.c. Sexual Harassment and Research Participants

Researchers do not condone or subject research participants to sexual harassment.

G.4. Reporting Results

G.4.a. Accurate Results

Counselors plan, conduct, and report research accurately. Counselors do not engage in misleading or fraudulent research, distort data, misrepresent data, or deliberately bias their results. They describe the extent to which results are applicable for diverse populations.

G.4.b. Obligation to Report Unfavorable Results

Counselors report the results of any research of professional value. Results that reflect unfavorably on institutions, programs, services, prevailing opinions, or vested interests are not withheld.

G.4.c. Reporting Errors

If counselors discover significant errors in their published research, they take reasonable steps to correct such errors in a correction erratum or through other appropriate publication means.

G.4.d. Identity of Participants

Counselors who supply data, aid in the research of another person, report research results, or make original data available take due care to disguise the identity of respective participants in the absence of specific authorization from the participants to do otherwise. In situations where participants self-identify their involvement in research studies, researchers take active steps to ensure that data are adapted/changed to protect the identity and welfare of all parties and that discussion of results does not cause harm to participants.

G.4.e. Replication Studies

Counselors are obligated to make available sufficient original research information to qualified professionals who may wish to replicate or extend the study.

G.5. Publications and Presentations

G.5.a. Use of Case Examples

The use of participants', clients', students', or supervisees' information for the purpose of case examples in a presentation or publication is permissible only when (a) participants, clients, students, or supervisees have reviewed the material and agreed to its presentation or publication or (b) the information has been sufficiently modified to obscure identity.

G.5.b. Plagiarism

Counselors do not plagiarize; that is, they do not present another person's work as their own.

G.5.c. Acknowledging Previous Work

In publications and presentations, counselors acknowledge and give recognition to previous work on the topic by others or self.

G.5.d. Contributors

Counselors give credit through joint authorship, acknowledgment, foot-note statements, or other appropriate means to those who have contributed significantly to research or concept development in accordance with such contributions. The principal contributor is listed first, and minor technical or professional contributions are acknowledged in notes or introductory statements.

G.5.e. Agreement of Contributors

Counselors who conduct joint research with colleagues or students/supervisors establish agreements in advance regarding allocation of tasks, publication credit, and types of acknowledgment that will be received.

G.5.f. Student Research

Manuscripts or professional presentations in any medium that are substantially based on a student's course papers, projects, dissertations, or theses are used only with the student's permission and list the student as lead author.

G.5.g. Duplicate Submissions

Counselors submit manuscripts for consideration to only one journal at a time. Manuscripts that are published in whole or in substantial part in one journal or published work are not submitted for publication to another publisher without acknowledgment and permission from the original publisher.

G.5.h. Professional Review

Counselors who review material submitted for publication, research, or other scholarly purposes respect the confidentiality and proprietary rights of those who submitted it. Counselors make publication decisions based on valid and defensible standards. Counselors review article submissions in a timely manner and based on their scope and competency in research methodologies. Counselors who serve as reviewers at the request of editors or publishers make every effort to only review materials that are within their scope of competency and avoid personal biases.

SECTION H: DISTANCE COUNSELING, TECHNOLOGY, AND SOCIAL MEDIA

Introduction

Counselors understand that the profession of counseling may no longer be limited to in-person, face-to-face interactions. Counselors actively attempt to understand the evolving nature of the profession with regard to distance counseling, technology, and social media and how such resources may be used to better serve their clients. Counselors strive to become knowledgeable about these resources. Counselors understand the additional concerns related to the use of distance counseling, technology, and social media and make every attempt to protect confidentiality and meet any legal and ethical requirements for the use of such resources.

H.1. Knowledge and Legal Considerations

H.1.a. Knowledge and Competency

Counselors who engage in the use of distance counseling, technology, and/or social media develop knowledge and skills regarding related technical, ethical, and legal considerations (e.g., special certifications, additional course work).

H.1.b. Laws and Statutes

Counselors who engage in the use of distance counseling, technology, and social media within their counseling practice understand that they may be subject to laws and regulations of both the counselor's practicing location and the client's place of residence. Counselors ensure that their clients are aware of pertinent legal rights and limitations governing the practice of counseling across state lines or international boundaries.

H.2. Informed Consent and Security

H.2.a. Informed Consent and Disclosure

Clients have the freedom to choose whether to use distance counseling, social media, and/or technology within the counseling process. In addition to the usual and customary protocol of informed consent between counselor and client for face-to-face counseling, the following issues, unique to the use of distance counseling, technology, and/or social media, are addressed in the informed consent process:

- distance counseling credentials, physical location of practice, and contact information;
- risks and benefits of engaging in the use of distance counseling, technology, and/or social media;
- possibility of technology failure and alternate methods of service delivery;
- anticipated response time;
- emergency procedures to follow when the counselor is not available;
- time zone differences;
- cultural and/or language differences that may affect delivery of services;
- possible denial of insurance benefits; and
- social media policy.

H.2.b. Confidentiality Maintained by the Counselor

Counselors acknowledge the limitations of maintaining the confidentiality of electronic records and transmissions. They inform clients that individuals might have authorized or unauthorized access to such records or transmissions (e.g., colleagues, supervisors, employees, information technologists).

H.2.c. Acknowledgment of Limitations

Counselors inform clients about the inherent limits of confidentiality when using technology. Counselors urge clients to be aware of authorized and/or unauthorized access to information disclosed using this medium in the counseling process.

H.2.d. Security

Counselors use current encryption standards within their websites and/or technology-based communications that meet applicable legal requirements. Counselors take reasonable precautions to ensure the confidentiality of information transmitted through any electronic means.

H.3. Client Verification

Counselors who engage in the use of distance counseling, technology, and/or social media to interact with clients take steps to verify the client's identity at the beginning and throughout the therapeutic process. Verification can include, but is not limited to, using code words, numbers, graphics, or other nondescript identifiers.

H.4. Distance Counseling Relationship

H.4.a. Benefits and Limitations

Counselors inform clients of the benefits and limitations of using technology applications in the provision of counseling services. Such technologies include, but are not limited to, computer hardware and/or software, telephones and applications, social media and Internet-based applications and other audio and/or video communication, or data storage devices or media.

H.4.b. Professional Boundaries in Distance Counseling

Counselors understand the necessity of maintaining a professional relationship with their clients. Counselors discuss and establish professional boundaries with clients regarding the appropriate use and/or application of technology and the limitations of its use within the counseling relationship (e.g., lack of confidentiality, times when not appropriate to use).

H.4.c. Technology-Assisted Services

When providing technology-assisted services, counselors make reasonable efforts to determine that clients are intellectually, emotionally, physically, linguistically, and functionally capable of using the application and that the application is appropriate for the needs of the client. Counselors verify that clients understand the purpose and operation of technology applications and follow up with clients to correct possible misconceptions, discover appropriate use, and assess subsequent steps.

H.4.d. Effectiveness of Services

When distance counseling services are deemed ineffective by the counselor or client, counselors consider delivering services face-to-face. If the counselor is not able to provide face-to-face services (e.g., lives in another state), the counselor assists the client in identifying appropriate services.

H.4.e. Access

Counselors provide information to clients regarding reasonable access to pertinent applications when providing technology-assisted services.

H.4.f. Communication Differences in Electronic Media

Counselors consider the differences between face-to-face and electronic communication (nonverbal and verbal cues) and how these may affect the counseling process. Counselors educate clients on how to prevent and address potential misunderstandings arising from the lack of visual cues and voice intonations when communicating electronically.

H.5. Records and Web Maintenance

H.5.a. Records

Counselors maintain electronic records in accordance with relevant laws and statutes. Counselors inform clients on how records are maintained electronically. This includes, but is not limited to, the type of encryption and security assigned to the records, and if/for how long archival storage of transaction records is maintained.

H.5.b. Client Rights

Counselors who offer distance counseling services and/or maintain a professional website provide electronic links to relevant licensure and professional certification boards to protect consumer and client rights and address ethical concerns.

H.5.c. Electronic Links

Counselors regularly ensure that electronic links are working and are professionally appropriate.

H.5.d. Multicultural and Disability Considerations

Counselors who maintain websites provide accessibility to persons with disabilities. They provide translation capabilities for clients who have a different primary language, when feasible. Counselors acknowledge the imperfect nature of such translations and accessibilities.

H.6. Social Media

H.6.a. Virtual Professional Presence

In cases where counselors wish to maintain a professional and personal presence for social media use, separate professional and personal web pages and profiles are created to clearly distinguish between the two kinds of virtual presence.

H.6.b. Social Media as Part of Informed Consent

Counselors clearly explain to their clients, as part of the informed consent procedure, the benefits, limitations, and boundaries of the use of social media.

H.6.c. Client Virtual Presence

Counselors respect the privacy of their clients' presence on social media unless given consent to view such information.

H.6.d. Use of Public Social Media

Counselors take precautions to avoid disclosing confidential information through public social media.

SECTION I: RESOLVING ETHICAL ISSUES

Introduction

Professional counselors behave in an ethical and legal manner. They are aware that client welfare and trust in the profession depend on a high level of professional conduct. They hold other counselors to the same standards and are willing to take appropriate action to ensure that standards are upheld. Counselors strive to resolve ethical dilemmas with direct and open communication among all parties involved and seek consultation with colleagues and supervisors when necessary. Counselors incorporate ethical practice into their daily professional work and engage in ongoing professional development regarding current topics in ethical and legal issues in counseling. Counselors become familiar with the ACA Policy and Procedures for Processing Complaints of Ethical Violations[1] and use it as a reference for assisting in the enforcement of the *ACA Code of Ethics*.

I.1. Standards and the Law

I.1.a. Knowledge

Counselors know and understand the *ACA Code of Ethics* and other applicable ethics codes from professional organizations or certification and licensure bodies of which they are members. Lack of knowledge or misunderstanding of an ethical responsibility is not a defense against a charge of unethical conduct.

I.1.b. Ethical Decision Making

When counselors are faced with an ethical dilemma, they use and document, as appropriate, an ethical decision-making model that may include, but is not limited to, consultation; consideration of relevant ethical standards, principles, and laws; generation of potential courses of action; deliberation of risks and benefits; and selection of an objective decision based on the circumstances and welfare of all involved.

I.1.c. Conflicts Between Ethics and Laws

If ethical responsibilities conflict with the law, regulations, and/or other governing legal authority, counselors make known their commitment to the *ACA Code of Ethics* and take steps to

---

[1]See the American Counseling Association web site at http://www.counseling.org/knowledge-center/ethics

resolve the conflict. If the conflict cannot be resolved using this approach, counselors, acting in the best interest of the client, may adhere to the requirements of the law, regulations, and/or other governing legal authority.

I.2. Suspected Violations

I.2.a. Informal Resolution

When counselors have reason to believe that another counselor is violating or has violated an ethical standard and substantial harm has not occurred, they attempt to first resolve the issue informally with the other counselor if feasible, provided such action does not violate confidentiality rights that may be involved.

I.2.b. Reporting Ethical Violations

If an apparent violation has substantially harmed or is likely to substantially harm a person or organization and is not appropriate for informal resolution or is not resolved properly, counselors take further action depending on the situation. Such action may include referral to state or national committees on professional ethics, voluntary national certification bodies, state licensing boards, or appropriate institutional authorities. The confidentiality rights of clients should be considered in all actions. This standard does not apply when counselors have been retained to review the work of another counselor whose professional conduct is in question (e.g., consultation, expert testimony).

I.2.c. Consultation

When uncertain about whether a particular situation or course of action may be in violation of the *ACA Code of Ethics*, counselors consult with other counselors who are knowledgeable about ethics and the *ACA Code of Ethics*, with colleagues, or with appropriate authorities, such as the ACA Ethics and Professional Standards Department.

I.2.d. Organizational Conflicts

If the demands of an organization with which counselors are affiliated pose a conflict with the *ACA Code of Ethics*, counselors specify the nature of such conflicts and express to their supervisors or other responsible officials their commitment to the *ACA Code of Ethics* and, when possible, work through the appropriate channels to address the situation.

I.2.e. Unwarranted Complaints

Counselors do not initiate, participate in, or encourage the filing of ethics complaints that are retaliatory in nature or are made with reckless disregard or willful ignorance of facts that would disprove the allegation.

I.2.f. Unfair Discrimination Against Complainants and Respondents

Counselors do not deny individuals employment, advancement, admission to academic or other programs, tenure, or promotion based solely on their having made or their being the subject of an ethics complaint. This does not preclude taking action based on the outcome of such proceedings or considering other appropriate information.

I.3. Cooperation With Ethics Committees

Counselors assist in the process of enforcing the *ACA Code of Ethics*. Counselors cooperate with investigations, proceedings, and requirements of the ACA Ethics Committee or ethics committees of other duly constituted associations or boards having jurisdiction over those charged with a violation.

Glossary of Terms

Abandonment – the inappropriate ending or arbitrary termination of a counseling relationship that puts the client at risk.

Advocacy – promotion of the well-being of individuals, groups, and the counseling profession within systems and organizations. Advocacy seeks to remove barriers and obstacles that inhibit access, growth, and development.

Assent – to demonstrate agreement when a person is otherwise not capable or competent to give formal consent (e.g., informed consent) to a counseling service or plan.

Assessment – the process of collecting in-depth information about a person in order to develop a comprehensive plan that will guide the collaborative counseling and service provision process.

Bartering – accepting goods or services from clients in exchange for counseling services.

Client – an individual seeking or referred to the professional services of a counselor.

Confidentiality – the ethical duty of counselors to protect a client's identity, identifying characteristics, and private communications.

Consultation – a professional relationship that may include, but is not limited to, seeking advice, information, and/or testimony.

Counseling – a professional relationship that empowers diverse individuals, families, and groups to accomplish mental health, wellness, education, and career goals.

Counselor Educator – a professional counselor engaged primarily in developing, implementing, and supervising the educational preparation of professional counselors.

Counselor Supervisor – a professional counselor who engages in a formal relationship with a practicing counselor or counselor-in-training for the purpose of overseeing that individual's counseling work or clinical skill development.

Culture – membership in a socially constructed way of living, which incorporates collective values, beliefs, norms, boundaries, and lifestyles that are cocreated with others who share similar worldviews comprising biological, psychosocial, historical, psychological, and other factors.

Discrimination – the prejudicial treatment of an individual or group based on their actual or perceived membership in a particular group, class, or category.

Distance Counseling – The provision of counseling services by means other than face-to-face meetings, usually with the aid of technology.

Diversity – the similarities and differences that occur within and across cultures, and the intersection of cultural and social identities.

Documents – any written, digital, audio, visual, or artistic recording of the work within the counseling relationship between counselor and client.

Encryption – process of encoding information in such a way that limits access to authorized users.

Examinee – a recipient of any professional counseling service that includes educational, psychological, and career appraisal, using qualitative or quantitative techniques.

Exploitation – actions and/or behaviors that take advantage of another for one's own benefit or gain.

Fee Splitting – the payment or acceptance of fees for client referrals (e.g., percentage of fee paid for rent, referral fees).

Forensic Evaluation – the process of forming professional opinions for court or other legal proceedings, based on professional knowledge and expertise, and supported by appropriate data.

Gatekeeping – the initial and ongoing academic, skill, and dispositional assessment of students' competency for professional practice, including remediation and termination as appropriate.

Impairment – a significantly diminished capacity to perform professional functions.

Incapacitation – an inability to perform professional functions.

Informed Consent – a process of information sharing associated with possible actions clients may choose to take, aimed at assisting clients in acquiring a full appreciation and understanding of the facts and implications of a given action or actions.

Instrument – a tool, developed using accepted research practices, that measures the presence and strength of a specified construct or constructs.

Interdisciplinary Teams – teams of professionals serving clients that may include individuals who may not share counselors' responsibilities regarding confidentiality.

Minors – generally, persons under the age of 18 years, unless otherwise designated by statute or regulation. In some jurisdictions, minors may have the right to consent to counseling without consent of the parent or guardian.

Multicultural/Diversity Competence – counselors' cultural and diversity awareness and knowledge about self and others, and how this awareness and knowledge are applied effectively in practice with clients and client groups.

Multicultural/Diversity Counseling – counseling that recognizes diversity and embraces approaches that support the worth, dignity, potential, and uniqueness of individuals within their historical, cultural, economic, political, and psychosocial contexts.

Personal Virtual Relationship – engaging in a relationship via technology and/or social media that blurs the professional boundary (e.g., friending on social networking sites); using personal accounts as the connection point for the virtual relationship.

Privacy – the right of an individual to keep oneself and one's personal information free from unauthorized disclosure.

Privilege – a legal term denoting the protection of confidential information in a legal proceeding (e.g., subpoena, deposition, testimony).

Pro bono publico – contributing to society by devoting a portion of professional activities for little or no financial return (e.g., speaking to groups, sharing professional information, offering reduced fees).

Professional Virtual Relationship – using technology and/or social media in a professional manner and maintaining appropriate professional boundaries; using business accounts that cannot be linked back to personal accounts as the connection point for the virtual relationship (e.g., a business page versus a personal profile).

Records – all information or documents, in any medium, that the counselor keeps about the client, excluding personal and psychotherapy notes.

Records of an Artistic Nature – products created by the client as part of the counseling process.

Records Custodian – a professional colleague who agrees to serve as the caretaker of client records for another mental health professional.

Self-Growth – a process of self-examination and challenging of a counselor's assumptions to enhance professional effectiveness.

Serious and Foreseeable – when a reasonable counselor can anticipate significant and harmful possible consequences.

Sexual Harassment – sexual solicitation, physical advances, or verbal/nonverbal conduct that is sexual in nature; occurs in connection with professional activities or roles; is unwelcome, offensive, or creates a hostile workplace or learning environment; and/or is sufficiently severe or intense to be perceived as harassment by a reasonable person.

Social Justice – the promotion of equity for all people and groups for the purpose of ending oppression and injustice affecting clients, students, counselors, families, communities, schools, workplaces, governments, and other social and institutional systems.

Social Media – technology-based forms of communication of ideas, beliefs, personal histories, etc. (e.g., social networking sites, blogs).

Student – an individual engaged in formal graduate-level counselor education.

Supervisee – a professional counselor or counselor-in-training whose counseling work or clinical skill development is being overseen in a formal supervisory relationship by a qualified trained professional.

Supervision – a process in which one individual, usually a senior member of a given profession designated as the supervisor, engages in a collaborative relationship with another individual or group, usually a junior member(s) of a given profession designated as the supervisee(s) in order to (a) promote the growth and development of the supervisee(s), (b) protect the welfare of the clients seen by the supervisee(s), and (c) evaluate the performance of the supervisee(s).

Supervisor – counselors who are trained to oversee the professional clinical work of counselors and counselors-in-training.

Teaching – all activities engaged in as part of a formal educational program that is designed to lead to a graduate degree in counseling.

Training – the instruction and practice of skills related to the counseling profession. Training contributes to the ongoing proficiency of students and professional counselors.

Virtual Relationship – a non–face-to-face relationship (e.g., through social media).

Ethics-Related Resources From ACA

- Free consultation on ethics for ACA members
- Bestselling publications revised in accordance with the 2014 *Code of Ethics*, including *ACA Ethical Standards Casebook, Boundary Issues in Counseling, Ethics Desk Reference for Counselors,* and *The Counselor and the Law*
- Podcast and six-part webinar series on the 2014 *Code of Ethics*
- The latest information on ethics at *counseling.org/ethics*

Source: American Counseling Association, (2014). ACA Code of Ethics. Alexandria, VA.

Appendix B: American School Counselor Association Ethical Standards for School Counselors

(Adopted 1984; revised 1992, 1998, 2004, and 2010)

Preamble

The American School Counselor Association (ASCA) is a professional organization whose members are school counselors certified/licensed in school counseling with unique qualifications and skills to address all students' academic, personal/social and career development needs. Members are also school counseling program directors/supervisors and counselor educators. These ethical standards are the ethical responsibility of school counselors. School counseling program directors/supervisors should know them and provide support for practitioners to uphold them. School counselor educators should know them, teach them to their students and provide support for school counseling candidates to uphold them.

Professional school counselors are advocates, leaders, collaborators and consultants who create opportunities for equity in access and success in educational opportunities by connecting their programs to the mission of schools and subscribing to the following tenets of professional responsibility:

- Each person has the right to be respected, be treated with dignity and have access to a comprehensive school counseling program that advocates for and affirms all students from diverse populations including: ethnic/racial identity, age, economic status, abilities/disabilities, language, immigration status, sexual orientation, gender, gender identity/expression, family type, religious/spiritual identity and appearance.
- Each person has the right to receive the information and support needed to move toward self-direction and self-development and affirmation within one's group identities, with special care being given to students who have historically not received adequate educational services, e.g., students of color, students living at a low socioeconomic status, students with disabilities and students from non-dominant language backgrounds.

- Each person has the right to understand the full magnitude and meaning of his/her educational choices and how those choices will affect future opportunities.
- Each person has the right to privacy and thereby the right to expect the school-counselor/student relationship to comply with all laws, policies and ethical standards pertaining to confidentiality in the school setting.
- Each person has the right to feel safe in school environments that school counselors help create, free from abuse, bullying, neglect, harassment or other forms of violence.

In this document, ASCA specifies the principles of ethical behavior necessary to maintain the high standards of integrity, leadership and professionalism among its members. The Ethical Standards for School Counselors were developed to clarify the nature of ethical responsibilities held in common by school counselors, supervisors/directors of school counseling programs and school counselor educators. The purposes of this document are to:

- Serve as a guide for the ethical practices of all professional school counselors, supervisors/directors of school counseling programs and school counselor educators regardless of level, area, population served or membership in this professional association;
- Provide self-appraisal and peer evaluations regarding school counselors' responsibilities to students, parents/guardians, colleagues and professional associates, schools, communities and the counseling profession; and
- Inform all stakeholders, including students, parents and guardians, teachers, administrators, community members and courts of justice, of best ethical practices, values and expected behaviors of the school counseling professional.

A.1. Responsibilities to Students

Professional school counselors:

a. Have a primary obligation to the students, who are to be treated with dignity and respect as unique individuals.

b. Are concerned with the educational, academic, career, personal and social needs and encourage the maximum development of every student.

c. Respect students' values, beliefs and cultural background and do not impose the school counselor's personal values on students or their families.

d. Are knowledgeable of laws, regulations and policies relating to students and strive to protect and inform students regarding their rights.

e. Promote the welfare of individual students and collaborate with them to develop an action plan for success.

f. Consider the involvement of support networks valued by the individual students.

g. Understand that professional distance with students is appropriate, and any sexual or romantic relationship with students whether illegal in the state of practice is considered a grievous breach of ethics and is prohibited regardless of a student's age.

h. Consider the potential for harm before entering into a relationship with former students or one of their family members.

A.2. Confidentiality

Professional school counselors:

a. Inform individual students of the purposes, goals, techniques and rules of procedure under which they may receive counseling. Disclosure includes the limits of confidentiality in a developmentally appropriate manner. Informed consent requires competence on the part of students to understand the limits of confidentiality and therefore, can be difficult to obtain from students of a certain developmental level. Professionals are aware that even though every attempt is made to obtain informed consent it is not always possible and when needed will make counseling decisions on students' behalf.

b. Explain the limits of confidentiality in appropriate ways such as classroom guidance lessons, the student handbook, school counseling brochures, school Web site, verbal notice or other methods of student, school and community communication in addition to oral notification to individual students.

c. Recognize the complicated nature of confidentiality in schools and consider each case in context. Keep information confidential unless legal requirements demand that confidential information be revealed or a breach is required to prevent serious and foreseeable harm to the student. Serious and foreseeable harm is different for each minor in schools and is defined by students' developmental and chronological age, the setting, parental rights and the nature of the harm. School counselors consult with appropriate professionals when in doubt as to the validity of an exception.

d. Recognize their primary obligation for confidentiality is to the students but balance that obligation with an understanding of parents'/guardians' legal and inherent rights to be the guiding voice in their children's lives, especially in value-laden issues. Understand the need to balance students' ethical rights to make choices, their capacity to give consent or assent and parental or familial legal rights and responsibilities to protect these students and make decisions on their behalf.

e. Promote the autonomy and independence of students to the extent possible and use the most appropriate and least intrusive method of breach. The developmental age and the circumstances requiring the breach are considered and as appropriate students are engaged in a discussion about the method and timing of the breach.

f. In absence of state legislation expressly forbidding disclosure, consider the ethical responsibility to provide information to an identified third party who, by his/her relationship with the student, is at a high risk of contracting a disease that is commonly known to be communicable and fatal. Disclosure requires satisfaction of all of the following conditions:

- Student identifies partner or the partner is highly identifiable
- School counselor recommends the student notify partner and refrain from further high-risk behavior
- Student refuses
- School counselor informs the student of the intent to notify the partner
- School counselor seeks legal consultation from the school district's legal representative in writing as to the legalities of informing the partner

g. Request of the court that disclosure not be required when the release of confidential information may potentially harm a student or the counseling relationship.

h. Protect the confidentiality of students' records and release personal data in accordance with prescribed federal and state laws and school policies including the laws within the Family Education Rights and Privacy Act (FERPA). Student information stored and transmitted electronically is treated with the same care as traditional student records. Recognize the vulnerability of confidentiality in electronic communications and only transmit sensitive information electronically in a way that is untraceable to students' identity. Critical information such as a student who has a history of suicidal ideation must be conveyed to the receiving school in a personal contact such as a phone call.

A.3. Academic, Career/College/Post-Secondary Access and Personal/Social Counseling Plans

Professional school counselors:

a. Provide students with a comprehensive school counseling program that parallels the ASCA National Model with emphasis on working jointly with all students to develop personal/social, academic and career goals.

b. Ensure equitable academic, career, post-secondary access and personal/social opportunities for all students through the use of data to help close achievement gaps and opportunity gaps.

c. Provide and advocate for individual students' career awareness, exploration and post-secondary plans supporting the students' right to choose from the wide array of options when they leave secondary education.

A.4. Dual Relationships

Professional school counselors:

a. Avoid dual relationships that might impair their objectivity and increase the risk of harm to students (*e.g.*, counseling one's family members or the children of close friends or associates). If a dual relationship is unavoidable, the school counselor is responsible for taking action to eliminate or reduce the potential for harm to the student through use of safeguards, which might include informed consent, consultation, supervision and documentation.

b. Maintain appropriate professional distance with students at all times.

c. Avoid dual relationships with students through communication mediums such as social networking sites.

d. Avoid dual relationships with school personnel that might infringe on the integrity of the school counselor/student relationship.

A.5. Appropriate Referrals

Professional school counselors:

a. Make referrals when necessary or appropriate to outside resources for student and/or family support. Appropriate referrals may necessitate informing both parents/guardians and students of applicable resources and making proper plans for transitions with minimal interruption of services. Students retain the right to discontinue the counseling relationship at any time.

b. Help educate about and prevent personal and social concerns for all students within the school counselor's scope of education and competence and make necessary referrals when the counseling needs are beyond the individual school counselor's education and training. Every attempt is made to find appropriate specialized resources for clinical therapeutic topics that are difficult or inappropriate to address in a school setting such as eating disorders, sexual trauma, chemical dependency and other addictions needing sustained clinical duration or assistance.

c. Request a release of information signed by the student and/or parents/guardians when attempting to develop a collaborative relationship with other service providers assigned to the student.

d. Develop a reasonable method of termination of counseling when it becomes apparent that counseling assistance is no longer needed or a referral is necessary to better meet the student's needs.

A.6. Group Work

Professional school counselors:

a. Screen prospective group members and maintain an awareness of participants' needs, appropriate fit and personal goals in relation to the group's intention and focus. The school counselor takes reasonable precautions to protect members from physical and psychological harm resulting from interaction within the group.

b. Recognize that best practice is to notify the parents/guardians of children participating in small groups.

c. Establish clear expectations in the group setting, and clearly state that confidentiality in group counseling cannot be guaranteed. Given the developmental and chronological ages of minors in schools, recognize the tenuous nature of confidentiality for minors renders some topics inappropriate for group work in a school setting.

d. Provide necessary follow up with group members, and document proceedings as appropriate.

e. Develop professional competencies, and maintain appropriate education, training and supervision in group facilitation and any topics specific to the group.

f. Facilitate group work that is brief and solution-focused, working with a variety of academic, career, college and personal/social issues.

A.7. Danger to Self or Others

Professional school counselors:

a. Inform parents/guardians and/or appropriate authorities when a student poses a danger to self or others. This is to be done after careful deliberation and consultation with other counseling professionals.

b. Report risk assessments to parents when they underscore the need to act on behalf of a child at risk; never negate a risk of harm as students sometimes deceive in order to avoid further scrutiny and/or parental notification.

c. Understand the legal and ethical liability for releasing a student who is in danger to self or others without proper and necessary support for that student.

A.8. Student Records

Professional school counselors:

a. Maintain and secure records necessary for rendering professional services to the student as required by laws, regulations, institutional procedures and confidentiality guidelines.

b. Keep sole-possession records or individual student case notes separate from students' educational records in keeping with state laws.

c. Recognize the limits of sole-possession records and understand these records are a memory aid for the creator and in absence of privileged communication may be subpoenaed and may become educational records when they are shared or are accessible to others in either verbal or written form or when they include information other than professional opinion or personal observations.

d. Establish a reasonable timeline for purging sole-possession records or case notes. Suggested guidelines include shredding sole possession records when the student transitions to the next level, transfers to another school or graduates. Apply careful discretion and deliberation before destroying sole-possession records that may be needed by a court of law such as notes on child abuse, suicide, sexual harassment or violence.

e. Understand and abide by the Family Education Rights and Privacy Act (FERPA, 1974), which safeguards student's records and allows parents to have a voice in what and how information is shared with others regarding their child's educational records.

A.9. Evaluation, Assessment and Interpretation

Professional school counselors:

a. Adhere to all professional standards regarding selecting, administering and interpreting assessment measures and only utilize assessment measures that are within the scope of practice for school counselors and for which they are trained and competent.

b. Consider confidentiality issues when utilizing evaluative or assessment instruments and electronically based programs.

c. Consider the developmental age, language skills and level of competence of the student taking the assessments before assessments are given.

d. Provide interpretation of the nature, purposes, results and potential impact of assessment/evaluation measures in language the students can understand.

e. Monitor the use of assessment results and interpretations, and take reasonable steps to prevent others from misusing the information.

f. Use caution when utilizing assessment techniques, making evaluations and interpreting the performance of populations not represented in the norm group on which an instrument is standardized.

g. Assess the effectiveness of their program in having an impact on students' academic, career and personal/social development through accountability measures especially examining efforts to close achievement, opportunity and attainment gaps.

A.10. Technology

Professional school counselors:

a. Promote the benefits of and clarify the limitations of various appropriate technological applications. Professional school counselors promote technological applications (1) that are appropriate for students' individual needs, (2) that students understand how to use and (3) for which follow-up counseling assistance is provided.

b. Advocate for equal access to technology for all students, especially those historically underserved.

c. Take appropriate and reasonable measures for maintaining confidentiality of student information and educational records stored or transmitted through the use of computers, facsimile machines, telephones, voicemail, answering machines and other electronic or computer technology.

d. Understand the intent of FERPA and its impact on sharing electronic student records.

e. Consider the extent to which cyberbullying is interfering with students' educational process and base guidance curriculum and intervention programming for this pervasive and potentially dangerous problem on research-based and best practices.

A.11. Student Peer Support Program

Professional school counselors:

a. Have unique responsibilities when working with peer-helper or student-assistance programs and safeguard the welfare of students participating in peer-to-peer programs under their direction.

b. Are ultimately responsible for appropriate training and supervision for students serving as peer-support individuals in their school counseling programs.

B. Responsibilities to Parents/Guardians

B.1. Parent Rights and Responsibilities

Professional school counselors:

a. Respect the rights and responsibilities of parents/guardians for their children and endeavor to establish, as appropriate, a collaborative relationship with parents/guardians to facilitate students' maximum development.

b. Adhere to laws, local guidelines and ethical standards of practice when assisting parents/guardians experiencing family difficulties interfering with the student's effectiveness and welfare.

c. Are sensitive to diversity among families and recognize that all parents/guardians, custodial and noncustodial, are vested with certain rights and responsibilities for their children's welfare by virtue of their role and according to law.

d. Inform parents of the nature of counseling services provided in the school setting.

e. Adhere to the FERPA act regarding disclosure of student information.

f. Work to establish, as appropriate, collaborative relationships with parents/guardians to best serve student.

B.2. Parents/Guardians and Confidentiality

Professional school counselors:

a. Inform parents/guardians of the school counselor's role to include the confidential nature of the counseling relationship between the counselor and student.

b. Recognize that working with minors in a school setting requires school counselors to collaborate with students' parents/guardians to the extent possible.

c. Respect the confidentiality of parents/guardians to the extent that is reasonable to protect the best interest of the student being counseled.

d. Provide parents/guardians with accurate, comprehensive and relevant information in an objective and caring manner, as is appropriate and consistent with ethical responsibilities to the student.

e. Make reasonable efforts to honor the wishes of parents/guardians concerning information regarding the student unless a court order expressly forbids the involvement of a parent(s). In cases of divorce or separation, school counselors exercise a good-faith effort to keep both parents informed, maintaining focus on the student and avoiding supporting one parent over another in divorce proceedings.

C. Responsibilities to Colleagues and Professional Associates

C.1. Professional Relationships

Professional school counselors, the school counseling program director/site supervisor and the school counselor educator:

a. Establish and maintain professional relationships with faculty, staff and administration to facilitate an optimum counseling program.

b. Treat colleagues with professional respect, courtesy and fairness.

c. Recognize that teachers, staff and administrators who are high-functioning in the personal and social development skills can be powerful allies in supporting student success. School counselors work to develop relationships with all faculty and staff in order to advantage students.

d. Are aware of and utilize related professionals, organizations and other resources to whom the student may be referred.

C.2. Sharing Information With Other Professionals

Professional school counselors:

a. Promote awareness and adherence to appropriate guidelines regarding confidentiality, the distinction between public and private information and staff consultation.

b. Provide professional personnel with accurate, objective, concise and meaningful data necessary to adequately evaluate, counsel and assist the student.

c. Secure parental consent and develop clear agreements with other mental health professionals when a student is receiving services from another counselor or other mental health professional in order to avoid confusion and conflict for the student and parents/guardians.

d. Understand about the "release of information" process and parental rights in sharing information and attempt to establish a cooperative and collaborative relationship with other professionals to benefit students.

e. Recognize the powerful role of ally that faculty and administration who function high in personal/social development skills can play in supporting students in stress, and carefully filter confidential information to give these allies what they "need to know" in order to advantage the student. Consultation with other members of the school counseling profession is helpful in determining need-to-know information. The primary focus and obligation is always on the student when it comes to sharing confidential information.

f. Keep appropriate records regarding individual students, and develop a plan for transferring those records to another professional school counselor should the need occur. This documentation transfer will protect the confidentiality and benefit the needs of the student for whom the records are written.

C.3. Collaborating and Educating Around the Role of the School Counselor

The school counselor, school counseling program supervisor/director and school counselor educator:

a. Share the role of the school counseling program in ensuring data-driven academic, career/college and personal/social success competencies for every student, resulting in specific outcomes/indicators with all stakeholders.

b. Broker services internal and external to the schools to help ensure every student receives the benefits of a school counseling program and specific academic, career/college and personal/social competencies.

D. Responsibilities to School, Communities and Families

D.1. Responsibilities to the School

Professional school counselors:

a. Support and protect students' best interest against any infringement of their educational program.

b. Inform appropriate officials, in accordance with school policy, of conditions that may be potentially disruptive or damaging to the school's mission, personnel and property while honoring the confidentiality between the student and the school counselor.

c. Are knowledgeable and supportive of their school's mission, and connect their program to the school's mission.

d. Delineate and promote the school counselor's role, and function as a student advocate in meeting the needs of those served. School counselors will notify appropriate officials of systemic conditions that may limit or curtail their effectiveness in providing programs and services.

e. Accept employment only for positions for which they are qualified by education, training, supervised experience, state and national professional credentials and appropriate professional experience.

f. Advocate that administrators hire only qualified, appropriately trained and competent individuals for professional school counseling positions.

g. Assist in developing: (1) curricular and environmental conditions appropriate for the school and community; (2) educational procedures and programs to meet students' developmental needs; (3) a systematic evaluation process for comprehensive, developmental, standards-based school counseling programs, services and personnel; and (4) a data-driven evaluation process guiding the comprehensive, developmental school counseling program and service delivery.

D.2. Responsibility to the Community

Professional school counselors:

a. Collaborate with community agencies, organizations and individuals in students' best interest and without regard to personal reward or remuneration.

b. Extend their influence and opportunity to deliver a comprehensive school counseling program to all students by collaborating with community resources for student success.

c. Promote equity for all students through community resources.

d. Are careful not to use their professional role as a school counselor to benefit any type of private therapeutic or consultative practice in which they might be involved outside of the school setting.

E. Responsibilities to Self

E.1. Professional Competence

Professional school counselors:

a. Function within the boundaries of individual professional competence and accept responsibility for the consequences of their actions.

b. Monitor emotional and physical health and practice wellness to ensure optimal effectiveness. Seek physical or mental health referrals when needed to ensure competence at all times.

c. Monitor personal responsibility and recognize the high standard of care a professional in this critical position of trust must maintain on and off the job and are cognizant of and refrain from activity that may lead to inadequate professional services or diminish their effectiveness with school community members. Professional and personal growth are ongoing throughout the counselor's career.

d. Strive through personal initiative to stay abreast of current research and to maintain professional competence in advocacy, teaming and collaboration, culturally competent counseling and school counseling program coordination, knowledge and use of technology, leadership, and equity assessment using data.

e. Ensure a variety of regular opportunities for participating in and facilitating professional development for self and other educators and school counselors through continuing education opportunities annually including: attendance at professional school counseling conferences; reading *Professional School Counseling* journal articles; facilitating workshops for education staff on issues school counselors are uniquely positioned to provide.

f. Enhance personal self-awareness, professional effectiveness and ethical practice by regularly attending presentations on ethical decision-making. Effective school counselors will seek supervision when ethical or professional questions arise in their practice.

g. Maintain current membership in professional associations to ensure ethical and best practices.

E.2. Multicultural and Social Justice Advocacy and Leadership

Professional school counselors:

a. Monitor and expand personal multicultural and social justice advocacy awareness, knowledge and skills. School counselors strive for exemplary cultural competence by ensuring personal beliefs or values are not imposed on students or other stakeholders.

b. Develop competencies in how prejudice, power and various forms of oppression, such as ableism, ageism, classism, familyism, genderism, heterosexism, immigrationism, linguicism, racism, religionism and sexism, affect self, students and all stakeholders.

c. Acquire educational, consultation and training experiences to improve awareness, knowledge, skills and effectiveness in working with diverse populations: ethnic/racial status, age, economic status, special needs, ESL or ELL, immigration status, sexual orientation, gender, gender identity/expression, family type, religious/spiritual identity and appearance.

d. Affirm the multiple cultural and linguistic identities of every student and all stakeholders. Advocate for equitable school and school counseling program policies and practices for every student and all stakeholders including use of translators and bilingual/multilingual school counseling program materials that represent all languages used by families in the school community, and advocate for appropriate accommodations and accessibility for students with disabilities.

e. Use inclusive and culturally responsible language in all forms of communication.

f. Provide regular workshops and written/digital information to families to increase understanding, collaborative two-way communication and a welcoming school climate between families and the school to promote increased student achievement.

g. Work as advocates and leaders in the school to create equity-based school counseling programs that help close any achievement, opportunity and attainment gaps that deny all students the chance to pursue their educational goals.

F. Responsibilities to the Profession

F.1. Professionalism

Professional school counselors:

a. Accept the policies and procedures for handling ethical violations as a result of maintaining membership in the American School Counselor Association.

b. Conduct themselves in such a manner as to advance individual ethical practice and the profession.

c. Conduct appropriate research, and report findings in a manner consistent with acceptable educational and psychological research practices. School counselors advocate for the protection of individual students' identities when using data for research or program planning.

d. Seek institutional and parent/guardian consent before administering any research, and maintain security of research records.

e. Adhere to ethical standards of the profession, other official policy statements, such as ASCA's position statements, role statement and the ASCA National Model and relevant statutes established by federal, state and local governments, and when these are in conflict work responsibly for change.

f. Clearly distinguish between statements and actions made as a private individual and those made as a representative of the school counseling profession.

g. Do not use their professional position to recruit or gain clients, consultees for their private practice or to seek and receive unjustified personal gains, unfair advantage, inappropriate relationships or unearned goods or services.

F.2. Contribution to the Profession

Professional school counselors:

a. Actively participate in professional associations and share results and best practices in assessing, implementing and annually evaluating the outcomes of data-driven school counseling programs with measurable academic, career/college and personal/social competencies for every student.

b. Provide support, consultation and mentoring to novice professionals.

c. Have a responsibility to read and abide by the ASCA Ethical Standards and adhere to the applicable laws and regulations.

F.3. Supervision of School Counselor Candidates Pursuing Practicum and Internship Experiences:

Professional school counselors:

a. Provide support for appropriate experiences in academic, career, college access and personal/social counseling for school counseling interns.

b. Ensure school counselor candidates have experience in developing, implementing and evaluating a data-driven school counseling program model, such as the ASCA National Model.

c. Ensure the school counseling practicum and internship have specific, measurable service delivery, foundation, management and accountability systems.

d. Ensure school counselor candidates maintain appropriate liability insurance for the duration of the school counseling practicum and internship experiences.

e. Ensure a site visit is completed by a school counselor education faculty member for each practicum or internship student, preferably when both the school counselor trainee and site supervisor are present.

F.4. Collaboration and Education about School Counselors and School Counseling Programs with other Professionals

School counselors and school counseling program directors/supervisors collaborate with special educators, school nurses, school social workers, school psychologists, college counselors/admissions officers, physical therapists, occupational therapists and speech pathologists to advocate for optimal services for students and all other stakeholders.

G. Maintenance of Standards

Professional school counselors are expected to maintain ethical behavior at all times.

G.1. When there exists serious doubt as to the ethical behavior of a colleague(s) the following procedure may serve as a guide:

1. The school counselor should consult confidentially with a professional colleague to discuss the nature of a complaint to see if the professional colleague views the situation as an ethical violation.

2. When feasible, the school counselor should directly approach the colleague whose behavior is in question to discuss the complaint and seek resolution.

3. The school counselor should keep documentation of all the steps taken.

4. If resolution is not forthcoming at the personal level, the school counselor shall utilize the channels established within the school, school district, the state school counseling association and ASCA's Ethics Committee.

5. If the matter still remains unresolved, referral for review and appropriate action should be made to the Ethics Committees in the following sequence:

   • State school counselor association
   • American School Counselor Association

6. The ASCA Ethics Committee is responsible for:

   • Educating and consulting with the membership regarding ethical standards
   • Periodically reviewing and recommending changes in code
   • Receiving and processing questions to clarify the application of such standards. Questions must be submitted in writing to the ASCA Ethics Committee chair.
   • Handling complaints of alleged violations of the ASCA Ethical Standards for School Counselors. At the national level, complaints should be submitted in writing to the ASCA Ethics Committee, c/o the Executive Director, American School Counselor Association, 1101 King St., Suite 625, Alexandria, VA 22314.

G.2. When school counselors are forced to work in situations or abide by policies that do not reflect the ethics of the profession, the school counselor works responsibly through the correct channels to try and remedy the condition.

G.3. When faced with any ethical dilemma school counselors, school counseling program directors/supervisors and school counselor educators use an ethical decision-making model such as Solutions to Ethical Problems in Schools (STEPS) (Stone, 2001):

1. *Define the problem emotionally and intellectually*

2. *Apply the ASCA Ethical Standards and the law*

3. *Consider the students' chronological and developmental levels*

4. *Consider the setting, parental rights and minors' rights*

5. *Apply the moral principles*

6. *Determine your potential courses of action and their consequences*

7. *Evaluate the selected action*

8. *Consult*

9. *Implement the course of action*

Source: American School Counselor Association, (2010). Ethical Standards for School Counselors, American School Counselor Association.

Appendix C: American Association for Marriage and Family Therapy Code of Ethics

Preamble

The Board of Directors of the American Association for Marriage and Family Therapy (AAMFT) hereby promulgates, pursuant to Article 2, Section 2.01.3 of the Association's Bylaws, the Revised AAMFT Code of Ethics, effective January 1, 2015.

Honoring Public Trust

The AAMFT strives to honor the public trust in marriage and family therapists by setting standards for ethical practice as described in this Code. The ethical standards define professional expectations and are enforced by the AAMFT Ethics Committee.

Commitment to Service, Advocacy and Public Participation

Marriage and family therapists are defined by an enduring dedication to professional and ethical excellence, as well as the commitment to service, advocacy, and public participation. The areas of service, advocacy, and public participation are recognized as responsibilities to the profession equal in importance to all other aspects. Marriage and family therapists embody these aspirations by participating in activities that contribute to a better community and society, including devoting a portion of their professional activity to services for which there is little or no financial return. Additionally, marriage and family therapists are concerned with developing laws and regulations pertaining to marriage and family therapy that serve the public interest, and with altering such laws and regulations that are not in the public interest. Marriage and family therapists also encourage public participation in the design and delivery of professional services and in the regulation of practitioners. Professional competence in these areas is essential to the character of the field, and to the well-being of clients and their communities.

Seeking Consultation

The absence of an explicit reference to a specific behavior or situation in the Code does not mean that the behavior is ethical or unethical. The standards are not exhaustive. Marriage and family therapists who are uncertain about the ethics of a particular course of action are encouraged to seek counsel from consultants, attorneys, supervisors, colleagues, or other appropriate authorities.

Ethical Decision-Making

Both law and ethics govern the practice of marriage and family therapy. When making decisions regarding professional behavior, marriage and family therapists must consider the AAMFT Code of Ethics and applicable laws and regulations. If the AAMFT Code of Ethics prescribes a standard higher than that required by law, marriage and family therapists must meet the higher standard of the AAMFT Code of Ethics. Marriage and family therapists comply with the mandates of law, but make known their commitment to the AAMFT Code of Ethics and take steps to resolve the conflict in a responsible manner. The AAMFT supports legal mandates for reporting of alleged unethical conduct.

Marriage and family therapists remain accountable to the AAMFT Code of Ethics when acting as members or employees of organizations. If the mandates of an organization with which a marriage and family therapist is affiliated, through employment, contract or otherwise, conflict with the AAMFT Code of Ethics, marriage and family therapists make known to the organization their commitment to the AAMFT Code of Ethics and take reasonable steps to resolve the conflict in a way that allows the fullest adherence to the Code of Ethics.

Binding Expectations

The AAMFT Code of Ethics is binding on members of AAMFT in all membership categories, all AAMFT Approved Supervisors and all applicants for membership or the Approved Supervisor designation. AAMFT members have an obligation to be familiar with the AAMFT Code of Ethics and its application to their professional services. Lack of awareness or misunderstanding of an ethical standard is not a defense to a charge of unethical conduct.

Resolving Complaints

The process for filing, investigating, and resolving complaints of unethical conduct is described in the current AAMFT Procedures for Handling Ethical Matters. Persons accused are considered innocent by the Ethics Committee until proven guilty, except as otherwise provided, and are entitled to due process. If an AAMFT member resigns in anticipation of, or during the course of, an ethics investigation, the Ethics Committee will complete its investigation. Any publication of action taken by the Association will include the fact that the member attempted to resign during the investigation.

Aspirational Core Values

The following core values speak generally to the membership of AAMFT as a professional association, yet they also inform all the varieties of practice and service in which marriage and family therapists engage. These core values are aspirational in nature, and are distinct from ethical standards. These values are intended to provide an aspirational framework within which marriage and family therapists may pursue the highest goals of practice.

The core values of AAMFT embody:

1. Acceptance, appreciation, and inclusion of a diverse membership.

2. Distinctiveness and excellence in training of marriage and family therapists and those desiring to advance their skills, knowledge and expertise in systemic and relational therapies.

3. Responsiveness and excellence in service to members.

4. Diversity, equity and excellence in clinical practice, research, education and administration.

5. Integrity evidenced by a high threshold of ethical and honest behavior within Association governance and by members.

6. Innovation and the advancement of knowledge of systemic and relational therapies.

Ethical Standards

Ethical standards, by contrast, are rules of practice upon which the marriage and family therapist is obliged and judged. The introductory paragraph to each standard in the AAMFT Code of Ethics is an aspirational/explanatory orientation to the enforceable standards that follow.

Standard I

Responsibility to Clients

Marriage and family therapists advance the welfare of families and individuals and make reasonable efforts to find the appropriate balance between conflicting goals within the family system.

1.1 **Non-Discrimination.** Marriage and family therapists provide professional assistance to persons without discrimination on the basis of race, age, ethnicity, socioeconomic status, disability, gender, health status, religion, national origin, sexual orientation, gender identity or relationship status.

1.2 **Informed Consent.** Marriage and family therapists obtain appropriate informed consent to therapy or related procedures and use language that is reasonably understandable to clients. When persons, due to age or mental status, are legally incapable of giving informed consent, marriage and family therapists obtain informed permission from a legally authorized person, if such substitute consent is legally permissible. The content of informed consent may vary depending upon the client and treatment plan; however, informed consent generally necessitates that the client: (a) has the capacity to consent; (b) has been adequately informed of significant information concerning treatment processes and procedures; (c) has been adequately informed of potential risks and benefits of treatments for which generally recognized standards do not yet exist; (d) has freely and without undue influence expressed consent; and (e) has provided consent that is appropriately documented.

1.3 **Multiple Relationships.** Marriage and family therapists are aware of their influential positions with respect to clients, and they avoid exploiting the trust and dependency of such persons. Therapists, therefore, make every effort to avoid conditions and multiple relationships with clients that could impair professional judgment or increase the risk of exploitation. Such relationships include, but are not limited to, business or close personal relationships with a client or the client's immediate family. When the risk of impairment or exploitation exists due to conditions or multiple roles, therapists document the appropriate precautions taken.

1.4 **Sexual Intimacy With Current Clients and Others.** Sexual intimacy with current clients or with known members of the client's family system is prohibited.

1.5 **Sexual Intimacy With Former Clients and Others.** Sexual intimacy with former clients or with known members of the client's family system is prohibited.

1.6 **Reports of Unethical Conduct.** Marriage and family therapists comply with applicable laws regarding the reporting of alleged unethical conduct.

1.7 **Abuse of the Therapeutic Relationship.** Marriage and family therapists do not abuse their power in therapeutic relationships.

1.8 **Client Autonomy in Decision Making.** Marriage and family therapists respect the rights of clients to make decisions and help them to understand the consequences of these decisions. Therapists clearly advise clients that clients have the responsibility to make decisions regarding relationships such as cohabitation, marriage, divorce, separation, reconciliation, custody, and visitation.

1.9 **Relationship Beneficial to Client.** Marriage and family therapists continue therapeutic relationships only so long as it is reasonably clear that clients are benefiting from the relationship.

1.10 **Referrals.** Marriage and family therapists respectfully assist persons in obtaining appropriate therapeutic services if the therapist is unable or unwilling to provide professional help.

1.11 **Non-Abandonment.** Marriage and family therapists do not abandon or neglect clients in treatment without making reasonable arrangements for the continuation of treatment.

1.12 **Written Consent to Record.** Marriage and family therapists obtain written informed consent from clients before recording any images or audio or permitting third-party observation.

1.13 **Relationships With Third Parties.** Marriage and family therapists, upon agreeing to provide services to a person or entity at the request of a third party, clarify, to the extent feasible and at the outset of the service, the nature of the relationship with each party and the limits of confidentiality.

Standard II

Confidentiality

Marriage and family therapists have unique confidentiality concerns because the client in a therapeutic relationship may be more than one person. Therapists respect and guard the confidences of each individual client.

2.1 **Disclosing Limits of Confidentiality.** Marriage and family therapists disclose to clients and other interested parties at the outset of services the nature of confidentiality and possible limitations of the clients' right to confidentiality. Therapists review with clients the circumstances where confidential information may be requested and where disclosure of confidential information may be legally required. Circumstances may necessitate repeated disclosures.

2.2 **Written Authorization to Release Client Information.** Marriage and family therapists do not disclose client confidences except by written authorization or waiver, or where mandated or permitted by law. Verbal authorization will not be sufficient except in emergency situations, unless prohibited by law. When providing couple, family or group treatment, the therapist does not disclose information outside the treatment context without a written authorization from each individual competent to execute a waiver. In the context of couple, family or group treatment, the therapist may not reveal any individual's confidences to others in the client unit without the prior written permission of that individual.

2.3 **Client Access to Records.** Marriage and family therapists provide clients with reasonable access to records concerning the clients. When providing couple, family, or group treatment, the therapist does not provide access to records without a written authorization from each individual competent to execute a waiver. Marriage and family therapists limit client's access to their records only in exceptional circumstances when they are concerned, based on compelling evidence, that such access could cause serious harm to the client. The client's request and the rationale for withholding some or all of the record should be documented in the client's file. Marriage and family therapists take steps to protect the confidentiality of other individuals identified in client records.

2.4 **Confidentiality in Non-Clinical Activities.** Marriage and family therapists use client and/or clinical materials in teaching, writing, consulting, research, and public presentations only if a written waiver has been obtained in accordance with Standard 2.2, or when appropriate steps have been taken to protect client identity and confidentiality.

2.5 **Protection of Records.** Marriage and family therapists store, safeguard, and dispose of client records in ways that maintain confidentiality and in accord with applicable laws and professional standards.

2.6 **Preparation for Practice Changes.** In preparation for moving a practice, closing a practice, or death, marriage and family therapists arrange for the storage, transfer, or disposal of client records in conformance with applicable laws and in ways that maintain confidentiality and safeguard the welfare of clients.

2.7 **Confidentiality in Consultations.** Marriage and family therapists, when consulting with colleagues or referral sources, do not share confidential information that could reasonably lead to the identification of a client, research participant, supervisee, or other person with whom they have a confidential relationship unless they have obtained the prior written consent of the client, research participant, supervisee, or other person with whom they have a confidential relationship. Information may be shared only to the extent necessary to achieve the purposes of the consultation.

Standard III

Professional Competence and Integrity

Marriage and family therapists maintain high standards of professional competence and integrity.

3.1 **Maintenance of Competency.** Marriage and family therapists pursue knowledge of new developments and maintain their competence in marriage and family therapy through education, training, and/or supervised experience.

3.2 **Knowledge of Regulatory Standards.** Marriage and family therapists pursue appropriate consultation and training to ensure adequate knowledge of and adherence to applicable laws, ethics, and professional standards.

3.3 **Seek Assistance.** Marriage and family therapists seek appropriate professional assistance for issues that may impair work performance or clinical judgment.

3.4 **Conflicts of Interest.** Marriage and family therapists do not provide services that create a conflict of interest that may impair work performance or clinical judgment.

3.5 **Maintenance of Records.** Marriage and family therapists maintain accurate and adequate clinical and financial records in accordance with applicable law.

3.6 **Development of New Skills.** While developing new skills in specialty areas, marriage and family therapists take steps to ensure the competence of their work and to protect clients from possible harm. Marriage and family therapists practice in specialty areas new to them only after appropriate education, training, and/or supervised experience.

3.7 **Harassment.** Marriage and family therapists do not engage in sexual or other forms of harassment of clients, students, trainees, supervisees, employees, colleagues, or research subjects.

3.8 **Exploitation.** Marriage and family therapists do not engage in the exploitation of clients, students, trainees, supervisees, employees, colleagues, or research subjects.

3.9 **Gifts.** Marriage and family therapists attend to cultural norms when considering whether to accept gifts from or give gifts to clients. Marriage and family therapists consider the potential effects that receiving or giving gifts may have on clients and on the integrity and efficacy of the therapeutic relationship.

3.10 **Scope of Competence.** Marriage and family therapists do not diagnose, treat, or advise on problems outside the recognized boundaries of their competencies.

3.11 **Public Statements.** Marriage and family therapists, because of their ability to influence and alter the lives of others, exercise special care when making public their professional recommendations and opinions through testimony or other public statements.

3.12 **Professional Misconduct.** Marriage and family therapists may be in violation of this Code and subject to termination of membership or other appropriate action if they: (a) are convicted of any felony; (b) are convicted of a misdemeanor related to their qualifications or functions; (c) engage in conduct which could lead to conviction of a felony, or a misdemeanor related to their qualifications or functions; (d) are expelled from or disciplined by other professional organizations; (e) have their licenses or certificates suspended or revoked or are otherwise disciplined by regulatory bodies; (f) continue to practice marriage and family therapy while no longer competent to do so because they are impaired by physical or mental causes or the abuse of alcohol or other substances; or (g) fail to cooperate with the Association at any point from the inception of an ethical complaint through the completion of all proceedings regarding that complaint.

Standard IV

Responsibility to Students and Supervisees

Marriage and family therapists do not exploit the trust and dependency of students and supervisees.

4.1 **Exploitation.** Marriage and family therapists who are in a supervisory role are aware of their influential positions with respect to students and supervisees, and they avoid exploiting the trust and dependency of such persons. Therapists, therefore, make every effort to avoid conditions and multiple relationships that could impair professional objectivity or increase the risk of exploitation. When the risk of impairment or exploitation exists due to conditions or multiple roles, therapists take appropriate precautions.

4.2 **Therapy With Students or Supervisees.** Marriage and family therapists do not provide therapy to current students or supervisees.

4.3 **Sexual Intimacy With Students or Supervisees.** Marriage and family therapists do not engage in sexual intimacy with students or supervisees during the evaluative or training relationship between the therapist and student or supervisee.

4.4 **Oversight of Supervisee Competence.** Marriage and family therapists do not permit students or supervisees to perform or to hold themselves out as competent to perform professional services beyond their training, level of experience, and competence.

4.5 **Oversight of Supervisee Professionalism.** Marriage and family therapists take reasonable measures to ensure that services provided by supervisees are professional.

4.6 **Existing Relationship With Students or Supervisees.** Marriage and family therapists are aware of their influential positions with respect to supervisees, and they avoid exploiting the trust and dependency of such persons. Supervisors, therefore, make every effort to avoid conditions and multiple relationships with supervisees that could impair professional judgment or increase the risk of exploitation. Examples of such relationships include, but are not limited to, business or close personal relationships with supervisees or the supervisee's immediate family. When the risk of impairment or exploitation exists due to conditions or multiple roles, supervisors document the appropriate precautions taken.

4.7 **Confidentiality With Supervisees.** Marriage and family therapists do not disclose supervisee confidences except by written authorization or waiver, or when mandated or permitted by law. In educational or training settings where there are multiple supervisors, disclosures are permitted only to other professional colleagues, administrators, or employers who share responsibility for training of the supervisee. Verbal authorization will not be sufficient except in emergency situations, unless prohibited by law.

4.8 **Payment for Supervision.** Marriage and family therapists providing clinical supervision shall not enter into financial arrangements with supervisees through deceptive or exploitative practices, nor shall marriage and family therapists providing clinical supervision exert undue influence over supervisees when establishing supervision fees. Marriage and family therapists shall also not engage in other exploitative practices of supervisees.

Standard V

Research and Publication

Marriage and family therapists respect the dignity and protect the welfare of research participants, and are aware of applicable laws, regulations, and professional standards governing the conduct of research.

5.1 **Institutional Approval.** When institutional approval is required, marriage and family therapists submit accurate information about their research proposals and obtain appropriate approval prior to conducting the research.

5.2 **Protection of Research Participants.** Marriage and family therapists are responsible for making careful examinations of ethical acceptability in planning research. To the extent that services to research participants may be compromised by participation in research, marriage and family therapists seek the ethical advice of qualified professionals not directly involved in the investigation and observe safeguards to protect the rights of research participants.

5.3 **Informed Consent to Research.** Marriage and family therapists inform participants about the purpose of the research, expected length, and research procedures. They also inform participants of the aspects of the research that might reasonably be expected to influence willingness to participate such as potential risks, discomforts, or adverse effects. Marriage and family therapists are especially sensitive to the possibility of diminished consent when participants are also receiving clinical services, or have impairments which limit understanding and/or communication, or when participants are children. Marriage and family therapists inform participants about any potential research benefits, the limits of confidentiality, and whom to contact concerning questions about the research and their rights as research participants.

5.4 **Right to Decline or Withdraw Participation.** Marriage and family therapists respect each participant's freedom to decline participation in or to withdraw from a research study at any time. This obligation requires special thought and consideration when investigators or other members of the research team are in positions of authority or influence over participants. Marriage and family therapists, therefore, make every effort to avoid multiple relationships with research participants that could impair professional judgment or increase the risk of exploitation. When offering inducements for research participation, marriage and family therapists make reasonable efforts to avoid offering inappropriate or excessive inducements when such inducements are likely to coerce participation.

5.5   **Confidentiality of Research Data.** Information obtained about a research participant during the course of an investigation is confidential unless there is a waiver previously obtained in writing. When the possibility exists that others, including family members, may obtain access to such information, this possibility, together with the plan for protecting confidentiality, is explained as part of the procedure for obtaining informed consent.

5.6   **Publication.** Marriage and family therapists do not fabricate research results. Marriage and family therapists disclose potential conflicts of interest and take authorship credit only for work they have performed or to which they have contributed. Publication credits accurately reflect the relative contributions of the individual involved.

5.7   **Authorship of Student Work.** Marriage and family therapists do not accept or require authorship credit for a publication based from student's research, unless the marriage and family therapist made a substantial contribution beyond being a faculty advisor or research committee member. Co-authorship on student research should be determined in accordance with principles of fairness and justice.

5.8   **Plagiarism.** Marriage and family therapists who are the authors of books or other materials that are published or distributed do not plagiarize or fail to cite persons to whom credit for original ideas or work is due.

5.9   **Accuracy in Publication.** Marriage and family therapists who are authors of books or other materials published or distributed by an organization take reasonable precautions to ensure that the published materials are accurate and factual.

Standard VI

Technology-Assisted Professional Services

Therapy, supervision, and other professional services engaged in by marriage and family therapists take place over an increasing number of technological platforms. There are great benefits and responsibilities inherent in both the traditional therapeutic and supervision contexts, as well as in the utilization of technologically-assisted professional services. This standard addresses basic ethical requirements of offering therapy, supervision, and related professional services using electronic means.

6.1   **Technology Assisted Services.** Prior to commencing therapy or supervision services through electronic means (including but not limited to phone and Internet), marriage and family therapists ensure that they are compliant with all relevant laws for the delivery of such services. Additionally, marriage and family therapists must: (a) determine that technologically-assisted services or supervision are appropriate for clients or supervisees, considering professional, intellectual, emotional, and physical needs; (b) inform clients or supervisees of the potential risks and benefits associated with technologically-assisted services; (c) ensure the security of their communication medium; and (d) only commence electronic therapy or supervision after appropriate education, training, or supervised experience using the relevant technology.

6.2 **Consent to Treat or Supervise.** Clients and supervisees, whether contracting for services as individuals, dyads, families, or groups, must be made aware of the risks and responsibilities associated with technology-assisted services. Therapists are to advise clients and supervisees in writing of these risks, and of both the therapist's and clients'/supervisees' responsibilities for minimizing such risks.

6.3 **Confidentiality and Professional Responsibilities.** It is the therapist's or supervisor's responsibility to choose technological platforms that adhere to standards of best practices related to confidentiality and quality of services, and that meet applicable laws. Clients and supervisees are to be made aware in writing of the limitations and protections offered by the therapist's or supervisor's technology.

6.4 **Technology and Documentation.** Therapists and supervisors are to ensure that all documentation containing identifying or otherwise sensitive information which is electronically stored and/or transferred is done using technology that adhere to standards of best practices related to confidentiality and quality of services, and that meet applicable laws. Clients and supervisees are to be made aware in writing of the limitations and protections offered by the therapist's or supervisor's technology.

6.5 **Location of Services and Practice.** Therapists and supervisors follow all applicable laws regarding location of practice and services, and do not use technologically-assisted means for practicing outside of their allowed jurisdictions.

6.6 **Training and Use of Current Technology.** Marriage and family therapists ensure that they are well trained and competent in the use of all chosen technology-assisted professional services. Careful choices of audio, video, and other options are made in order to optimize quality and security of services, and to adhere to standards of best practices for technology-assisted services. Furthermore, such choices of technology are to be suitably advanced and current so as to best serve the professional needs of clients and supervisees.

Standard VII

Professional Evaluations

Marriage and family therapists aspire to the highest of standards in providing testimony in various contexts within the legal system.

7.1 **Performance of Forensic Services.** Marriage and family therapists may perform forensic services which may include interviews, consultations, evaluations, reports, and assessments both formal and informal, in keeping with applicable laws and competencies.

7.2 **Testimony in Legal Proceedings.** Marriage and family therapists who provide expert or fact witness testimony in legal proceedings avoid misleading judgments, base conclusions and opinions on appropriate data, and avoid inaccuracies insofar as possible. When offering testimony, as marriage and family therapy experts, they shall strive to be accurate, objective, fair, and independent.

7.3 **Competence.** Marriage and family therapists demonstrate competence via education and experience in providing testimony in legal systems.

7.4 **Informed Consent.** Marriage and family therapists provide written notice and make reasonable efforts to obtain written consents of persons who are the subject(s) of evaluations and inform clients about the evaluation process, use of information and recommendations, financial arrangements, and the role of the therapist within the legal system.

7.5 **Avoiding Conflicts.** Clear distinctions are made between therapy and evaluations. Marriage and family therapists avoid conflict in roles in legal proceedings wherever possible and disclose potential conflicts. As therapy begins, marriage and family therapists clarify roles and the extent of confidentiality when legal systems are involved.

7.6 **Avoiding Dual Roles.** Marriage and family therapists avoid providing therapy to clients for whom the therapist has provided a forensic evaluation and avoid providing evaluations for those who are clients, unless otherwise mandated by legal systems.

7.7 **Separation of Custody Evaluation From Therapy.** Marriage and family therapists avoid conflicts of interest in treating minors or adults involved in custody or visitation actions by not performing evaluations for custody, residence, or visitation of the minor. Marriage and family therapists who treat minors may provide the court or mental health professional performing the evaluation with information about the minor from the marriage and family therapist's perspective as a treating marriage and family therapist, so long as the marriage and family therapist obtains appropriate consents to release information.

7.8 **Professional Opinions.** Marriage and family therapists who provide forensic evaluations avoid offering professional opinions about persons they have not directly interviewed. Marriage and family therapists declare the limits of their competencies and information.

7.9 **Changes in Service.** Clients are informed if changes in the role of provision of services of marriage and family therapy occur and/or are mandated by a legal system.

7.10 **Familiarity With Rules.** Marriage and family therapists who provide forensic evaluations are familiar with judicial and/or administrative rules prescribing their roles.

Standard VIII

Financial Arrangements

Marriage and family therapists make financial arrangements with clients, third-party payors, and supervisees that are reasonably understandable and conform to accepted professional practices.

8.1 **Financial Integrity.** Marriage and family therapists do not offer or accept kickbacks, rebates, bonuses, or other remuneration for referrals. Fee-for-service arrangements are not prohibited.

8.2 **Disclosure of Financial Policies.** Prior to entering into the therapeutic or supervisory relationship, marriage and family therapists clearly disclose and explain to clients and supervisees: (a) all financial arrangements and fees related to professional services, including charges for canceled or missed appointments; (b) the use of collection agencies or legal measures for nonpayment; and (c) the procedure for obtaining payment from the client, to the extent allowed by law, if payment is denied by the third-party payor. Once services have begun, therapists provide reasonable notice of any changes in fees or other charges.

8.3 **Notice of Payment Recovery Procedures.** Marriage and family therapists give reasonable notice to clients with unpaid balances of their intent to seek collection by agency or legal recourse. When such action is taken, therapists will not disclose clinical information.

8.4 **Truthful Representation of Services.** Marriage and family therapists represent facts truthfully to clients, third-party payors, and supervisees regarding services rendered.

8.5 **Bartering.** Marriage and family therapists ordinarily refrain from accepting goods and services from clients in return for services rendered. Bartering for professional services may be conducted only if: (a) the supervisee or client requests it; (b) the relationship is not exploitative; (c) the professional relationship is not distorted; and (d) a clear written contract is established.

8.6 **Withholding Records for Non-Payment.** Marriage and family therapists may not withhold records under their immediate control that are requested and needed for a client's treatment solely because payment has not been received for past services, except as otherwise provided by law.

Standard IX

Advertising

Marriage and family therapists engage in appropriate informational activities, including those that enable the public, referral sources, or others to choose professional services on an informed basis.

9.1 **Accurate Professional Representation.** Marriage and family therapists accurately represent their competencies, education, training, and experience relevant to their practice of marriage and family therapy in accordance with applicable law.

9.2 **Promotional Materials.** Marriage and family therapists ensure that advertisements and publications in any media are true, accurate, and in accordance with applicable law.

9.3 **Professional Affiliations.** Marriage and family therapists do not hold themselves out as being partners or associates of a firm if they are not.

9.4 **Professional Identification.** Marriage and family therapists do not use any professional identification (such as a business card, office sign, letterhead, Internet, or telephone or association directory listing) if it includes a statement or claim that is false, fraudulent, misleading, or deceptive.

9.5 **Educational Credentials.** Marriage and family therapists claim degrees for their clinical services only if those degrees demonstrate training and education in marriage and family therapy or related fields.

9.6 **Employee or Supervisee Qualifications.** Marriage and family therapists make certain that the qualifications of their employees and supervisees are represented in a manner that is true, accurate, and in accordance with applicable law.

9.7 **Specialization.** Marriage and family therapists represent themselves as providing specialized services only after taking reasonable steps to ensure the competence of their work and to protect clients, supervisees, and others from harm.

9.8 **Correction of Misinformation.** Marriage and family therapists correct, wherever possible, false, misleading, or inaccurate information and representations made by others concerning the therapist's qualifications, services, or products.

Source: American Association for Marriage and Family Therapy, (2015). AAMFT Code of Ethics.

Appendix D: American Psychological Association Ethical Principles of Psychologists and Code of Conduct

Contents

9.   *Assessment*

9.01   Bases for Assessments

9.02   Use of Assessments

9.03   Informed Consent in Assessments

9.04   Release of Test Data

9.05   Test Construction

9.06   Interpreting Assessment Results

9.07   Assessment by Unqualified Persons

9.08   Obsolete Tests and Outdated Test Results

9.09   Test Scoring and Interpretation Services

9.10   Explaining Assessment Results

9.11   Maintaining Test Security

10.   *Therapy*

10.01   Informed Consent to Therapy

10.02   Therapy Involving Couples or Families

10.03   Group Therapy

10.04   Providing Therapy to Those Served by Others

10.05   Sexual Intimacies With Current Therapy Clients/Patients

10.06   Sexual Intimacies With Relatives or Significant Others of Current Therapy Clients/Patients

10.07   Therapy With Former Sexual Partners

10.08   Sexual Intimacies With Former Therapy Clients/Patients

10.09   Interruption of Therapy

10.10   Terminating Therapy

Effective June 1, 2003, as amended 2010

2010 Amendments to the 2002 "Ethical Principles of Psychologists and Code of Conduct"

Introduction and Applicability

The American Psychological Association's (APA's) Ethical Principles of Psychologists and Code of Conduct (hereinafter referred to as the Ethics Code) consists of an Introduction, a Preamble, five General Principles (A–E), and specific Ethical Standards. The Introduction discusses the intent, organization, procedural considerations, and scope of application of the Ethics Code. The Preamble and General Principles are aspirational goals to guide psychologists toward the highest ideals of psychology. Although the Preamble and General Principles are not themselves enforceable rules, they should be considered by psychologists in arriving at an ethical course of action. The Ethical Standards set forth enforceable rules for conduct as psychologists. Most of the Ethical Standards are written broadly, in order to apply to psychologists in varied roles, although the application of an Ethical Standard may vary depending on the context. The Ethical Standards are not exhaustive. The fact that a given conduct is not specifically addressed by an Ethical Standard does not mean that it is necessarily either ethical or unethical.

This Ethics Code applies only to psychologists' activities that are part of their scientific, educational, or professional roles as psychologists. Areas covered include but are not limited to the clinical, counseling, and school practice of psychology; research; teaching; supervision of trainees; public service; policy development; social intervention; development of assessment instruments; conducting assessments; educational counseling; organizational consulting; forensic activities; program design and evaluation; and administration. This Ethics Code applies to these activities across a variety of contexts, such as in person, postal, telephone, Internet, and other electronic transmissions. These activities shall be distinguished from the purely private conduct of psychologists, which is not within the purview of the Ethics Code.

Membership in the APA commits members and student affiliates to comply with the standards of the APA Ethics Code and to the rules and procedures used to enforce them. Lack of awareness or misunderstanding of an Ethical Standard is not itself a defense to a charge of unethical conduct.

The procedures for filing, investigating, and resolving complaints of unethical conduct are described in the current Rules and Procedures of the APA Ethics Committee. APA may impose sanctions on its members for violations of the standards of the Ethics Code, including termination of APA membership, and may notify other bodies and individuals of its actions. Actions that violate the standards of the Ethics Code may also lead to the imposition of sanctions on psychologists or students whether or not they are APA members by bodies other than APA, including state psychological associations, other professional groups, psychology boards, other state or federal agencies, and payors for health services. In addition, APA may take action against a member after his or her conviction of a felony, expulsion or suspension from an affiliated state psychological association, or suspension or loss of licensure. When the sanction to be imposed by APA is less than expulsion, the 2001 Rules and Procedures do not guarantee an opportunity for an in-person hearing, but generally provide that complaints will be resolved only on the basis of a submitted record.

The Ethics Code is intended to provide guidance for psychologists and standards of professional conduct that can be applied by the APA and by other bodies that choose to adopt them. The Ethics Code is not intended to be a basis of civil liability. Whether a psychologist has violated the Ethics Code standards does not by itself determine whether the psychologist is legally liable in a court action, whether a contract is enforceable, or whether other legal consequences occur.

The modifiers used in some of the standards of this Ethics Code (e.g., *reasonably, appropriate, potentially*) are included in the standards when they would (1) allow professional judgment on the part of psychologists, (2) eliminate injustice or inequality that would occur without the modifier, (3) ensure applicability across the broad range of activities conducted by psychologists, or (4) guard against a set of rigid rules that might be quickly outdated. As used in this Ethics Code, the term *reasonable* means the prevailing professional judgment of psychologists engaged in similar activities in similar circumstances, given the knowledge the psychologist had or should have had at the time.

The American Psychological Association's Council of Representatives adopted this version of the APA Ethics Code during its meeting on August 21, 2002. The Code became effective on June 1, 2003. The Council of Representatives amended this version of the Ethics Code on February 20, 2010. The amendments became effective on June 1, 2010 (see p. 15 of this pamphlet). Inquiries concerning the substance or interpretation of the APA Ethics Code should be addressed to the Director, Office of Ethics, American Psychological Association, 750 First Street, NE, Washington, DC 20002-4242. The Ethics Code and information regarding the Code can be found on the APA website, http://www.apa.org/ethics. The standards in this Ethics Code will be used to adjudicate complaints brought concerning alleged conduct occurring on or after the effective date. Complaints will be adjudicated on the basis of the version of the Ethics Code that was in effect at the time the conduct occurred.

The APA has previously published its Ethics Code as follows:

American Psychological Association. (1953). *Ethical standards of psychologists*. Washington, DC: Author.

American Psychological Association. (1959). Ethical standards of psychologists. *American Psychologist, 14,* 279–282.

American Psychological Association. (1963). Ethical standards of psychologists. *American Psychologist, 18,* 56–60.

American Psychological Association. (1968). Ethical standards of psychologists. *American Psychologist, 23,* 357–361.

American Psychological Association. (1977, March). Ethical standards of psychologists. *APA Monitor,* 22–23.

American Psychological Association. (1979). *Ethical standards of psychologists*. Washington, DC: Author.

American Psychological Association. (1981). Ethical principles of psychologists. *American Psychologist, 36,* 633–638.

American Psychological Association. (1990). Ethical principles of psychologists (Amended June 2, 1989). *American Psychologist, 45,* 390–395.

American Psychological Association. (1992). Ethical principles of psychologists and code of conduct. *American Psychologist, 47,* 1597–1611.

American Psychological Association. (2002). Ethical principles of psychologists and code of conduct. *American Psychologist, 57,* 1060-1073.

Request copies of the APA's Ethical Principles of Psychologists and Code of Conduct from the APA Order Department, 750 First Street, NE, Washington, DC 20002-4242, or phone (202) 336-5510.

In the process of making decisions regarding their professional behavior, psychologists must consider this Ethics Code in addition to applicable laws and psychology board regulations. In applying the Ethics Code to their professional work, psychologists may consider other materials and guidelines that have been adopted or endorsed by scientific and professional psychological organizations and the dictates of their own conscience, as well as consult with others within the field. If this Ethics Code establishes a higher standard of conduct than is required by law, psychologists must meet the higher ethical standard. If psychologists' ethical responsibilities conflict with law, regulations, or other governing legal authority, psychologists make known their commitment to this Ethics Code and take steps to resolve the conflict in a responsible manner in keeping with basic principles of human rights.

Preamble

Psychologists are committed to increasing scientific and professional knowledge of behavior and people's understanding of themselves and others and to the use of such knowledge to improve the condition of individuals, organizations, and society. Psychologists respect and protect civil and human rights and the central importance of freedom of inquiry and expression in research, teaching, and publication. They strive to help the public in developing informed judgments and choices concerning human behavior. In doing so, they perform many roles, such as researcher, educator, diagnostician, therapist, supervisor, consultant, administrator, social interventionist, and expert witness. This Ethics Code provides a common set of principles and standards upon which psychologists build their professional and scientific work.

This Ethics Code is intended to provide specific standards to cover most situations encountered by psychologists. It has as its goals the welfare and protection of the individuals and groups with whom psychologists work and the education of members, students, and the public regarding ethical standards of the discipline.

The development of a dynamic set of ethical standards for psychologists' work-related conduct requires a personal commitment and lifelong effort to act ethically; to encourage ethical behavior by students, supervisees, employees, and colleagues; and to consult with others concerning ethical problems.

General Principles

This section consists of General Principles. General Principles, as opposed to Ethical Standards, are aspirational in nature. Their intent is to guide and inspire psychologists toward the very highest ethical ideals of the profession. General Principles, in contrast to Ethical Standards, do not represent obligations and should not form the basis for imposing sanctions. Relying upon General Principles for either of these reasons distorts both their meaning and purpose.

Principle A: Beneficence and Nonmaleficence

Psychologists strive to benefit those with whom they work and take care to do no harm. In their professional actions, psychologists seek to safeguard the welfare and rights of those with whom they interact professionally and other affected persons, and the welfare of animal subjects of research. When conflicts occur among psychologists' obligations or concerns, they attempt to resolve these conflicts in a responsible fashion that avoids or minimizes harm. Because psychologists' scientific and professional judgments and actions may affect the lives of others, they are alert to and guard against personal, financial, social, organizational, or political factors that might lead to misuse of their influence. Psychologists strive to be aware of the possible effect of their own physical and mental health on their ability to help those with whom they work.

Principle B: Fidelity and Responsibility

Psychologists establish relationships of trust with those with whom they work. They are aware of their professional and scientific responsibilities to society and to the specific communities in which they work. Psychologists uphold professional standards of conduct, clarify their professional roles and obligations, accept appropriate responsibility for their behavior, and seek to manage conflicts of interest that could lead to exploitation or harm. Psychologists consult with, refer to, or cooperate with other professionals and institutions to the extent needed to serve the best interests of those with whom they work. They are concerned about the ethical compliance of their colleagues' scientific and professional conduct. Psychologists strive to contribute a portion of their professional time for little or no compensation or personal advantage.

Principle C: Integrity

Psychologists seek to promote accuracy, honesty, and truthfulness in the science, teaching, and practice of psychology. In these activities psychologists do not steal, cheat, or engage in fraud, subterfuge, or intentional misrepresentation of fact. Psychologists strive to keep their promises and to avoid unwise or unclear commitments. In situations in which deception may be ethically justifiable to maximize benefits and minimize harm, psychologists have a serious obligation to consider the need for, the possible consequences of, and their responsibility to correct any resulting mistrust or other harmful effects that arise from the use of such techniques.

Principle D: Justice

Psychologists recognize that fairness and justice entitle all persons to access to and benefit from the contributions of psychology and to equal quality in the processes, procedures, and services being conducted by psychologists. Psychologists exercise reasonable judgment and take precautions to ensure that their potential biases, the boundaries of their competence, and the limitations of their expertise do not lead to or condone unjust practices.

Principle E: Respect for People's Rights and Dignity

Psychologists respect the dignity and worth of all people, and the rights of individuals to privacy, confidentiality, and self-determination. Psychologists are aware that special safeguards may be necessary to protect the rights and welfare of persons or communities whose vulnerabilities impair autonomous decision making. Psychologists are aware of and respect cultural, individual, and role differences, including those based on age, gender, gender identity, race, ethnicity, culture, national origin, religion, sexual orientation, disability, language, and socioeconomic status, and consider these factors when working with members of such groups. Psychologists try to eliminate the effect on their work of biases based on those factors, and they do not knowingly participate in or condone activities of others based upon such prejudices.

Ethical Standards

1. Resolving Ethical Issues

1.01 Misuse of Psychologists' Work

If psychologists learn of misuse or misrepresentation of their work, they take reasonable steps to correct or minimize the misuse or misrepresentation.

1.02 Conflicts Between Ethics and Law, Regulations, or Other Governing Legal Authority

If psychologists' ethical responsibilities conflict with law, regulations, or other governing legal authority, psychologists clarify the nature of the conflict, make known their commitment to the Ethics Code, and take reasonable steps to resolve the conflict consistent with the General Principles and Ethical Standards of the Ethics Code. Under no circumstances may this standard be used to justify or defend violating human rights.

1.03 Conflicts Between Ethics and Organizational Demands

If the demands of an organization with which psychologists are affiliated or for whom they are working are in conflict with this Ethics Code, psychologists clarify the nature of the conflict, make known their commitment to the Ethics Code, and take reasonable steps to resolve the conflict consistent with the General Principles and Ethical Standards of the Ethics Code. Under no circumstances may this standard be used to justify or defend violating human rights.

1.04 Informal Resolution of Ethical Violations

When psychologists believe that there may have been an ethical violation by another psychologist, they attempt to resolve the issue by bringing it to the attention of that individual, if an informal resolution appears appropriate and the intervention does not violate any confidentiality rights that may be involved. (See also Standards 1.02, Conflicts Between Ethics and Law, Regulations, or Other Governing Legal Authority, and 1.03, Conflicts Between Ethics and Organizational Demands.)

1.05 Reporting Ethical Violations

If an apparent ethical violation has substantially harmed or is likely to substantially harm a person or organization and is not appropriate for informal resolution under Standard 1.04, Informal Resolution of Ethical Violations, or is not resolved properly in that fashion, psychologists take further action appropriate to the situation. Such action might include referral to state or national committees on professional ethics, to state licensing boards, or to the appropriate institutional authorities. This standard does not apply when an intervention would violate confidentiality rights or when psychologists have been retained to review the work of another psychologist whose professional conduct is in question. (See also Standard 1.02, Conflicts Between Ethics and Law, Regulations, or Other Governing Legal Authority.)

1.06 Cooperating With Ethics Committees

Psychologists cooperate in ethics investigations, proceedings, and resulting requirements of the APA or any affiliated state psychological association to which they belong. In doing so, they address any confidentiality issues. Failure to cooperate is itself an ethics violation. However, making a request for deferment of adjudication of an ethics complaint pending the outcome of litigation does not alone constitute noncooperation.

1.07 Improper Complaints

Psychologists do not file or encourage the filing of ethics complaints that are made with reckless disregard for or willful ignorance of facts that would disprove the allegation.

1.08 Unfair Discrimination Against Complainants and Respondents

Psychologists do not deny persons employment, advancement, admissions to academic or other programs, tenure, or promotion, based solely upon their having made or their being the subject of an ethics complaint. This does not preclude taking action based upon the outcome of such proceedings or considering other appropriate information.

2. Competence

2.01 Boundaries of Competence

a. Psychologists provide services, teach, and conduct research with populations and in areas only within the boundaries of their competence, based on their education, training, supervised experience, consultation, study, or professional experience.

b. Where scientific or professional knowledge in the discipline of psychology establishes that an understanding of factors associated with age, gender, gender identity, race, ethnicity, culture, national origin, religion, sexual orientation, disability, language, or socioeconomic status is essential for effective implementation of their services or research, psychologists have or obtain the training, experience, consultation, or supervision necessary to ensure the competence of their services, or they make appropriate referrals, except as provided in Standard 2.02, Providing Services in Emergencies.

c. Psychologists planning to provide services, teach, or conduct research involving populations, areas, techniques, or technologies new to them undertake relevant education, training, supervised experience, consultation, or study.

d. When psychologists are asked to provide services to individuals for whom appropriate mental health services are not available and for which psychologists have not obtained the competence necessary, psychologists with closely related prior training or experience may provide such services in order to ensure that services are not denied if they make a reasonable effort to obtain the competence required by using relevant research, training, consultation, or study.

e. In those emerging areas in which generally recognized standards for preparatory training do not yet exist, psychologists nevertheless take reasonable steps to ensure the competence of their work and to protect clients/patients, students, supervisees, research participants, organizational clients, and others from harm.

f. When assuming forensic roles, psychologists are or become reasonably familiar with the judicial or administrative rules governing their roles.

2.02 Providing Services in Emergencies

In emergencies, when psychologists provide services to individuals for whom other mental health services are not available and for which psychologists have not obtained the necessary training, psychologists may provide such services in order to ensure that services are not denied. The services are discontinued as soon as the emergency has ended or appropriate services are available.

2.03 Maintaining Competence

Psychologists undertake ongoing efforts to develop and maintain their competence.

2.04 Bases for Scientific and Professional Judgments

Psychologists' work is based upon established scientific and professional knowledge of the discipline. (See also Standards 2.01e, Boundaries of Competence, and 10.01b, Informed Consent to Therapy.)

2.05 Delegation of Work to Others

Psychologists who delegate work to employees, supervisees, or research or teaching assistants or who use the services of others, such as interpreters, take reasonable steps to (1) avoid delegating such work to persons who have a multiple relationship with those being served that would likely lead to exploitation or loss of objectivity; (2) authorize only those responsibilities that such persons can be expected to perform competently on the basis of their education, training, or experience, either independently or with the level of supervision being provided; and (3) see that such persons perform these services competently. (See also Standards 2.02, Providing Services in Emergencies; 3.05, Multiple Relationships; 4.01, Maintaining Confidentiality; 9.01, Bases for Assessments; 9.02, Use of Assessments; 9.03, Informed Consent in Assessments; and 9.07, Assessment by Unqualified Persons.)

2.06 Personal Problems and Conflicts

a. Psychologists refrain from initiating an activity when they know or should know that there is a substantial likelihood that their personal problems will prevent them from performing their work-related activities in a competent manner.

b. When psychologists become aware of personal problems that may interfere with their performing work-related duties adequately, they take appropriate measures, such as obtaining professional consultation or assistance, and determine whether they should limit, suspend, or terminate their work-related duties. (See also Standard 10.10, Terminating Therapy.)

3. Human Relations

3.01 Unfair Discrimination

In their work-related activities, psychologists do not engage in unfair discrimination based on age, gender, gender identity, race, ethnicity, culture, national origin, religion, sexual orientation, disability, socioeconomic status, or any basis proscribed by law.

3.02 Sexual Harassment

Psychologists do not engage in sexual harassment. Sexual harassment is sexual solicitation, physical advances, or verbal or nonverbal conduct that is sexual in nature, that occurs in connection with the psychologist's activities or roles as a psychologist, and that either (1) is unwelcome, is offensive, or creates a hostile workplace or educational environment, and the psychologist knows or is told this or (2) is sufficiently severe or intense to be abusive to a reasonable person in the context. Sexual harassment can consist of a single intense or severe act or of multiple persistent or pervasive acts. (See also Standard 1.08, Unfair Discrimination Against Complainants and Respondents.)

3.03 Other Harassment

Psychologists do not knowingly engage in behavior that is harassing or demeaning to persons with whom they interact in their work based on factors such as those persons' age, gender, gender identity, race, ethnicity, culture, national origin, religion, sexual orientation, disability, language, or socioeconomic status.

3.04 Avoiding Harm

Psychologists take reasonable steps to avoid harming their clients/patients, students, supervisees, research participants, organizational clients, and others with whom they work, and to minimize harm where it is foreseeable and unavoidable.

3.05 Multiple Relationships

a. A multiple relationship occurs when a psychologist is in a professional role with a person and (1) at the same time is in another role with the same person, (2) at the same time is in a relationship with a person closely associated with or related to the person with whom the psychologist has the professional relationship, or (3) promises to enter into another relationship in the future with the person or a person closely associated with or related to the person.

   A psychologist refrains from entering into a multiple relationship if the multiple relationship could reasonably be expected to impair the psychologist's objectivity, competence, or effectiveness in performing his or her functions as a psychologist, or otherwise risks exploitation or harm to the person with whom the professional relationship exists.

   Multiple relationships that would not reasonably be expected to cause impairment or risk exploitation or harm are not unethical.

b. If a psychologist finds that, due to unforeseen factors, a potentially harmful multiple relationship has arisen, the psychologist takes reasonable steps to resolve it with due regard for the best interests of the affected person and maximal compliance with the Ethics Code.

c. When psychologists are required by law, institutional policy, or extraordinary circumstances to serve in more than one role in judicial or administrative proceedings, at the outset they clarify role expectations and the extent of confidentiality and thereafter as changes occur. (See also Standards 3.04, Avoiding Harm, and 3.07, Third-Party Requests for Services.)

3.06 Conflict of Interest

Psychologists refrain from taking on a professional role when personal, scientific, professional, legal, financial, or other interests or relationships could reasonably be expected to (1) impair their objectivity, competence, or effectiveness in performing their functions as psychologists or (2) expose the person or organization with whom the professional relationship exists to harm or exploitation.

3.07 Third-Party Requests for Services

When psychologists agree to provide services to a person or entity at the request of a third party, psychologists attempt to clarify at the outset of the service the nature of the relationship with all individuals or organizations involved. This clarification includes the role of the psychologist (e.g., therapist, consultant, diagnostician, or expert witness), an identification of who is the client, the probable uses of the services provided or the information obtained, and the fact that there may be limits to confidentiality. (See also Standards 3.05, Multiple Relationships, and 4.02, Discussing the Limits of Confidentiality.)

3.08 Exploitative Relationships

Psychologists do not exploit persons over whom they have supervisory, evaluative, or other authority such as clients/patients, students, supervisees, research participants, and employees. (See also Standards 3.05, Multiple Relationships; 6.04, Fees and Financial Arrangements; 6.05, Barter With Clients/Patients; 7.07, Sexual Relationships With Students and Supervisees; 10.05, Sexual Intimacies With Current Therapy Clients/Patients; 10.06, Sexual Intimacies With Relatives or Significant Others of Current Therapy Clients/ Patients; 10.07, Therapy With Former Sexual Partners; and 10.08, Sexual Intimacies With Former Therapy Clients/Patients.)

3.09 Cooperation With Other Professionals

When indicated and professionally appropriate, psychologists cooperate with other professionals in order to serve their clients/patients effectively and appropriately. (See also Standard 4.05, Disclosures.)

3.10 Informed Consent

a. When psychologists conduct research or provide assessment, therapy, counseling, or consulting services in person or via electronic transmission or other forms of communication, they obtain the informed consent of the individual or individuals using language that is reasonably understandable to that person or persons except when conducting such activities without consent is mandated by law or governmental regulation or as otherwise provided in this Ethics Code. (See also Standards 8.02, Informed Consent to Research; 9.03, Informed Consent in Assessments; and 10.01, Informed Consent to Therapy.)

b. For persons who are legally incapable of giving informed consent, psychologists nevertheless (1) provide an appropriate explanation, (2) seek the individual's assent, (3) consider such persons' preferences and best interests, and (4) obtain appropriate permission from a legally authorized person, if such substitute consent is permitted or required by law. When consent by a legally authorized person is not permitted or required by law, psychologists take reasonable steps to protect the individual's rights and welfare.

c. When psychological services are court ordered or otherwise mandated, psychologists inform the individual of the nature of the anticipated services, including whether the services are court ordered or mandated and any limits of confidentiality, before proceeding.

d. Psychologists appropriately document written or oral consent, permission, and assent. (See also Standards 8.02, Informed Consent to Research; 9.03, Informed Consent in Assessments; and 10.01, Informed Consent to Therapy.)

3.11 Psychological Services Delivered to or Through Organizations

a. Psychologists delivering services to or through organizations provide information beforehand to clients and when appropriate those directly affected by the services about (1) the nature and objectives of the services, (2) the intended recipients, (3) which of the individuals are clients, (4) the relationship the psychologist will have with each person and the organization, (5) the probable uses of services provided and information obtained, (6) who will have access to the information, and (7) limits of confidentiality. As soon as feasible, they provide information about the results and conclusions of such services to appropriate persons.

b. If psychologists will be precluded by law or by organizational roles from providing such information to particular individuals or groups, they so inform those individuals or groups at the outset of the service.

3.12 Interruption of Psychological Services

Unless otherwise covered by contract, psychologists make reasonable efforts to plan for facilitating services in the event that psychological services are interrupted by factors such as the psychologist's illness, death, unavailability, relocation, or retirement or by the client's/patient's relocation or financial limitations. (See also Standard 6.02c, Maintenance, Dissemination, and Disposal of Confidential Records of Professional and Scientific Work.)

4. Privacy and Confidentiality

4.01 Maintaining Confidentiality

Psychologists have a primary obligation and take reasonable precautions to protect confidential information obtained through or stored in any medium, recognizing that the extent and limits of confidentiality may be regulated by law or established by institutional rules or professional or scientific relationship. (See also Standard 2.05, Delegation of Work to Others.)

4.02 Discussing the Limits of Confidentiality

a. Psychologists discuss with persons (including, to the extent feasible, persons who are legally incapable of giving informed consent and their legal representatives) and organizations with whom they establish a scientific or professional relationship (1) the relevant limits of confidentiality and (2) the foreseeable uses of the information generated through their psychological activities. (See also Standard 3.10, Informed Consent.)

b. Unless it is not feasible or is contraindicated, the discussion of confidentiality occurs at the outset of the relationship and thereafter as new circumstances may warrant.

c. Psychologists who offer services, products, or information via electronic transmission inform clients/patients of the risks to privacy and limits of confidentiality.

4.03 Recording

Before recording the voices or images of individuals to whom they provide services, psychologists obtain permission from all such persons or their legal representatives. (See also Standards 8.03, Informed Consent for Recording Voices and Images in Research; 8.05, Dispensing With Informed Consent for Research; and 8.07, Deception in Research.)

4.04 Minimizing Intrusions on Privacy

a. Psychologists include in written and oral reports and consultations, only information germane to the purpose for which the communication is made.

b. Psychologists discuss confidential information obtained in their work only for appropriate scientific or professional purposes and only with persons clearly concerned with such matters.

4.05 Disclosures

a. Psychologists may disclose confidential information with the appropriate consent of the organizational client, the individual client/patient, or another legally authorized person on behalf of the client/patient unless prohibited by law.

b. Psychologists disclose confidential information without the consent of the individual only as mandated by law, or where permitted by law for a valid purpose such as to (1) provide needed professional services; (2) obtain appropriate professional consultations; (3) protect the client/patient, psychologist, or others from harm; or (4) obtain payment for services from a client/patient, in which instance disclosure is limited to the minimum that is necessary to achieve the purpose. (See also Standard 6.04e, Fees and Financial Arrangements.)

4.06 Consultations

When consulting with colleagues, (1) psychologists do not disclose confidential information that reasonably could lead to the identification of a client/patient, research participant, or other person or organization with whom they have a confidential relationship unless they have obtained the prior consent of the person or organization or the disclosure cannot be avoided, and (2) they disclose information only to the extent necessary to achieve the purposes of the consultation. (See also Standard 4.01, Maintaining Confidentiality.)

4.07 Use of Confidential Information for Didactic or Other Purposes

Psychologists do not disclose in their writings, lectures, or other public media, confidential, personally identifiable information concerning their clients/patients, students, research participants, organizational clients, or other recipients of their services that they obtained during the course of their work, unless (1) they take reasonable steps to disguise the person or organization, (2) the person or organization has consented in writing, or (3) there is legal authorization for doing so.

5. Advertising and Other Public Statements

5.01 Avoidance of False or Deceptive Statements

a. Public statements include but are not limited to paid or unpaid advertising, product endorsements, grant applications, licensing applications, other credentialing applications, brochures, printed matter, directory listings, personal resumes or curricula vitae, or comments for use in media such as print or electronic transmission, statements in legal proceedings, lectures and public oral presentations, and published materials. Psychologists do not knowingly make public statements that are false, deceptive, or fraudulent concerning their research, practice, or other work activities or those of persons or organizations with which they are affiliated.

b. Psychologists do not make false, deceptive, or fraudulent statements concerning (1) their training, experience, or competence; (2) their academic degrees; (3) their credentials; (4) their institutional or association affiliations; (5) their services; (6) the scientific or clinical basis for, or results or degree of success of, their services; (7) their fees; or (8) their publications or research findings.

c. Psychologists claim degrees as credentials for their health services only if those degrees (1) were earned from a regionally accredited educational institution or (2) were the basis for psychology licensure by the state in which they practice.

5.02 Statements by Others

a. Psychologists who engage others to create or place public statements that promote their professional practice, products, or activities retain professional responsibility for such statements.

b. Psychologists do not compensate employees of press, radio, television, or other communication media in return for publicity in a news item. (See also Standard 1.01, Misuse of Psychologists' Work.)

c. A paid advertisement relating to psychologists' activities must be identified or clearly recognizable as such.

5.03 Descriptions of Workshops and Non-Degree-Granting Educational Programs

To the degree to which they exercise control, psychologists responsible for announcements, catalogs, brochures, or advertisements describing workshops, seminars, or other non-degree-granting educational programs ensure that they accurately describe the audience for which the program is intended, the educational objectives, the presenters, and the fees involved.

5.04 Media Presentations

When psychologists provide public advice or comment via print, Internet, or other electronic transmission, they take precautions to ensure that statements (1) are based on their professional knowledge, training, or experience in accord with appropriate psychological literature and practice; (2) are otherwise consistent with this Ethics Code; and (3) do not indicate that a professional relationship has been established with the recipient. (See also Standard 2.04, Bases for Scientific and Professional Judgments.)

5.05 Testimonials

Psychologists do not solicit testimonials from current therapy clients/patients or other persons who because of their particular circumstances are vulnerable to undue influence.

5.06 In-Person Solicitation

Psychologists do not engage, directly or through agents, in uninvited in-person solicitation of business from actual or potential therapy clients/patients or other persons who because of their particular circumstances are vulnerable to undue influence. However, this prohibition does not preclude (1) attempting to implement appropriate collateral contacts for the purpose of benefiting an already engaged therapy client/patient or (2) providing disaster or community outreach services.

6. Record Keeping and Fees

6.01 Documentation of Professional and Scientific Work and Maintenance of Records

Psychologists create, and to the extent the records are under their control, maintain, disseminate, store, retain, and dispose of records and data relating to their professional and scientific work in order to (1) facilitate provision of services later by them or by other professionals, (2) allow for replication of research design and analyses, (3) meet institutional requirements, (4) ensure accuracy of billing and payments, and (5) ensure compliance with law. (See also Standard 4.01, Maintaining Confidentiality.)

6.02 Maintenance, Dissemination, and Disposal of Confidential Records of Professional and Scientific Work

a. Psychologists maintain confidentiality in creating, storing, accessing, transferring, and disposing of records under their control, whether these are written, automated, or in any other medium. (See also Standards 4.01, Maintaining Confidentiality, and 6.01, Documentation of Professional and Scientific Work and Maintenance of Records.)

b. If confidential information concerning recipients of psychological services is entered into databases or systems of records available to persons whose access has not been consented to by the recipient, psychologists use coding or other techniques to avoid the inclusion of personal identifiers.

c. Psychologists make plans in advance to facilitate the appropriate transfer and to protect the confidentiality of records and data in the event of psychologists' withdrawal from positions or practice. (See also Standards 3.12, Interruption of Psychological Services, and 10.09, Interruption of Therapy.)

6.03 Withholding Records for Nonpayment

Psychologists may not withhold records under their control that are requested and needed for a client's/patient's emergency treatment solely because payment has not been received.

6.04 Fees and Financial Arrangements

a. As early as is feasible in a professional or scientific relationship, psychologists and recipients of psychological services reach an agreement specifying compensation and billing arrangements.

b. Psychologists' fee practices are consistent with law.

c. Psychologists do not misrepresent their fees.

d. If limitations to services can be anticipated because of limitations in financing, this is discussed with the recipient of services as early as is feasible. (See also Standards 10.09, Interruption of Therapy, and 10.10, Terminating Therapy.)

e. If the recipient of services does not pay for services as agreed, and if psychologists intend to use collection agencies or legal measures to collect the fees, psychologists first inform the person that such measures will be taken and provide that person an opportunity to make prompt payment. (See also Standards 4.05, Disclosures; 6.03, Withholding Records for Nonpayment; and 10.01, Informed Consent to Therapy.)

6.05 Barter With Clients/Patients

Barter is the acceptance of goods, services, or other nonmonetary remuneration from clients/patients in return for psychological services. Psychologists may barter only if (1) it is not clinically contraindicated, and (2) the resulting arrangement is not exploitative. (See also Standards 3.05, Multiple Relationships, and 6.04, Fees and Financial Arrangements.)

6.06 Accuracy in Reports to Payors and Funding Sources

In their reports to payors for services or sources of research funding, psychologists take reasonable steps to ensure the accurate reporting of the nature of the service provided or research conducted, the fees, charges, or payments, and where applicable, the identity of the provider, the findings, and the diagnosis. (See also Standards 4.01, Maintaining Confidentiality; 4.04, Minimizing Intrusions on Privacy; and 4.05, Disclosures.)

6.07 Referrals and Fees

When psychologists pay, receive payment from, or divide fees with another professional, other than in an employer–employee relationship, the payment to each is based on the services provided (clinical, consultative, administrative, or other) and is not based on the referral itself. (See also Standard 3.09, Cooperation With Other Professionals.)

7. Education and Training

7.01 Design of Education and Training Programs

Psychologists responsible for education and training programs take reasonable steps to ensure that the programs are designed to provide the appropriate knowledge and proper experiences, and to meet the requirements for licensure, certification, or other goals for which claims are made by the program. (See also Standard 5.03, Descriptions of Workshops and Non-Degree-Granting Educational Programs.)

7.02 Descriptions of Education and Training Programs

Psychologists responsible for education and training programs take reasonable steps to ensure that there is a current and accurate description of the program content (including participation in required course or program-related counseling, psychotherapy, experiential groups, consulting projects, or community service), training goals and objectives, stipends and benefits, and requirements that must be met for satisfactory completion of the program. This information must be made readily available to all interested parties.

7.03 Accuracy in Teaching

a. Psychologists take reasonable steps to ensure that course syllabi are accurate regarding the subject matter to be covered, bases for evaluating progress, and the nature of course experiences. This standard does not preclude an instructor from modifying course content or requirements when the instructor considers it pedagogically necessary or desirable, so long as students are made aware of these modifications in a manner that enables them to fulfill course requirements. (See also Standard 5.01, Avoidance of False or Deceptive Statements.)

b. When engaged in teaching or training, psychologists present psychological information accurately. (See also Standard 2.03, Maintaining Competence.)

7.04 Student Disclosure of Personal Information

Psychologists do not require students or supervisees to disclose personal information in course- or program-related activities, either orally or in writing, regarding sexual history, history of abuse and neglect, psychological treatment, and relationships with parents, peers, and spouses or significant others except if (1) the program or training facility has clearly identified this requirement in its admissions and program materials or (2) the information is necessary to evaluate or obtain assistance for students whose personal problems could reasonably be judged to be preventing them from performing their training- or professionally related activities in a competent manner or posing a threat to the students or others.

7.05 Mandatory Individual or Group Therapy

a. When individual or group therapy is a program or course requirement, psychologists responsible for that program allow students in undergraduate and graduate programs the option of selecting such therapy from practitioners unaffiliated with the program. (See also Standard 7.02, Descriptions of Education and Training Programs.)

b. Faculty who are or are likely to be responsible for evaluating students' academic performance do not themselves provide that therapy. (See also Standard 3.05, Multiple Relationships.)

7.06 Assessing Student and Supervisee Performance

a. In academic and supervisory relationships, psychologists establish a timely and specific process for providing feedback to students and supervisees. Information regarding the process is provided to the student at the beginning of supervision.

b. Psychologists evaluate students and supervisees on the basis of their actual performance on relevant and established program requirements.

7.07 Sexual Relationships With Students and Supervisees

Psychologists do not engage in sexual relationships with students or supervisees who are in their department, agency, or training center or over whom psychologists have or are likely to have evaluative authority. (See also Standard 3.05, Multiple Relationships.)

8. Research and Publication

8.01 Institutional Approval

When institutional approval is required, psychologists provide accurate information about their research proposals and obtain approval prior to conducting the research. They conduct the research in accordance with the approved research protocol.

8.02 Informed Consent to Research

a. When obtaining informed consent as required in Standard 3.10, Informed Consent, psychologists inform participants about (1) the purpose of the research, expected duration, and procedures; (2) their right to decline to participate and to withdraw from the research once participation has begun; (3) the foreseeable consequences of declining or withdrawing; (4) reasonably foreseeable factors that may be expected to influence their willingness to participate such as potential risks, discomfort, or adverse effects; (5) any prospective research benefits; (6) limits of confidentiality; (7) incentives for participation; and (8) whom to contact for questions about the research and research participants' rights. They provide opportunity for the prospective participants to ask questions and receive answers. (See also Standards 8.03, Informed Consent for Recording Voices and Images in Research; 8.05, Dispensing With Informed Consent for Research; and 8.07, Deception in Research.)

b. Psychologists conducting intervention research involving the use of experimental treatments clarify to participants at the outset of the research (1) the experimental nature of the treatment; (2) the services that will or will not be available to the control group(s) if appropriate; (3) the means by which assignment to treatment and control groups will be made; (4) available treatment alternatives if an individual does not wish to participate in the research or wishes to withdraw once a study has begun; and (5) compensation for or monetary costs of participating including, if appropriate, whether reimbursement from the participant or a third-party payor will be sought. (See also Standard 8.02a, Informed Consent to Research.)

8.03 Informed Consent for Recording Voices and Images in Research

Psychologists obtain informed consent from research participants prior to recording their voices or images for data collection unless (1) the research consists solely of naturalistic observations in public places, and it is not anticipated that the recording will be used in a manner that could cause personal identification or harm, or (2) the research design includes deception, and consent for the use of the recording is obtained during debriefing. (See also Standard 8.07, Deception in Research.)

8.04 Client/Patient, Student, and Subordinate Research Participants

a. When psychologists conduct research with clients/patients, students, or subordinates as participants, psychologists take steps to protect the prospective participants from adverse consequences of declining or withdrawing from participation.

b. When research participation is a course requirement or an opportunity for extra credit, the prospective participant is given the choice of equitable alternative activities.

8.05 Dispensing With Informed Consent for Research

Psychologists may dispense with informed consent only (1) where research would not reasonably be assumed to create distress or harm and involves (a) the study of normal educational practices, curricula, or classroom management methods conducted in educational settings; (b) only anonymous questionnaires, naturalistic observations, or archival research for which disclosure of responses would not place participants at risk of criminal or civil liability or damage their financial standing, employability, or reputation, and confidentiality is protected; or (c) the study of factors related to job or organization effectiveness conducted in organizational settings for which there is no risk to participants' employability, and confidentiality is protected or (2) where otherwise permitted by law or federal or institutional regulations.

8.06 Offering Inducements for Research Participation

a. Psychologists make reasonable efforts to avoid offering excessive or inappropriate financial or other inducements for research participation when such inducements are likely to coerce participation.

b. When offering professional services as an inducement for research participation, psychologists clarify the nature of the services, as well as the risks, obligations, and limitations. (See also Standard 6.05, Barter With Clients/Patients.)

8.07 Deception in Research

a. Psychologists do not conduct a study involving deception unless they have determined that the use of deceptive techniques is justified by the study's significant prospective scientific, educational, or applied value and that effective nondeceptive alternative procedures are not feasible.

b. Psychologists do not deceive prospective participants about research that is reasonably expected to cause physical pain or severe emotional distress.

c. Psychologists explain any deception that is an integral feature of the design and conduct of an experiment to participants as early as is feasible, preferably at the conclusion of their participation, but no later than at the conclusion of the data collection, and permit participants to withdraw their data. (See also Standard 8.08, Debriefing.)

8.08 Debriefing

a. Psychologists provide a prompt opportunity for participants to obtain appropriate information about the nature, results, and conclusions of the research, and they take reasonable steps to correct any misconceptions that participants may have of which the psychologists are aware.

b. If scientific or humane values justify delaying or withholding this information, psychologists take reasonable measures to reduce the risk of harm.

c. When psychologists become aware that research procedures have harmed a participant, they take reasonable steps to minimize the harm.

8.09 Humane Care and Use of Animals in Research

a. Psychologists acquire, care for, use, and dispose of animals in compliance with current federal, state, and local laws and regulations, and with professional standards.

b. Psychologists trained in research methods and experienced in the care of laboratory animals supervise all procedures involving animals and are responsible for ensuring appropriate consideration of their comfort, health, and humane treatment.

c. Psychologists ensure that all individuals under their supervision who are using animals have received instruction in research methods and in the care, maintenance, and handling of the species being used, to the extent appropriate to their role. (See also Standard 2.05, Delegation of Work to Others.)

d. Psychologists make reasonable efforts to minimize the discomfort, infection, illness, and pain of animal subjects.

e. Psychologists use a procedure subjecting animals to pain, stress, or privation only when an alternative procedure is unavailable and the goal is justified by its prospective scientific, educational, or applied value.

f. Psychologists perform surgical procedures under appropriate anesthesia and follow techniques to avoid infection and minimize pain during and after surgery.

g. When it is appropriate that an animal's life be terminated, psychologists proceed rapidly, with an effort to minimize pain and in accordance with accepted procedures.

8.10 Reporting Research Results

a. Psychologists do not fabricate data. (See also Standard 5.01a, Avoidance of False or Deceptive Statements.)

b. If psychologists discover significant errors in their published data, they take reasonable steps to correct such errors in a correction, retraction, erratum, or other appropriate publication means.

8.11 Plagiarism

Psychologists do not present portions of another's work or data as their own, even if the other work or data source is cited occasionally.

8.12 Publication Credit

a. Psychologists take responsibility and credit, including authorship credit, only for work they have actually performed or to which they have substantially contributed. (See also Standard 8.12b, Publication Credit.)

b. Principal authorship and other publication credits accurately reflect the relative scientific or professional contributions of the individuals involved, regardless of their relative status. Mere possession of an institutional position, such as department chair, does not justify authorship credit. Minor contributions to the research or to the writing for publications are acknowledged appropriately, such as in footnotes or in an introductory statement.

c. Except under exceptional circumstances, a student is listed as principal author on any multiple-authored article that is substantially based on the student's doctoral dissertation. Faculty advisors discuss publication credit with students as early as feasible and throughout the research and publication process as appropriate. (See also Standard 8.12b, Publication Credit.)

8.13 Duplicate Publication of Data

Psychologists do not publish, as original data, data that have been previously published. This does not preclude republishing data when they are accompanied by proper acknowledgment.

8.14 Sharing Research Data for Verification

a. After research results are published, psychologists do not withhold the data on which their conclusions are based from other competent professionals who seek to verify the substantive claims through reanalysis and who intend to use such data only for that purpose, provided that the confidentiality of the participants can be protected and unless legal rights concerning proprietary data preclude their release. This does not preclude psychologists from requiring that such individuals or groups be responsible for costs associated with the provision of such information.

b. Psychologists who request data from other psychologists to verify the substantive claims through reanalysis may use shared data only for the declared purpose. Requesting psychologists obtain prior written agreement for all other uses of the data.

8.15 Reviewers

Psychologists who review material submitted for presentation, publication, grant, or research proposal review respect the confidentiality of and the proprietary rights in such information of those who submitted it.

9. Assessment

9.01 Bases for Assessments

a. Psychologists base the opinions contained in their recommendations, reports, and diagnostic or evaluative statements, including forensic testimony, on information and techniques sufficient to substantiate their findings. (See also Standard 2.04, Bases for Scientific and Professional Judgments.)

b. Except as noted in 9.01c, psychologists provide opinions of the psychological characteristics of individuals only after they have conducted an examination of the individuals adequate to support their statements or conclusions. When, despite reasonable efforts, such an examination is not practical, psychologists document the efforts they made and the result of those efforts, clarify the probable impact of their limited information on the reliability and validity of their opinions, and appropriately limit the nature and extent of their conclusions or recommendations. (See also Standards 2.01, Boundaries of Competence, and 9.06, Interpreting Assessment Results.)

c. When psychologists conduct a record review or provide consultation or supervision and an individual examination is not warranted or necessary for the opinion, psychologists explain this and the sources of information on which they based their conclusions and recommendations.

9.02 Use of Assessments

a. Psychologists administer, adapt, score, interpret, or use assessment techniques, interviews, tests, or instruments in a manner and for purposes that are appropriate in light of the research on or evidence of the usefulness and proper application of the techniques.

b. Psychologists use assessment instruments whose validity and reliability have been established for use with members of the population tested. When such validity or reliability has not been established, psychologists describe the strengths and limitations of test results and interpretation.

c. Psychologists use assessment methods that are appropriate to an individual's language preference and competence, unless the use of an alternative language is relevant to the assessment issues.

9.03 Informed Consent in Assessments

a. Psychologists obtain informed consent for assessments, evaluations, or diagnostic services, as described in Standard 3.10, Informed Consent, except when (1) testing is mandated by law or governmental regulations; (2) informed consent is implied because testing is conducted as a routine educational, institutional, or organizational activity (e.g., when participants voluntarily agree to assessment when applying for a job); or (3) one purpose of the testing is to evaluate decisional capacity. Informed consent includes an explanation of the nature and purpose of the assessment, fees, involvement of third parties, and limits of confidentiality and sufficient opportunity for the client/patient to ask questions and receive answers.

b. Psychologists inform persons with questionable capacity to consent or for whom testing is mandated by law or governmental regulations about the nature and purpose of the proposed assessment services, using language that is reasonably understandable to the person being assessed.

c. Psychologists using the services of an interpreter obtain informed consent from the client/ patient to use that interpreter, ensure that confidentiality of test results and test security are maintained, and include in their recommendations, reports, and diagnostic or evaluative statements, including forensic testimony, discussion of any limitations on the data obtained. (See also Standards 2.05, Delegation of Work to Others; 4.01, Maintaining Confidentiality; 9.01, Bases for Assessments; 9.06, Interpreting Assessment Results; and 9.07, Assessment by Unqualified Persons.)

9.04 Release of Test Data

a. The term *test data* refers to raw and scaled scores, client/patient responses to test questions or stimuli, and psychologists' notes and recordings concerning client/patient statements and behavior during an examination. Those portions of test materials that include client/patient responses are included in the definition of *test data*. Pursuant to a client/patient release, psychologists provide test data to the client/patient or other persons identified in the release. Psychologists may refrain from releasing test data to protect a client/patient or others from substantial harm or misuse or misrepresentation of the data or the test, recognizing that in many instances release of confidential information under these circumstances is regulated by law. (See also Standard 9.11, Maintaining Test Security.)

b. In the absence of a client/patient release, psychologists provide test data only as required by law or court order.

9.05 Test Construction

Psychologists who develop tests and other assessment techniques use appropriate psychometric procedures and current scientific or professional knowledge for test design, standardization, validation, reduction or elimination of bias, and recommendations for use.

9.06 Interpreting Assessment Results

When interpreting assessment results, including automated interpretations, psychologists take into account the purpose of the assessment as well as the various test factors, test-taking abilities, and other characteristics of the person being assessed, such as situational, personal, linguistic, and cultural differences, that might affect psychologists' judgments or reduce the accuracy of their interpretations. They indicate any significant limitations of their interpretations. (See also Standards 2.01b and c, Boundaries of Competence, and 3.01, Unfair Discrimination.)

9.07 Assessment by Unqualified Persons

Psychologists do not promote the use of psychological assessment techniques by unqualified persons, except when such use is conducted for training purposes with appropriate supervision. (See also Standard 2.05, Delegation of Work to Others.)

9.08 Obsolete Tests and Outdated Test Results

a. Psychologists do not base their assessment or intervention decisions or recommendations on data or test results that are outdated for the current purpose.

b. Psychologists do not base such decisions or recommendations on tests and measures that are obsolete and not useful for the current purpose.

9.09 Test Scoring and Interpretation Services

a. Psychologists who offer assessment or scoring services to other professionals accurately describe the purpose, norms, validity, reliability, and applications of the procedures and any special qualifications applicable to their use.

b. Psychologists select scoring and interpretation services (including automated services) on the basis of evidence of the validity of the program and procedures as well as on other appropriate considerations. (See also Standard 2.01b and c, Boundaries of Competence.)

c. Psychologists retain responsibility for the appropriate application, interpretation, and use of assessment instruments, whether they score and interpret such tests themselves or use automated or other services.

9.10 Explaining Assessment Results

Regardless of whether the scoring and interpretation are done by psychologists, by employees or assistants, or by automated or other outside services, psychologists take reasonable steps to ensure that explanations of results are given to the individual or designated representative unless the nature of the relationship precludes provision of an explanation of results (such as in some organizational consulting, preemployment or security screenings, and forensic evaluations), and this fact has been clearly explained to the person being assessed in advance.

9.11 Maintaining Test Security

The term *test materials* refers to manuals, instruments, protocols, and test questions or stimuli and does not include *test data* as defined in Standard 9.04, Release of Test Data. Psychologists make reasonable efforts to maintain the integrity and security of test materials and other assessment techniques consistent with law and contractual obligations, and in a manner that permits adherence to this Ethics Code.

10. Therapy

10.01 Informed Consent to Therapy

a. When obtaining informed consent to therapy as required in Standard 3.10, Informed Consent, psychologists inform clients/patients as early as is feasible in the therapeutic relationship about the nature and anticipated course of therapy, fees, involvement of third parties, and limits of confidentiality and provide sufficient opportunity for the client/patient to ask questions and receive answers. (See also Standards 4.02, Discussing the Limits of Confidentiality, and 6.04, Fees and Financial Arrangements.)

b. When obtaining informed consent for treatment for which generally recognized techniques and procedures have not been established, psychologists inform their clients/patients of the developing nature of the treatment, the potential risks involved, alternative treatments that may be available, and the voluntary nature of their participation. (See also Standards 2.01e, Boundaries of Competence, and 3.10, Informed Consent.)

c. When the therapist is a trainee and the legal responsibility for the treatment provided resides with the supervisor, the client/patient, as part of the informed consent procedure, is informed that the therapist is in training and is being supervised and is given the name of the supervisor.

10.02 Therapy Involving Couples or Families

a. When psychologists agree to provide services to several persons who have a relationship (such as spouses, significant others, or parents and children), they take reasonable steps to clarify at the outset (1) which of the individuals are clients/patients and (2) the relationship the psychologist will have with each person. This clarification includes the psychologist's role and the probable uses of the services provided or the information obtained. (See also Standard 4.02, Discussing the Limits of Confidentiality.)

b. If it becomes apparent that psychologists may be called on to perform potentially conflicting roles (such as family therapist and then witness for one party in divorce proceedings), psychologists take reasonable steps to clarify and modify, or withdraw from, roles appropriately. (See also Standard 3.05c, Multiple Relationships.)

10.03 Group Therapy

When psychologists provide services to several persons in a group setting, they describe at the outset the roles and responsibilities of all parties and the limits of confidentiality.

10.04 Providing Therapy to Those Served by Others

In deciding whether to offer or provide services to those already receiving mental health services elsewhere, psychologists carefully consider the treatment issues and the potential client's/patient's welfare. Psychologists discuss these issues with the client/patient or another legally authorized person on behalf of the client/patient in order to minimize the risk of confusion and conflict, consult with the other service providers when appropriate, and proceed with caution and sensitivity to the therapeutic issues.

10.05 Sexual Intimacies With Current Therapy Clients/Patients

Psychologists do not engage in sexual intimacies with current therapy clients/patients.

10.06 Sexual Intimacies With Relatives or Significant Others of Current Therapy Clients/Patients

Psychologists do not engage in sexual intimacies with individuals they know to be close relatives, guardians, or significant others of current clients/patients. Psychologists do not terminate therapy to circumvent this standard.

10.07 Therapy With Former Sexual Partners

Psychologists do not accept as therapy clients/patients persons with whom they have engaged in sexual intimacies.

10.08 Sexual Intimacies With Former Therapy Clients/Patients

a. Psychologists do not engage in sexual intimacies with former clients/patients for at least two years after cessation or termination of therapy.

b. Psychologists do not engage in sexual intimacies with former clients/patients even after a two-year interval except in the most unusual circumstances. Psychologists who engage in such activity after the two years following cessation or termination of therapy and of having no sexual contact with the former client/patient bear the burden of demonstrating that there has been no exploitation, in light of all relevant factors, including (1) the amount of time that has passed since therapy terminated; (2) the nature, duration, and intensity of the therapy; (3) the circumstances of termination; (4) the client's/patient's personal history; (5) the client's/patient's current mental status; (6) the likelihood of adverse impact on the client/patient; and (7) any statements or actions made by the therapist during the course of therapy suggesting or inviting the possibility of a posttermination sexual or romantic relationship with the client/patient. (See also Standard 3.05, Multiple Relationships.)

10.09 Interruption of Therapy

When entering into employment or contractual relationships, psychologists make reasonable efforts to provide for orderly and appropriate resolution of responsibility for client/patient care in the event that the employment or contractual relationship ends, with paramount consideration given to the welfare of the client/patient. (See also Standard 3.12, Interruption of Psychological Services.)

10.10 Terminating Therapy

a. Psychologists terminate therapy when it becomes reasonably clear that the client/patient no longer needs the service, is not likely to benefit, or is being harmed by continued service.

b. Psychologists may terminate therapy when threatened or otherwise endangered by the client/patient or another person with whom the client/patient has a relationship.

c. Except where precluded by the actions of clients/patients or third-party payors, prior to termination psychologists provide pretermination counseling and suggest alternative service providers as appropriate.

2010 AMENDMENTS TO THE 2002 "ETHICAL PRINCIPLES OF PSYCHOLOGISTS AND CODE OF CONDUCT"

The American Psychological Association's Council of Representatives adopted the following amendments to the 2002 "Ethical Principles of Psychologists and Code of Conduct" at its February 2010 meeting. Changes are indicated by underlining for additions and striking through for deletions. A history of amending the Ethics Code is provided in the "Report of the Ethics Committee, 2009" in the July-August 2010 issue of the *American Psychologist* (Vol. 65, No. 5).
Original Language With Changes Marked

Introduction and Applicability

If psychologists' ethical responsibilities conflict with law, regulations, or other governing legal authority, psychologists make known their commitment to this Ethics Code and take steps to resolve the conflict in a responsible manner. If the conflict is unresolvable via such means, psychologists may adhere to the requirements of the law, regulations, or other governing authority in keeping with basic principles of human rights.

(Continued)

(Continued)

1.02 Conflicts Between Ethics and Law, Regulations, or Other Governing Legal Authority

If psychologists' ethical responsibilities conflict with law, regulations, or other governing legal authority, psychologists clarify the nature of the conflict, make known their commitment to the Ethics Code, and take reasonable steps to resolve the conflict consistent with the General Principles and Ethical Standards of the Ethics Code. ~~If the conflict is unresolvable via such means, psychologists may adhere to the requirements of the law, regulations, or other governing legal authority.~~ Under no circumstances may this standard be used to justify or defend violating human rights.

1.03 Conflicts Between Ethics and Organizational Demands

If the demands of an organization with which psychologists are affiliated or for whom they are working are in conflict with this Ethics Code, psychologists clarify the nature of the conflict, make known their commitment to the Ethics Code, and ~~to the extent feasible, resolve the conflict in a way that permits adherence to the Ethics Code.~~ take reasonable steps to resolve the conflict consistent with the General Principles and Ethical Standards of the Ethics Code. Under no circumstances may this standard be used to justify or defend violating human rights.

Index

Page references followed by (table) indicate a table.